AFTER
CANCER
Care

D0469818

The Definitive Self-Care Guide
to Getting and Staying Well for
Patients after Cancer

AFTER
CANCER
Care

| GERALD M. | PALLAV K. | DWIGHT L. |
| LEMOLE, MD | MEHTA, MD | MCKEE, MD |

FOREWORD BY MEHMET C. OZ, MD

RODALE.

© 2015 by Gerald Lemole, MD, Pallav Mehta, MD, and Dwight McKee, MD

Rodale books may be purchased for business or promotional use or for special sales. For information, please write to:
Special Markets Department, Rodale Inc., 733 Third Avenue, New York, NY 10017

Printed in the United States of America

Rodale Inc. makes every effort to use acid-free ♾, recycled paper ♻.

Selected recipes courtesy of Conner Middelmann-Whitney, author of
Zest for Life: The Mediterranean Anti-Cancer Diet and modernmediterranean.com.

Book design by Amy C. King

Library of Congress Cataloging-in-Publication Data is on file with the publisher.

ISBN 978-1-62336-502-8 paperback

Distributed to the trade by Macmillan

2 4 6 8 10 9 7 5 3 1 paperback

We inspire and enable people to improve their lives and the world around them.
rodalebooks.com

To my wife, Emily Jane, whose ideas and
inspiration made this book possible.

—GERALD LEMOLE, MD

To all the patients and families I've had the good fortune
of meeting: Thank you for sharing your story as you
have taught me invaluable lessons about courage and hope.
I never forget what a privilege it is to take care of you.

To my wife, Neeta, and my three children, Isabel, Aidan, and Lily, for being
my primary source of love, support, humor, aggravation, and inspiration while
teaching me the importance of always staying present.

—PALLAV MEHTA, MD

To all of my patients with cancer challenges over the past 40 years
who have been the inspiration to me for acquiring more knowledge to assist
them, while teaching me deep lessons about compassion, love, healing,
living with uncertainty, and the transformational nature of the process
we call "cancer"—and for teaching me that healing is not always
the same as physical recovery from illness.

To my dearest wife, Jillellen; my daughter, Micaela Collins;
and my son, Luke, for supporting and loving me
even when my work takes me away from them.

—DWIGHT MCKEE, MD

CONTENTS

FOREWORD

BY DR. MEHMET C. OZ

A FEW YEARS AGO, I WAS ASKED TO OPERATE ON A 60-YEAR-OLD MAN (LET'S CALL him Mike) with a leaky heart valve. His 10-inch-thick hospital chart warned that he had a complex medical history. As I read more deeply into his background, I learned that, sadly, he had metastatic stomach cancer that appeared incurable. I realized that he was either unaware of his dire diagnosis or was ignoring the reality of his situation. Operating on the heart of a terminal patient makes no sense, so I felt compelled to have an uncomfortable conversation and turn down his request for life-saving heart surgery.

When I delicately broached the topic, he looked strangely amused. "Yes, I carried a diagnosis of advanced gastric cancer," he said. "Thankfully, I am better now," he added. I knew this was nearly impossible, especially with an aggressive cancer that had spread so widely, so I gently challenged him using the raw data in the chart itself and pointed out the overflowing negative reports. Just as I thought my point was made, he calmly noted that all the data was true, but the comments were also irrelevant since they were more than 5 years old. Stunned, I returned to the chart. He was right!

How did Mike survive metastatic stomach cancer? Like most patients in this predicament, he had struggled with surgery, radiation, and chemotherapy. He sheepishly explained that his full recovery was not solely because of these conventional approaches. He admitted those practices were essential but that he'd also sought alternative approaches, traveling the world in search of experienced practitioners who could help him walk away healthy. He consulted several guides, each of whom further crafted his game plan for full recovery. No food was overlooked. Every supplement was carefully reviewed. He was coached on groundbreaking stress management techniques. He tried new exercises and made new social connections. And he sat peacefully in front of me 5 years later—5 years after he should have passed away—healthy enough to undergo heart surgery.

––––––––––––––––––––––

No cancer has a 100 percent mortality rate. No matter how deadly, no matter what the odds, there are always survivors. Yet patients like Mike, who defy the odds, are exceedingly rare. After undergoing treatment, many cancer patients suffer unnecessarily and some face high risks—even failure of therapy—because of missed opportunities in *after* care. Hence, the need for this wonderful book that offers superbly organized and researched advice for the almost 50 percent of us who will develop cancer in our lifetimes.

Drs. Lemole, Mehta, and McKee are world-class experts in helping patients navigate cancer and the effects of necessary conventional therapy (such as chemotherapy, radiation, and surgery) with subsequent recovery of full vitality. They'll take you on an in-depth yet easy-to-digest journey through cancer protocols to understand how complementary approaches can accelerate recovery. They'll expand on foods that heal and foods that hurt, and they'll offer delicious, easy-to-prepare recipes to incorporate nourishing foods into your life. They'll explain and break down nutritional supplement strategies so you can feel confident talking to your doctor about what's right for you. Throughout the book, they'll offer cutting-edge insights on how after cancer care can dramatically alter patient outcomes—including yours—favorably.

They'll also introduce groundbreaking concepts like epigenetics, a proven mechanism by which our genes can adjust to environmental stresses and support. Now that we recognize we can influence the blueprint of our bodies, ignoring opportunities to nudge this code in the right direction is unwise, and *After Cancer Care* elegantly offers needed tools to do so. Now you can "turn on" hundreds of genes that fight cancer and "turn off" the ones that encourage cancer just by incorporating the lifestyle changes outlined in these pages.

Reducing overall inflammation has always been a goal of healing, but the authors argue that this simultaneously boosts immune surveillance. The tools you'll find in *After Cancer Care* also help reduce inflammation—something Drs. Lemole, Mehta, and McKee argue can promote overall health and boost immune surveillance. The docs will also teach you to read food and product labels and to avoid risky chemicals.

The result of all of this? A simple yet comprehensive manifesto that reduces the stress perceived by our bodies. Some of the tips appear subtle, like making social connections and practicing compassion and kindness, but each is powerful in its own way. The sweeping wisdom of these three wonderful doctors is abundantly clear, and you and your loved ones will reap the benefits in this book.

My patient Mike had to work tirelessly and research meticulously to gather the information and techniques that helped save his life. He didn't have this book. Now, *After Cancer Care* compiles the information you need to live your healthiest and most vibrant postcancer life. Take the first step by turning the page.

INTRODUCTION

WHEN KEN WAS 71 YEARS OLD, HE FELL OUT OF A TREE AND WAS INJURED. IN the emergency room, the doctors took an x-ray and saw a broken rib, as well as a mass in Ken's left lung accompanied by enlarged lymph nodes. He was immediately referred for a biopsy—which confirmed the mass was a small-cell cancer—and a total-body CT scan, which showed that it had not metastasized. Ken was referred for chemotherapy and radiation, and after 6 weeks of concurrent treatment, he was told the tumor had dissolved completely.

At Ken's final visit with his oncologist, he was told that he would be seen for a scan and blood work in 6 months. Ken asked, "So, Doc, what should I do now to decrease the chance of a recurrence?"

His doctor replied, "Do whatever you want!"

Ken's experience was not unique. The standard farewell given to patients by their oncologists after they've completed cancer care is "See you in a few months." When asked what they should do in the meantime, they are given a vague answer such as "Now you can get back to your old life!"

Ken, like many patients, was not satisfied with his doctor's answer. Other than his cancer, he was fit and healthy. He had a lot to live for, and he knew that only 20 percent of patients with his tumor type and grade made it to the 5-year mark following their diagnosis. He wanted to optimize his chances for survival, and he wanted a plan that would give him some semblance of control rather than just wait for his next appointment.

If Ken had had a heart attack, he would have left the hospital with an appointment for cardiac rehab. Depending on where he was being treated, at this first appointment, he might have been assigned a physical trainer, a nutritionist, and even a counselor. Over the course of 12 weeks, Ken would have seen these practitioners several times a week, learning how to handle stress, how to shop for and cook heart-healthy foods, and how to establish an exercise routine.

Over the last 20 years, heart disease has come to be accepted as at least partly a disease of lifestyle, and cardiac rehab has become an accepted part of its treatment. The cardiac rehab triad of better nutrition, exercise, and stress management leads to fewer repeat heart attacks and better patient outcomes. Better still, patients who go through rehab are less likely to develop diabetes, high blood pressure, and a host of other conditions. After 12 weeks of rehab, a high percentage of patients establish new habits and substantially change their lifestyles.

Cancer, however, is still treated as though it is a bolt of lightning out of the sky. Other than urging patients to stop using tobacco, oncologists rarely ask their patients to make direct connections between their lifestyle and their cancer. But we now know there are strong, documented ways to prevent recurrence. There are correlations, for example, between obesity and a sedentary lifestyle and certain types of cancer—so why aren't more patients being told to at least move more after their treatment is over? Why aren't more tactics presented to help patients live their healthiest lives post-treatment?

We three doctors—Gerald Lemole, Dwight McKee, and Pallav Mehta—have varied backgrounds and experiences, but we agree with Ken that cancer care should not stop with the final visit to your oncologist. Surgery, chemotherapy, radiation, and immunotherapy treatments for cancer are nothing less than extraordinary. Millions of lives have been saved through their use. But their focus is on destroying cancer cells, not strengthening healthy cells. Once their use is complete and treatment is over, there is still work to do.

There is now overwhelming data showing that exercise, good nutrition, and management of stress can improve the likelihood of cancer survival and prevent recurrence. And there is no dispute that strengthening your immune system through a healthy lifestyle will allow you to live a healthier life in general.

Yet 95 percent of people who have been treated for cancer either are not using or are underusing these powerful strategies. The main reason for this is simply lack of knowledge. Few cancer patients are aware of the research showing the correlations between lifestyle and cancer, and few oncologists are trained to provide advice to patients regarding after cancer care. Some patients, as was the case with Ken, do their own research and find the correlations between lifestyle and cancer on their own. Through various sources and advice from multiple practitioners—including an integrative oncologist, if they live in a place where there is a practitioner—they piece together a plan for after care. But we'd like to see this type of care for all cancer patients, not just those with the ability to access it.

ABOUT US

Dr. Pallav Mehta is a practicing oncologist and hematologist and director of integrative oncology, Dr. Dwight McKee is an integrative oncologist and hematologist with nearly 40 years of clinical experience, and Dr. Gerald Lemole is a world-renowned cardiothoracic surgeon and holistic practitioner. He's also a close friend of Ken, the 71-year-old we've been talking about. Dr. Lemole was troubled by Ken's experience and was inspired to do more for cancer patients following their treatment.

The three of us have experienced positive results when we've integrated better nutrition, exercise, and stress management into our patients' care. We know anecdotally that lifestyle changes affect cancer recurrence, and now the data back us up. It's a matter of time before the medical community and insurance providers catch up to the fact that lifestyle changes following cancer treatment save lives.

The fact that 95 percent of cancer patients are not embracing these methods is troubling to us. There is no downside to the type of lifestyle changes we are recommending. Even if the data were incorrect, we know through our practices and personal experiences that these changes improve the overall health and happiness of patients. With the exception of supplementation (which should be done under the advice of your primary care doctor, naturopath, or nutritionist), the light exercise, dietary adjustments, and stress-management suggestions made in this book are not contraindicated for any disease or treatment and will only stand to improve overall health.

In his book *Anticancer*, David Servan-Schreiber, MD, PhD, relates the story of a stage IV cancer patient with a terrible prognosis. The young man was a drug addict and alcoholic, and was estranged from his family and community. In the last 6 months of his life, he embraced Dr. Servan-Schreiber's ethos of changing his lifestyle, both physically and mentally. Although the changes did not extend his life, before he died he thanked Dr. Servan-Schreiber for saving him. He died content, knowing that he'd lived his final 6 months with purpose.

For patients in remission, we can do more than that. You can live your life with purpose, and you can extend your life. The added bonus is that you will also be less likely to die of another degenerative disease after making it through cancer treatment.

Our hope is that ultimately the medical community and insurance providers embrace the role of a cancer patient's lifestyle when advising about postcancer treatment. Rather than telling their patients "See you in 6 months," oncologists will be able to hand them an appointment card for their first visit to cancer rehab.

In the meantime, this book will be your after cancer guide. If you have difficult, important questions about what to do after your cancer therapy, you're not alone. In this book, you will learn how to confidently transition to a healthy lifestyle. By maintaining a positive attitude, eating right, and exercising effectively, you can optimize your chances for survival and take control of your health. With this knowledge in hand, you can live your strongest, healthiest postcancer life possible. While our book focuses primarily on patients who have completed their cancer treatments, we all fully acknowledge that there exists a population of patients who either were diagnosed with stage IV cancer or developed it at some point in their course of treatment. For these individuals, there is often no defined point at which therapy is complete, and they may perpetually remain on some sort of treatment. With the advances that have been made in the world of conventional oncology, it's not out of the ordinary to see some of these patients living for years with active cancer, often leading relatively normal lives while visiting with their oncologists periodically to receive their chemotherapy or refill the prescription for some new oral targeted medication, which is keeping their cancer at bay. Many of the approaches to lifestyle management apply to these patients, as well, but it is all the more important that they speak to their oncologists before embarking on a specific plan, particularly one that includes supplements and/or nutritional changes. Let's get started.

PART ONE

THRIVING POSTCANCER

CHAPTER ONE

WHAT NOW?

Y OU'VE JUST FINISHED TREATMENT FOR CANCER, AND YOU HAVE BEEN TOLD THAT you are cancer-free. After months or years of treatment—including major surgery and rounds of nauseating chemotherapy and scarring radiation— you've achieved your goal. You can go back to your old life as though none of this ever happened! Or can you?

When you go through treatment for cancer, there is a clear end goal: remission and beating your disease. But when the day comes that your oncologist bids you adieu, with just an appointment card for a 3- or 6-month follow-up appointment, that farewell can feel . . . anticlimactic. He's done what he can for you, and your cancer is in remission. You are essentially healthy again. Oh, you'll be coming back to see him once in a while for a checkup, but you can finally pick up your normal life and move on. This is a joyful moment!

But once the initial relief wears off, many patients find that instead of feeling ecstatic, they feel uncertain, frightened, and out of control. They've heard so many stories of recurrence, and they've heard the prognosis after recurrence can be dire. Instead of providing an action plan to fend off the threat of a relapse, few oncologists offer anything in the way of advice or care following the end of treatment. After fighting for your life with a team of experts, you are on your own with no compass to guide you.

For some patients, the time following their treatment for cancer can be more emotionally fraught than the time during treatment itself. During treatment, they are focused on getting better, and they have a team of passionate professionals working toward that goal. Co-workers rally around them, and friends and family show up with casseroles and offer rides. Everything is focused on killing the cancer.

When treatment is over, the team of professionals disappears. The need for rides and casseroles also disappears. Physically, you feel much better, and it's high time you got back to your life. But getting "back to your life" isn't always possible or even desirable; you've been through a life-changing experience. The fact is, the end of treatment may not mean going back to your old life at all. You aren't out of the woods yet and still have those follow-ups to contend with.

THE SWORD OF DAMOCLES

For many people, the stress they feel about their future health is debilitating. At least during cancer treatment, they were fighting it. Of course, it's natural to worry about the future. But excessive worry and anxiety about possible hazards in our path can prevent us from living life to its fullest.

There is an ancient story, told by the Roman orator Cicero, about a man named Damocles. Damocles was envious of the power and possessions of his ruler, Dionysius, whom he served at court. Dionysus was well aware of Damocles's jealousy. He shrewdly proposed that they switch places, to allow Damocles a firsthand taste of the fabulous benefits of royalty. Damocles greedily accepted the invitation. He was escorted to the throne room, where he was surrounded by treasures, exquisite food and wines, silk fabrics, precious metals, and beautiful courtiers.

As Damocles sat upon the great throne, the king advised him to look up toward the ceiling. There, above the chair, hanging solely by a single horse-tail hair, was a large and deadly sword. Damocles quickly jumped off the throne, declaring as he departed that he no longer wished to experience the luxuries of power if they were paired with such risks.

In his fifth *Disputations*, Cicero asks: "Does not Dionysius seem to have made it sufficiently clear that there can be nothing happy for the person over whom some fear always looms?" Imagine how differently Cicero's story would have been had Damocles stepped calmly from the throne, ordered the removal of the hanging sword, and then resumed his longed-for adventure.

Fortunately, we can remove the metaphorical swords that hang over our lives. Contrary to the advice of many oncologists, we now know there are things we can do to significantly reduce the risk of recurrence. In a pleasant irony, taking physical action to prevent recurrence can lead to a more positive outlook, and there is scientific evidence that our attitude affects our body's well-being, as well.

AFTER CANCER CARE

It is now well known that lifestyle does have an effect on some types of cancer. According to the World Health Organization, 30 percent of cancers are related to lifestyle or infections: "More than 30% of cancer could be prevented, mainly by not using tobacco, having a healthy diet, being physically active and moderating the use of alcohol."[1]

These are not the words of naturopaths, integrative oncologists, or vegan nutritionists. These are the words of one of the world's most established—and conventional—health organizations.

In our practices, we have seen how diet and lifestyle can also help individuals prevent recurrence of cancer. Significant medical research has established both theory and practical application of the links between nutrition, exercise, stress, and cancer recurrence. These principles are beginning to change the face of cancer treatment centers around this country and the world, and many hospitals currently have integrative cancer care centers as part of what they offer patients. However, there is more to be done.

Integrative oncology—the acknowledged term for cancer care that blends cancer-killing medicine with other lifestyle and immune-supporting practices—is actually an oxymoron. Oncology, the study of tumors and ways to attack them, is only a part of integrative cancer medicine. The rest is in the person who has the malignancy and that person's individual terrain—that is, the microenvironment within which tumor cells live. This microenvironment is finally beginning to be a focus of laboratory researchers; we are at the dawn of a new era. We use the term *integrative oncology* for convenience, and generally everyone knows what that means, but we prefer the term *integrative cancer medicine*.

THRIVING POSTCANCER

Most published data in oncology measure the value of a given intervention in terms of "survival." We don't just want our patients to survive; we want them to thrive.

All of the recommendations we have made in this book have scientific support. Some of the evidence-based studies required to achieve FDA approval are included, but also small clinical trials and epidemiologic, demographic, or laboratory studies that show evidence of benefit from lifestyle changes for those who have or have had cancer. Some examples of the latter include increasing immunity, regulating DNA and protein production in cancer, increasing psychological and spiritual well-being, and enhancing overall health.

The key to incorporating the advice given in this book is to apply the "risk-benefit ratio," a philosophy that lies at the heart of all good medicine. That is: How does the risk of using any given treatment or procedure balance with the benefits that might be achieved?

Doctors routinely use a risk-benefit ratio when performing surgery. Is the risk to the patient—of death, postoperative attack, disability, and cost—worth the benefit he or she will likely receive, such as a longer life and an improved quality of life? If the benefit outweighs the risk, we recommend surgery.

In the case of our basic recommendations in this book, there is minimal risk and the opportunity for great benefit. Light exercise, improved diet, and practicing stress-management techniques have universally positive benefits. When intensifying exercise, making drastic diet changes, adding supplementation, or taking medication for anxiety, the risk-benefit ratio may be more of a balance and should be undertaken under the supervision of a doctor. For example, a rigorous exercise regimen could lead to injuries for previously sedentary people; a vegan diet could lead to anemia if there is not sufficient B_{12} in the diet; certain supplements can be contraindicated with certain medications; and anti-anxiety drugs can have side effects.

Terrain

We also need to broaden our approach so that we don't only fight against cancer. We tend to think about cancer treatment as a war, but we can move from a nasty internal terrain that's in turmoil to one filled with relaxation, peace, hope, trust, empathy, and compassion.

We need to nurture our body, mind, and soul. *After Cancer Care* can provide a structure for a healthier diet and physical lifestyle, as well as support an informed decision-making process, enhance hope and utilize the wisdom and experiences of exceptional patients, reduce hopelessness and helplessness, reduce social isolation by providing support groups and other group activities, and offer instruction on stress-reduction practices.

From a conceptual viewpoint, we loosely associate the two approaches of conventional oncology and complementary and alternative medicine (CAM) with the left and right brain.

Conventional oncology is a military model of attack on tumors. It's very "left-brained"—logical, linear, and evaluated by statistical methods. It categorizes and systematizes, whereas CAM is a holistic approach designed to support multiple host systems with many types of intervention. CAM is thus more a product of the "right brain": Intuitive and nonlinear, it individualizes rather than systematizes. The goal of oncology is to destroy tumor cells in the body; the goal of CAM therapies is to increase host resistance to tumor cells by changing the internal terrain of the body. There is good evidence that we do better when we use both sides of our brain, which is the way we can view integrative cancer medicine.

Some early studies—the significance of which may not have been understood at the time—profoundly demonstrated the impact of terrain. In 1975 Beatrice Mintz showed that injecting teratocarcinoma cells into an adult mouse caused a lethal cancer, but when injected into a mouse embryo, the tumor genes were expressed but healthy mice developed. More than 30 years earlier, researchers had discovered that the Rous sarcoma virus, which creates lethal sarcomas when injected into adult chickens, had no effect on chicken embryos.[2] Dr. Mina Bissell repeated these experiments with the Rous sarcoma virus in the 1970s and found the same thing. She then went on to discover that the virus only forms a tumor in a wound, not in healthy tissue.[3] Clearly, the environment (terrain) of a tumor cell or a tumor-inducing virus has a profound effect on whether or not tumors form.

Similarly, tumor cells have been found in the bone marrow of patients with ductal carcinoma in situ, which can also be called stage 0 breast cancer.[4] This is an indication that even in the earliest precancer conditions, tumor cells far from the breast can also be present. The significance of this finding is that these non-invasive breast cancers are frequently treated by local excision +/- radiotherapy—both of which are local (within the breast) treatments. Whether individual tumor cells found in blood or bone marrow ever grow into dangerous tumors or not depends a great deal on their environment, or the internal "terrain," which is produced by the sum total of diet, lifestyle, metabolism, environmental exposures, and stress.

Traditional Chinese medicine (TCM) has had this view for millennia—that cancer is a systemic disease and the tumor is just a symptom of it. In TCM one must alter the underlying constitution in order to heal the disease. This may be the direction we are moving in integrative cancer medicine.

A metaphor illustrates this: We know how to look for the seeds, but we have not really learned how to assess the soil, the microenvironment, and the internal terrain. The study of terrain is beginning to gain traction in mainstream cancer research now. It may be that cancer cells with a permissive terrain equal a tumor, while cancer cells in a nonpermissive terrain never develop into a diagnosable tumor.

Dean Ornish, MD, a clinical professor of medicine at the University of California, San Francisco, did a groundbreaking study, published in 2008, in which prostate cancer patients on "active surveillance" changed their diets, exercised, did yoga, and meditated. It was very similar to the lifestyle and diet interventions that Dr. Ornish did in his original cardiovascular studies. After 3 months, patients' prostates were biopsied. After just a 3-month interval of this diet and lifestyle intervention, a shift was shown in the expression of more than 200 genes. The genes associated with biological aggressiveness "downregulated" (their expression was turned off), and the genes associated with less aggressive behavior "upregulated" (turned on). Inflammatory genes were also downregulated; it is well understood that cancer cells thrive in an environment of chronic inflammation, so this was also beneficial.[5]

We don't yet know how these effects are brought about. Maybe more available nutrients are directly affecting the tumor cells or are influencing the terrain or microenvironment; or maybe they are doing both. It is very likely that the changes are mediated through the process we call epigenetics—that is, the regulation of gene expression by our internal terrain. This is an entire area of study in itself and very much relates to what is done in integrative cancer medicine. In Part Two of this book, we undertake an in-depth discussion of the new science of epigenetics.

YOUR AFTER CANCER CARE

If you are very lucky, you have an oncologist who is fully or partly on board with the premise that your actions following your cancer treatment can affect your outcome. He or she may refer you to a nutritionist, advise you to alter your diet, recommend an exercise regimen, or refer you to a counselor or support group. But let's assume you are like most patients who are in remission. Your oncologist has given you a "clean bill of health" and asked you to call her or your primary doctor with any new problems. Otherwise, she'll see you back in her office in a few months. You are given little additional guidance as to what you should be doing in the meantime. It's up to you to create your own after cancer care plan. That's where we come in.

The first thing we recommend you do is make an assessment of where you are coming from, where you are now, and where you are going. It is time to take a look at some good habits—some may be new to you, some you may have adopted long ago—that will support and maintain your remission from cancer and promote your continued good health. We suggest you keep a journal when doing this.

Integrating these new ideas and actions into your life is not as difficult as it might sound at first. The suggestions we make in this book are gently presented and easy to follow. However, they do represent changes in your life, and we understand that a reassessment of your lifestyle is not always easy. It can encourage feelings of denial and anger, and we recognize that those feelings are real and need to be addressed. There may be things that you don't want to give up at first. It is easy to even deny the need to change at all. But the smoker needs to change into a committed nonsmoker. The couch potato must change into a person with regular, moderate exercise habits. The fast-food devotee or the heavy alcohol drinker is required to transform into a more health-conscious consumer of organic and other nutritious foods, and to enjoy the "guilty pleasures" in moderation. The negative thinker needs to cultivate a more positive attitude. Finally, the person who is out of touch with himself or herself now needs to connect with what's going on inside.

We ask you to take a hard and honest look at how you feel about making these sorts of adjustments in your life—changes that will help you maintain the good health you have just recovered from a long period of pain and hard work, intensive medical care, and constant guidance by health professionals.

You are on your own two feet once more. Your continued good health is no longer up to your doctor, it's up to you. You have to be the one to take charge now. Regardless of any guidance provided by a sympathetic oncologist or even an evangelistic natural healer, it is you who will moderate the old habits and learn new ones, and it is you who is responsible for making the changes.

Some patients feel some anger or reluctance at having to face this next step in a seemingly endless health journey. When you were ill, you may have longed to return to all your old ways. You've been through so much. Don't you deserve it? And now we three high-and-mighty docs are suggesting that returning to all your old ways may not be in your best interest.

You may also feel that you are not ready to make a commitment to the lifestyle suggestions we make in this book. For months or years, experts and technicians in white coats have controlled and ordered your life. They had all the expertise while you had none, and their decisions and actions throughout your treatment ruled with total authority over your life. You've reached a moment now when you are finally able to make decisions of your own.

This book does not and should not interfere with your autonomy. We

Lise's Story

For Lise, who was diagnosed with ovarian cancer and has been in remission for 6 years, having a plan developed with Dr. McKee felt like an invaluable lifeline following her cancer treatments. "After having been through all the necessary and horrific protocols, there was no way I was just going to sit there. I had a highly aggressive, high-grade cancer. So I felt like if I didn't do anything, I would literally be waiting for it to come back. Instead, I felt like I was working toward something rather than treading water waiting for the other shoe to fall."

applaud and encourage you to find your own way to lifestyle habits that will encourage long-term healing. We are presenting the evidence that research and our combined clinical experience tell us is likely to be effective in your health prognosis. Some of the changes we suggest may seem quite drastic, and we don't expect every person to embrace each and every practice. It's important that you be on board with your lifestyle changes, though. The evidence shows that the more of the recommended changes you embrace, the better your health will be and the less likely you will have a recurrence of your disease.

It is also normal for you to want a little break before starting this new regimen. Can't it wait? Surely you deserve at least a little time off for good behavior—especially if you were living a healthy lifestyle when you were diagnosed with cancer.

Think back to your initial diagnosis. You were likely confused and maybe even a little furious. You had already been doing everything possible in support of good health. You never smoked but ended up with lung cancer; you breastfed both your children and ended up with breast cancer. You may have been eating well, exercising regularly, practicing good mental and spiritual health—and still you were struck down by this terrible disease. How could this have happened to you?

Unfortunately, there is no good answer. Your specific cancer, no matter which kind, is not necessarily the result of anything you did. And as successful as we are in being able to live healthfully today, there is always more to learn. Even if your efforts in the past were positive, constructive habits to support a healthy body, almost certainly more is available that you can add to build on your good history—especially given that your body has been so seriously compromised and still needs additional support.

Instead of thinking about the deprivations of a healthier lifestyle or the unfairness of your cancer, think of what your body has been through—from the onset of your cancer to finishing your treatment—and the miraculous job your body has done for you in bringing you to this state of remission. Try to think of these changes we're recommending as rewards that you give your body for the incredible work it has done.

Nothing we recommend will cause you pain in the way chemo, radiation, or surgery may have. You will not have pain from anything we suggest (other than some mildly sore muscles if you push your exercise). In contrast, you will feel good, mentally and physically. Yes, we are asking you to make some changes, but what we are suggesting in exchange will feel so much better.

With each new step you take toward better nutrition, exercise, and overall healthy living, you give one more gift to your body—in effect, saying "thanks for what has been" and making a promise for further gifts that are yet to come.

(continued on page 14)

Margaret's Story

When Dr. Mehta considers the benefits of applying healthy lifestyle precepts to a patient's after cancer care, one patient's story of survival against the odds stands out. Dr. Mehta recalled:

"I walked out of the exam room that afternoon thoroughly exhausted, nearing the end of another long day. My thoughts were starting to drift to my upcoming vacation. I hadn't taken one in quite some time, much to the chagrin of my wife and children. Methodically, I went to the nearest sink and washed my hands, and then moved over to the sparkling new computers that housed our recently implemented electronic medical records system. After punching in my ID and password, I pulled up the information on my next patient.

"From the physician's notes, I could gather that Margaret was a 43-year-old woman who had noted a lump in her left breast a few months ago, not long after her 8-year-old son accidentally bumped into her. Because it did not recede, she sought some guidance from her gynecologist, who ordered a mammogram and ultrasound—which confirmed a suspicious mass. This was followed up with a biopsy that confirmed a diagnosis of breast cancer.

"After an extensive conversation with the surgeon and with her husband, she elected to proceed with a bilateral mastectomy (removing both breasts). Two weeks after her surgery, she was referred to a medical oncologist—me. I carefully reviewed the pathology and radiology reports, and then formulated an outline of a plan in my head.

"I took a breath before I opened the door to the exam room. I see hundreds of breast cancer patients every year, but whenever I meet someone for the first time, I try to appreciate and acknowledge the trauma that particular person is undergoing.

"Giving her as much time to answer as she needed, I went through my usual battery of questions, starting with how she noticed the lump all the way to her decision making about the mastectomy. In the process, I heard all about how rambunctious her younger son, Colin, could be and how he'd had multiple inadvertent run-ins with family, friends, and furniture.

"One month after her first visit with me, we began chemotherapy. As expected, a few weeks later, Margaret had the usual panoply of side effects, including hair loss. Overall, however, she did quite well. On our routine visits, we would talk briefly about the treatments and their impact on her, but more about her children, the grand party she was planning to

(continued)

throw once she was done with her treatment, and her upcoming 15th wedding anniversary and planned trip to Paris. 'The first time without the kids!' she said multiple times. 'Chemo brain' made her forget she had told me this 3 weeks earlier.

"She completed her chemotherapy on a sweltering day in July, and came into the office with a feather boa around her neck and a tiara adorning her beautifully shaven head. I congratulated her on finishing a very difficult therapy relatively unscathed.

"We then entered into our obligatory 5-year period of surveillance—as if nature has somehow agreed that 5 years is the magic number subsequent to which we can all cast away our fears. Her follow-up involved routine visits with me every few months, with blood tests. Her hair grew back, as it always does, though not quite the same. 'You didn't tell me it was going to be so kinky, Dr. Mehta,' she told me.

"A year later, her oldest son, Jack, was graduating high school, and they were going to celebrate with a vacation to a Caribbean island. She came in before the big day for a routine visit and once again looked and felt great. Three days after her visit, as I was reviewing her blood work, I noticed something unusual. One of the blood tests—something known as the 'tumor marker'—was slightly abnormal. This can happen for all sorts of reasons and often means absolutely nothing.

"I called to let her know that we would need to repeat the tests in about a month. She picked up the phone and then hesitated a second before she acknowledged me. I had never called her after a visit. 'What's wrong?' she asked, getting right to the point. I told her about the blood test and tried to reassure her that it was probably nothing. Needless to say, such a reassurance is almost always ineffective (it likely serves to reassure the physician more than the patient). I told her to enjoy her vacation, and I would see her after her next blood tests.

"Margaret called me a few weeks later. She wanted to let me know about some pain she had been having in her ribs. She said she did all sorts of things while away, and at one point got thrown in the water while trying Jet Skiing. She thought that must be the culprit. I told her I agreed, but of course we both had the tumor markers on our minds. A week or two later, she came in for the blood work as I'd requested.

"As I was reviewing the laboratory results from that day, I stopped when I came across Margaret's tumor markers. Given the volume of patients an oncologist sees, some find it hard to fathom that our hearts sink when we know something is awry. Mine did that morning. The markers were now significantly abnormal. I waited until she came in for her appointment to let her know that I wanted to investigate further. This would involve the head-to-toe scan test known as the PET scan, and if something was 'lighting up,' it would be followed by a biopsy. Something did light up, and I did have her get the biopsy.

"On a blustery winter afternoon, I told Margaret she had incurable cancer—and I remember, as I do with many of my patients, the moment of contact and the visit. I recall how I felt when I saw her name on my patient list that day and opening the door to the room once again, this time being faced with Margaret and several family members who were there to offer their support for what was undoubtedly bad news. I explained in great detail the diagnosis of recurrence and the fact that her fight now began anew. She was ready as she ever was and, in fact, seemed to be the one comforting her family.

"That was 4 years ago. I know this because her oldest son is now graduating college, and she is mighty proud.

"She has attributed her remarkable survival to her attention to activity and nutrition. I am not inclined to disagree, as I have seen this time and time again. From my office window, I've seen her take a slow jog from her car to the chemotherapy infusion suite. I always smile.

"Today, Margaret remains a vibrant and productive mother, wife, and friend who also happens to have metastatic cancer and is on intermittent treatment. Throughout her journey, which I fully believe will continue for years to come, she has been mindful of staying active and following a nutrition and supplement plan that makes sense to her. She comes into appointments often with articles and reports of 'this new supplement' or 'that new exercise' for patients with cancer. I suspect she brings this information in so that I can learn and then share this with other patients who may benefit both now and in the future. She has also done her darndest to diminish stress in her day-to-day life and keep a truly positive outlook.

"I believe with full conviction that it is not simply my chemotherapy that has kept Margaret alive all this time, despite a diagnosis that statistically should have led to her demise many years ago. She, and patients like her, have taught me a considerable amount about the tremendous value of a healthy lifestyle after cancer."

In addition to decreasing your chance of a recurrence, you will gain much more: an increase in your energy and your confidence and an inner joy at being in control of your own health. You will also gain a vastly improved ability to fight off your cancer again should it recur. Your new, stronger body will be better able to weaken cancer's grip and handle the treatment to rid your body of it.

Today really is the first day of the rest of your life. The quality of that remaining span of your life may be very much in your own hands.

MOVING BEYOND THE SWORD OF DAMOCLES

The Sword of Damocles hangs over many heads today—not in a throne room surrounded by treasure, but from the fear of cancer recurrence for those who have completed their cancer therapy. This fear is like a prison wall preventing its victims from joining in the celebration of life and drinking deeply of its joy. Unless this fear is at least faced courageously and appropriately addressed—if not totally overcome—it controls your future and your present, and severely diminishes the quality and quantity of your life.

We have all seen patients do well when the three vital components—nutrition, exercise, and stress management—are practiced with awareness. They can have a truly miraculous impact on the well-being and vitality of patients with cancer and in preventing recurrence for patients who are in remission.

People who have had cancer are often looking for a way to make a change, but they have not had good guidelines about what to do or how to do it. That is why we like to think of cancer as a lifestyle coach once patients get to the end of their treatment. It's sitting on the patient's shoulder every day saying, "You need to get out and exercise. You need to do relaxation and meditation. You need to eat this and not that. You need to take a supplement." That will protect you. Use the cancer and the knowledge that the cancer could relapse to optimize your wellness—and to thrive, not just survive.

CHAPTER TWO

"SEE YOU IN 6 MONTHS"

F OR PATIENTS WHO HAVE COMPLETED THEIR CANCER TREATMENT AND ARE SENT BACK to their "regular lives," there is a constant stressor: the knowledge that in 3, 6, or 12 months, they will be back in their oncologist's office hearing the results of blood tests or CT scans. Yet few patients are even sure what their oncologists are looking for during those visits—and often neither patient nor oncologist wants to broach the question of why they are looking at blood work and scans at all—or what will happen if the cancer does, in fact, come back.

Ashley was diagnosed with stage I breast cancer at the age of 33. Because of several factors, she was advised to have a double mastectomy and undergo chemotherapy and radiation. When her treatment concluded, she wondered what would happen next. "I was scheduled every 3 months, and I guess I thought more would happen. But instead they'd look at my blood work and would go through a list of questions . . . and it was a lot of 'yes, yes.' I just kept waiting for there to be something more. At the second appointment, I was finally like, 'Oh, I think this is all there is.'

"It wouldn't have even needed to come from the oncologist. Even if the nurse had sat down and said, 'Okay, you're done with chemo and here's what your next year looks like.' But no one ever explained it to me. People would ask, 'What's your ongoing care?' and I'd say, 'I don't know—what is my ongoing care?'"

Unfortunately, Ashley's experience is more typical than not. While oncologists are very good at ridding your body of cancer and explaining that process to you, they often don't explain what comes next.

ABOUT YOUR ONCOLOGIST

Although you have been working with your oncologist for months or years to combat your cancer, few oncologists have information to offer their patients once conventional treatment concludes. Why is this so?

In truth, few oncologists are trained to provide guidance for life after treatment. And many oncologists are reluctant to discuss improvising or changing any protocol, adding any supplements, or making any recommendations as to lifestyle while the patient is undergoing standard cancer treatment. If a patient pushes the oncologist to add alternative treatments to the regimen, some combination of resistance and rejection will be the likely response.

Unfortunately, an atmosphere of competition exists between the oncologist's legitimate need for strict, uncompromising protocol and the patient's equally important need for wide-open options and life choices. Positive recommendations that could be helpful after treatment are often lost in this adversarial atmosphere.

Most oncologists are only practicing what they have learned—often from long experience—and what they think is best for their patients. They follow the guidelines of the National Comprehensive Cancer Network and the American Society of Clinical Oncology. A specific protocol has been painstakingly formulated to treat each different cancer type. By following these directives, physicians have access to databanks from across the nation, so they are able to enroll their patients, as well as get statistics on the survival of patients with similar diseases nationally. This process is called the "standard of care." By following the conventional standard of care, the doctors are doing what they feel is right for the patient and are protected when facing litigation, are reimbursed by the insurance companies, and are eligible for affiliation with local medical schools. They may also participate in clinical research projects.

Staying within the prescribed guidelines of the standard of care is much like receiving a sort of "merit badge" from your peers. Deviating from this established protocol puts doctors in uncharted waters, often on thin ice with no backup. They jeopardize their insurance, reimbursement, peer standing, and their much-needed support in case of litigation.

In addition to all this, they are simply not well trained to discuss complementary or alternative therapies, even those as simple as increasing exercise. The bulk of their nutrition and exercise training often amounts to a grand total of

2 to 4 weeks during medical school (so about one-half of 1 percent of the total time spent in medical training). There is also something we call "the specialist's syndrome." If someone is a specialist in a particular field—oncology, cardiology, cardiac surgery, or neurology, for example—and is among the best in his specialty, he likely feels that he should know virtually everything there is to know about that very finite universe of medical information, and should be the source of information to you, the patient, and not vice versa. If you go to your oncologist with research or information on a new treatment he is unfamiliar with, he might assume that it is speculative and untested. After all, he is being paid to provide your treatment and information, not the other way around!

So the forces of human psychology combined with the risks that arise within our litigious society all stifle the physician's inquisitive and curious nature. In addition, the exigencies of daily work—with crowded schedules, forms to fill out, patients to see, and squabbles with insurance companies—put pressure on all doctors to be as efficient as possible in order to have some hope of finishing the office and hospital practice at a halfway reasonable time of day.

This situation is only exacerbated by the many books, manuals, and manuscripts about alternative, complementary, or integrative therapies that are downright hostile to the practicing oncologist. They are frequently written to suggest, often dogmatically, what should be done in lieu of orthodox therapy, not in addition to it. These recommendations are, more often than not, presented as an assault to the entire oncology profession. Of course, this creates an adversarial relationship with the medical professionals, and cooperation is difficult, even in areas where complementary therapies may enhance treatment, protect the patient's normal tissue, or minimize the side effects of orthodox treatment. Due to this approach, complementary information on cancer treatment often falls on deaf ears.

Because of their scientific orientation, it is the position of those in the oncology specialty—in accordance with the National Cancer Institute and the American Cancer Society—that they will only incorporate complementary treatments that are evidence-based and scientifically proven. These are the same guidelines used for chemotherapeutic agents. This means approval by the FDA comes only after long, multi-hundred-million-dollar studies have successfully shown benefits reaching the level of statistical significance.

Oncologists are also very concerned that the addition of a food or a supplement could be a confounding component, affecting the results of an outcome study. This is actually good, solid scientific thinking—pro forma, if you're doing an experiment in a laboratory. But we're talking about people's lives here. We have to examine these nontraditional therapies in light of the risks taken versus the benefits received. Much of the resistance to adding vitamins and minerals to the patient's diet during radiation or chemotherapy has been on a purely hypothetical basis. Little research has been done to prove or disprove the efficacy of many of these substances.

A good example of this is the controversy over adding vitamin C therapy during conventional treatments for cancer. While several papers show the possible efficacy of vitamin C during treatment—and indeed some oncologists are incorporating this into their regimen—the standard thinking goes like this: Tumor therapy works by creating oxidative stress in the cancer cell, but antioxidants

THE TROUBLE WITH DOUBLE-BLIND STUDIES IN INTEGRATIVE MEDICINE

In conventional oncology, the gold standard of deciding on treatment efficacy is the double-blind randomized clinical trial that tries to "minimize variables." Essentially, a double-blind study means both the experimenter and the experiment are shielded from information that could lead to bias.

However, minimizing variables is largely an illusion, because many uncontrolled variables are still present in clinical trials. For example, researchers do not know or specify what patients are eating; they do not know about their relationships, their stressors, whether their lifestyle is physically active or sedentary, what is happening in their environment, and significant other factors. In addition, patients often change many of these things on their own, or with guidance from a natural medicine practitioner, without the awareness of the scientists running the clinical trials.

The double-blind randomized study takes the "healing" element of the healer-client relationship out of the equation—and that can be a very big part of the treatment itself. We don't know how to quantify it, but we know it exists and that it's very important.

It is especially difficult to study integrative cancer medicine (conventional oncology plus CAM therapies) by the double-blind randomized clinical trial method, because we are altering many variables intentionally, and we haven't come up with an ideal way of evaluating integrative treatments. It's also challenging to develop placebos and blinding methods for many of the CAM therapies.

In addition, conventional oncology is very suspicious of anecdotal evidence. A favorite saying in conventional medicine is "the plural of anecdote is not evidence." However, in CAM and integrative cancer medicine, anecdotes and the "best case series" are used to support evidence of efficacy.

At this point, looking carefully at outcomes is about the best we can do. A new field, called whole systems research, is rapidly developing and is badly needed for us to investigate and quantify which interventions work, and how well, within the field of integrative cancer medicine.

like vitamin C work to decrease oxidative stress, not only in the normal cells but potentially in the malignant ones as well. Therefore, vitamin C supplementation should not be used during treatment for cancer. Paradoxically, when vitamin C is given intravenously in large doses (10 to 100 grams), it actually acts as an oxidative therapy; most oncologists are unaware of this.

Although the idea that vitamin C will interfere with chemotherapy or radiation has never been substantiated, it is dogma for most physicians. Since some practitioners of alternative, nonorthodox therapies have actually prescribed such a regimen in lieu of orthodox treatment, one can understand the naturally adversarial relationship that can develop with the patient's oncologist. What responsible oncologist wouldn't be suspect of a therapy that prescribes the exact opposite of what she has been trained in?

It's clear why any effort to improve the general health of a patient during cancer therapy can lead to very real angst for that patient, who only wants to get well and do what's best for his or her overall health. Unfortunately, this struggle and confusion in patients' minds about what is best for them is not in their best interest. It sets up a poor emotional and psychological environment for optimizing their chances for complete and lasting recovery.

It is interesting to note that while orthodox oncologists are very precise and exacting about their demands for scientific evidence when it involves the possible use of certain foods, herbs, micronutrients, and other supplements, they tend to be laissez-faire in their attitude toward some of the softer and "fuzzier" alternative therapies such as Reiki, acupuncture, hypnosis, massage, yoga, and music therapy. These therapies are welcomed in many of the larger cancer centers, even though they lack the solid research-backed evidence of effectiveness demanded of other integrative and alternative therapies, such as supplements and diet.

Why is that? We believe there are three specific reasons. One, patients have advocated for it. Two, it brings in money for the treatment centers. Three, it doesn't step on the toes of conventional medicine or challenge, threaten, or detract from established treatment procedures nor present obvious ways that such therapies might interact or interfere with conventional oncology therapies.

It would be fortunate, indeed, to find that rare oncologist willing to work with an integrative practitioner, so that together they would develop an overarching program to include alternative treatments or supplementation, along with a carefully crafted post-therapy program. Failing that, it simply is not in the best interest of patients to challenge their oncologist's established routine. This is just not very likely to lead to success. Patients should not be required to participate in fractious areas hotly contested by physicians and health practitioners, as this inevitably creates stress for patients, which can be detrimental to their outcomes.

While it may take some time before conventional oncologists are willing to integrate complementary and alternative medicine into their treatment of cancer, most oncologists are far more willing to view such therapies favorably for their patients *after* completion of conventional treatment for their cancer. Most patients choose to stay with their oncologists after treatment, but we understand many of them harbor doubts about their prospects for overall wellness, as well as unanswered questions about how to optimize overall health and general confusion over whether or not they are making the best decisions.

Our goal with this book is to help create the best possible environment for helping you stay well after definitive cancer treatment has been completed. We hope this book will help you sidestep the war zone that sometimes occurs between orthodox and alternative oncology treatment by providing a blueprint for living that allows you to feel confident you are doing something positive about optimizing your health and, in the long run, about minimizing the chances for recurrence, with or without the involvement of your oncologist.

WORKING WITH YOUR ONCOLOGIST

Having said all that, what does conventional oncology actually offer the patient at the completion of the recommended therapy, and how do you work with your oncologist following your cancer treatment?

Ideally, you have a good enough relationship with your oncologist that you are comfortable talking about some of your concerns and posing your questions about things you should be doing after cancer treatment. Ideally, too, when you leave formal care under your oncologist, you have already thought about and started to talk to your oncologist about integrating some diet, exercise, and stress-management changes into your life. Then, when treatment concludes and you are feeling better, you can build on this work.

Jay was diagnosed with Ewing's sarcoma a few months shy of his 50th birthday. In January 2011, a tumor on his spine was removed, and he subsequently underwent 6 weeks of radiation and 12 cycles of chemotherapy—a total of 18 or 19 months of chemotherapy, including rest periods during which he received blood transfusions.

Although he was physically and mentally weakened due to surgeries, brutal rounds of chemotherapy, and radiation, he did several things for himself throughout his treatment. Primary among them was walking. "First I would walk, and I would walk farther and farther," he says. "It wasn't a linear progression. I'd walk farther and then there would be a day when I wasn't feeling as well, and then I'd walk farther the next day. I wanted my circulatory system to work

Sherry's Story

Sherry was first diagnosed with ductal carcinoma in situ in 2002 and had a mastectomy. In 2010, she was diagnosed with stage IV breast cancer. She has been in remission for 3½ years. Sherry was lucky to start the conversation about after care with her oncologist while still in treatment. "Personally, I think it needs to start in the first few visits. Patients need to understand the importance of lifestyle," she says. "They need to understand the glycemic index of food, watch their sugar and carbohydrate intake, and try to limit their exposure to toxins as much as they can. The most important things are diet, exercise, and stress management—and I think those are really important early. I think that a really thorough workup with your primary care doctor is critical because your body is so depleted. You've just got to find out where you are, what's your new baseline."

as hard as possible when I was doing chemo. I wanted the chemo to get into every nook and cranny."

When Jay finally finished chemo and was told that there was no evidence of disease, he began physical therapy for his spine—a year and a half after his surgery. "It was very challenging, very arduous, but I had been walking the whole time."

There are ways to begin preparing yourself for life after treatment even when you are still undergoing treatment. Dr. Mehta tries to do this with his breast cancer patients as much as possible by establishing a rapport with them and beginning a conversation about what they are looking toward at the end of their treatment. This way he has a sense of their current lifestyle, their interests, and their goals following treatment.

You can begin to have this same type of conversation with your own oncologist by asking specific questions about how lifestyle might fit in to or affect your treatment. "Is it okay if I take this supplement or eat this type of food?" "What are my limits as far as exercise while undergoing treatment?" "Is there anything you recommend I not do?"

Let your doctor know that you are looking to make a commitment to health moving forward and that you'd love her help with this. Oncologists want you to be healthy and will generally respond favorably if you approach them with questions that will help guide your after care and not compromise your treatment.

Dr. Mehta suggests that at the last visit with your oncologist when concluding treatment, you ask for a short interval follow-up appointment to discuss lifestyle if your doctor is comfortable with it. Rather than wait the standard

3 months, Dr. Mehta tries to schedule his patients' first follow-up at 1 month. He asks them to bring a food diary listing everything they ingest, everything they drink, and every pill they take. This is a proactive step that often helps open his patients' eyes to what they are actually ingesting versus what they think they are ingesting. At the visit, he discusses what they are eating, provides some tips for better nutrition, and offers some strategies for losing weight for those patients who need it. Because recent studies have shown a strong correlation between mortality and obesity in breast cancer, he can provide his patients with this information.

Assuming you are reading this book, you are likely reading other sources of information about your life postcancer. The caregivers in your life may also be reading information about postcancer care, which they may want to share with you. If you read an interesting article about the promising effects of a supplement, an exercise regimen, or some type of superfood, instead of photocopying it and sticking it under your doctor's nose at your next appointment, send it via e-mail with a note saying something like this: "I read this article and would like

Dr. Bouch's Story

Brian Bouch, MD, is both a doctor and a cancer patient. He was first diagnosed with head and neck cancer with lymph node metastases in 1997. "It's tough to say what oncologists should be saying to patients because their training doesn't take them there," says Dr. Bouch. "They don't know about nutrition. They don't know about mind-body practice. Unless there is something really obvious like smoking, they tell their patients to live their lives. If they had the training and knowledge, I'd like to see them say something like, 'You should detoxify now. You should eat a diet that is very low glycemic and low carbohydrate, and we want your emotional health to be as good as it can be. With a healthy immune system, you have a much better chance of not getting this cancer back and not getting another cancer.'"

When Dr. Bouch concluded his own treatment, he received the same advice most patients receive: Go back to your old life. But with his background in alternative medicine, he was able to formulate a plan for keeping himself healthy—something he now does for his own patients. He estimates 60 percent of the patients at his integrative clinic are oncology patients.

"Basically, from the mainstream providers, I got the same line—'You are finished with treatment, we want to keep an eye on you,'"—says Dr. Bouch. "But I was very much aware that this was a golden opportunity to work on preventing it from coming back."

to try their suggestions. Is there anything about my cancer that would preclude this supplement, exercise, or food? Could we discuss this at my next visit?"

Your oncologist may have a specific reaction right away. For example, if you had a kidney removed due to renal cancer, your doctor may recommend against an exercise regimen that includes contact sports. Or she may say that she'll read the article and discuss it with you when you come in. When you do go in for your appointment, rather than expecting your oncologist to have read the entire article and be instantly able to comment on it, bring the article with you and ask any specific questions it brings up. For example, "I sent you an article about the potential benefits of taking vitamin D after cancer. Do you think there is any merit to it, and is there any reason why I shouldn't take vitamin D at the dose the article suggests?" Posing the question in this way allows your oncologist to feel included in your treatment but doesn't put her in a position of being asked about a treatment or study that she isn't familiar with. At the same time, it provides you the medical information you need: Is this regimen advisable based on my personal history?

Most oncologists will be better able to address your questions if they are specific rather than open-ended. Instead of asking your oncologist what you should be eating, ask questions about your particular health status and a specific type of food. These questions might be: "Based on my current weight, should I reduce my weight to improve my outcome?" "Do you think there is a correlation between eating adequate fiber and my cancer?"

Even if oncologists are thinking about it, they will rarely address weight and cancer because they are neither trained for it nor comfortable bringing it up with patients who are overweight. They are more skilled in having difficult conversations about death and dying than they are in talking about lifestyle concerns.

Because oncology follow-up appointments tend to be short—no more than 15 minutes on average—patients may feel rushed and not address questions they have. If this is the case for you, ask your oncologist if you can follow up by e-mail or phone later, or if that's not possible, whether you can schedule an interval appointment.

YOUR FAMILY DOCTOR

In the chaos and panic that come with a cancer diagnosis, it can be easy to forget one of your most valuable resources in your overall health: your general practitioner (GP). You may not see him or her for a year or more while you undergo treatment. Everything becomes about the cancer. But following treatment, it's essential you reestablish a close connection with your primary care doctor's office. Dr. Mehta recommends that all of his patients see their internist for a comprehensive physical exam and follow-up within a few months following treatment.

Cancer treatment can wear down your immune system, leaving you vulnerable to infections and other physical ailments, and chemo and radiation can have physical side effects that are best addressed by your GP. And just because you had cancer doesn't mean you can't have other illnesses! Sometimes patients become so accustomed to seeing their oncologist, they assume that all of their functions are being monitored, but that's not the case. Generally, your oncologist will only run blood work pertinent to your cancer. For general health and for annual exams, including full blood work, you should see your primary physician. General questions about your nutrition, physical fitness, and stress management can also be posed to your GP.

There is some evidence that people who continue to see their primary care doctors have better outcomes than people who don't. Some hypothesize that this is because GPs pay attention to things that oncologists don't and may be more holistically minded when it comes to general health.

ALL THOSE TESTS: WHAT ARE THEY SEARCHING FOR?

Generally, your oncologist will do some type of follow-up exam every 3 to 6 months for a couple of years and then annually. This may include x-rays, CT scans, MRIs, mammograms, and blood studies. However, the new "standard of care" following treatment for some types of cancer is not to do any monitoring other than periodic follow-up physical exams. Instead, the patient is told to return if new symptoms appear. Then CT scans and blood work are done. This approach is based on studies that indicate there is not always survival advantage to treating recurrent cancers early, when they are first diagnosed through testing, as opposed to treating them when diagnosed later after symptoms develop.

Neither of these approaches to follow-up care constitutes treatment. In the first case, this is just surveillance and detection, not prevention. Waiting for a recurrence of symptoms isn't even surveillance. However, it may be that avoiding surveillance itself might be a positive step. According to the National Cancer Institute, about 2 percent of the cancers in the United States are created by overexposure to diagnostic radiation itself.[1] When you consider that a total-body CT scan (depending on the age and type of machine) exposes you to 50 to 500 times more radiation than a chest x-ray, you can recognize the possible severity of this problem.

Patients who have had one cancer are more prone to getting a second cancer than people who have *never* had cancer. Is it that immune-system suppression, an inherent outcome of chemo and radiation therapy, sets up the conditions for a recurrence of cancer or the development of a new one? Or could it be that the excessive use of CT scans, x-rays, and nuclear medicine studies, such as PET scans, causes recurrence or new tumor formation? Or does it mean the patient is predisposed to cancer? Unfortunately, we don't know that answer.

After the follow-up testing is done, your visit with your oncologist will likely be brief. She will review your blood work and/or scans, and discuss the results with you. Your oncologist is looking for signs that cancer has returned; in your blood work, she is specifically looking for tumor markers in the form of protein markers or circulating tumor markers. Any blood levels that are too high or too low might also indicate a second look. Cancer is rarely diagnosed by blood work alone, but abnormal results will lead to more diagnostic tests, such as additional blood work, scans, or a biopsy.

Computed tomography, or CT, essentially uses multiple x-rays from multiple cross sections to provide a 3-D view inside the body. Sometimes a contrast material, often iodine, will be used. A tumor will show up as an aberration. Positron-emission tomography, or PET, uses a small amount of a radiotracer that collects in the body and allows the oncologist to see cancers through the rate of their glucose uptake. (This may be illustrated best by picturing a brain scan. Active parts of the brain utilize more glucose than inactive parts, so it is easy to see which parts are the most active.) Cancer cells are highly metabolic and rapidly utilize glucose, so they show up on the scan.

As mentioned above, following treatment for some cancers, the trend in the last few years has been to do fewer or no scans. It's estimated that one CT scan exposes you to the same amount of radiation you would normally be exposed to in a year. If you get three or four scans a year, that's quite a bit. For breast cancer and prostate cancer, oncologists no longer do scans. For colon cancer, scans are done once a year, and with lymphoma, scans may be done once a year or every 3 years, depending on the type. For other cancers, oncologists now only do chest x-rays, or they limit the scan to a specific region.

Patients concerned about radiation should discuss this with their oncologist. There may be an option to do an ultrasound or MRI instead of a radiation-driven scan, or they may be able to take more time between scans. Oncologists anticipate that their patients will advocate for more scans rather than fewer scans, so your oncologist may be more willing to limit scans than you might expect.

Testing: What to Expect

There is little preparation needed for blood work or CT or PET scans. You may be asked to fast for 8 hours prior to blood work or scans, although you will be allowed to drink water. For blood work, a phlebotomist will draw your blood, then you will be done until you meet with your oncologist.

For a PET scan, you'll be asked to change into a hospital gown and remove any metal jewelry. Then you will be injected with a radiotracer—a small amount of radioactive material that is traced through your body. You will then lie on a narrow table that slides into the PET machine. The scan itself will only take a few minutes and is painless, although you will be asked not to move. If you are cold, you can usually ask for a blanket. Let the office know if you are claustrophobic, as you may be offered a sedative to relieve your anxiety. Unless you take a sedative, there is no recovery time. However, you should drink plenty of water to flush the radiotracer from your system.

A CT scan is generally a simple procedure. For a CT scan, you will be asked to change into a hospital gown and then lie on a narrow table, which slides into the doughnut-shaped CT machine. There is no pain, although the loud noise created by the machine can be jarring for some patients. Sometimes you will be given a contrast dye when receiving a CT scan, which allows some abnormalities to show up better. The dye is generally iodine and injected, swallowed, or given as an enema. Again, drink plenty of water afterward to flush out the iodine.

For an x-ray, you will lie down or stand while it is taken. There is no recovery time.

Depending on your oncologist, your office visit may be scheduled the same day as the tests or a few days later. The appointment is quite short, usually only 15 minutes. At that appointment, the doctor will review your tests with you. If she sees any markers in your blood work, she may ask to have it repeated in a few weeks. It's quite common for labs to show abnormalities that resolve upon retesting. If repeat blood work still indicates areas of concern, she may ask for a CT or PET scan. If anything suspicious is seen on the scan, the oncologist will likely order a biopsy.

Your oncologist may also see benign abnormalities or small changes that she'll note to you. For example, she may notice scar tissue, calcium buildups, or small nodules in your lungs or liver. Generally these are nothing to be concerned about, but you should feel very comfortable asking the oncologist to clarify her meaning: "You say there are two nodules in my lungs. What does this mean? Could this be a sign of recurrence? What is your plan in watching them?"

You should also feel comfortable asking your oncologist what she is looking for and why. Sometimes oncologists are looking for a side effect from an ongoing medication such as tamoxifen, while other times they are looking for tumor markers. Your oncologist may be willing to do blood work on things that are a particular concern to you: "Could you check my vitamin D level?" or "I'm feeling tired a lot. Could you check my thyroid function?"

After reviewing your blood work and scans, your doctor will generally ask whether you have any other concerns you'd like to discuss. Again, because of the brevity of these visits, prepare specific questions to produce better answers.

BRING THESE TO YOUR FOLLOW-UP VISIT

A PEN AND PAPER. Write down what your oncologist tells you. Follow-up visits are short, and it helps to be able to review information at your leisure after the appointment.

A FRIEND OR FAMILY MEMBER. Because follow-ups can be quite stressful, it can be helpful to bring someone to take notes for you. Patients do not always "hear" their doctors because of strong emotions or anxiety during the appointment. Encourage your companion to ask any questions that come to mind.

PRINTOUTS OF ANY ARTICLES YOU MAY HAVE SENT THE DOCTOR PREVIOUSLY. Don't spring new articles on your doctor, but do have copies of things you've sent before to jog her memory. You can also leave articles with her and ask whether you can follow up via e-mail or phone or at a future appointment.

YOUR NUTRITION AND EXERCISE JOURNALS. If your oncologist has questions about specific exercises or nutritional guidelines, you'll have the journals there for immediate reference.

ANY QUESTIONS YOU'VE BEEN THINKING ABOUT. Write down any questions that come up between appointments and go through the list with your doctor. (Of course, if you have any immediate concerns, don't hesitate to contact your oncologist between follow-ups.)

Many times patients are afraid to ask their oncologist too many questions. They may not want to know what is going to happen if a test is abnormal, or they may be concerned about taking too much of the doctor's time. However, a lot of the stress of having cancer is the loss of control and the not knowing. Arming yourself with knowledge about the disease can be empowering, as can understanding the next steps if there is a recurrence.

As Dr. Mehta points out, oncologists tend to have a captain-of-the-ship mentality, and that's for a good reason. Patients come into an oncologist's office scared. They want to see their doctor as knowledgeable, so even if oncologists have only seen a disease once, they will read up on it. They don't want patients to lose confidence in them. At the same time, if a patient brings up an alternative protocol or new research that the oncologist isn't experienced with, she might be dismissive of it at first. However, it's okay to continue that discussion at the next visit or to ask whether you could follow up on the discussion via e-mail or on the phone. It's also okay to ask for a referral to an oncologist who may have more interest in or knowledge on the subject. Most urban areas now have academic centers that have integrative clinics, and some patients may find it helpful to visit one.

In general, oncologists appreciate specific questions rather than open-ended ones. Here are a few of the type of questions you might pose to your oncologist:

> I'm having a lot of numbness around my scar. Is there anything I could do to relieve this?

> I have lymphedema in my arm. Are there any exercises that could help with this?

> I still feel like I have chemo brain. Can you suggest any supplements that might help with this?

> I'd like to try acupuncture for stress management, but I heard that it can spread cancer cells. Is this true?

Other questions might be more general:

> I read an article linking eating refined sugar to cancer. What are your thoughts on this? Can I leave the article with you to read?

> I've had a lot of fatigue since finishing my treatments. Do you have any suggestions for things I might do to combat this?

> I've heard that environmental toxins might affect cancer recurrence. Do you have any thoughts on things I could do around my home to limit my exposure to toxins? Are there specific toxins you think I should be concerned about?

It is common for people who have had cancer to assume that every ache and pain is a sign of recurrence. Talk to your oncologist about what symptoms you should be looking for. You don't want to go through anxiety over benign symptoms, but you do want to bring up questions about symptoms that may be pertinent, either as a possible sign of recurrence or an aftereffect of your treatment.

Although your oncologist may not initially offer a great deal of advice about your lifestyle following cancer treatment, most doctors want their patients to live the fullest, healthiest lives possible. If you engage with them in a way that respects their knowledge of the oncological field while asking specific questions that they can address (or refer you to someone who can), you will have the best luck.

PREPARING FOR FOLLOW-UPS

Follow-up tests are arguably the most stressful part of a cancer survivor's life. In the months, weeks, and days leading up to your appointment, you may find yourself thinking about it constantly and becoming increasingly fearful about the test results. This is normal. The unfortunate setup for cancer surveillance is that you hope for good news and deal with bad news if it comes—with very little conversation about what that really means. Despite the fact that many people do well after recurrence, few oncologists talk candidly about this possibility with their patients. This can only exacerbate the feelings of anxiety and stress that occur around follow-ups.

Over time, most people do feel less anxious about upcoming tests, but the anxiety never completely goes away—even after the magical 5-year mark.

Dr. McKee knows that all his patients feel some anxiety about follow-up appointments. He believes the ones who feel the least anxiety, however, are those who have confronted their mortality and—while working very hard to live healthily—have worked to diminish their fear around death and dying. Many counselors and psychologists work in this area, and your primary doctor or oncologist can suggest a professional if you feel like this would be helpful.

You may also find that engaging in relaxation methods and physical exercise helps relieve the stress of a follow-up visit. You are already doing one of the most helpful things to alleviate this stress: taking action by working to keep yourself healthy. By being proactive about staying healthy, being knowledgeable about what to expect in your follow-ups and in the event of recurrence, and going into your follow-ups with questions and goals, you are taking control of your own health, which will result in less stress and a more productive visit.

Your first evaluation is going to be stressful; there's no way around it. You'll be worried about how your scan will look. But you can use specific breathing techniques to calm yourself. You can also review the positive changes in your life to empower yourself. Finally, you can accept that there will be some anxiety, without letting it take over.

"Those visits are so fraught with terror," says Dr. Bouch. "But for the person going back for a visit, they should try to remain as calm as they can. To be able to hear anything that might come from the oncologist with any value, they should be calm and should have someone with them. Most people who come to see me bring someone with them. That person takes notes, and I encourage them to ask questions."

Like Dr. Bouch, Tara is a physician and a cancer survivor. She was diagnosed 5 years ago with breast cancer with lymph-node involvement. Like Dr. Bouch, she takes a philosophical approach to follow-ups. "I just came to expect that every single visit with the doctor was especially stressful, and it was for about the 2 weeks before," said Tara, adding that while there is little to do about the stress associated with follow-ups, she did actively work to protect herself from the effects of radiation from scans by taking antioxidants. "First there was the blood work, then the scan, then the visit, and then stress. I definitely didn't want more visits. Each visit was more stressful. I just chose to deal with the fear."

CHAPTER THREE

CANCER REHAB

WHEN BOB LEFT THE HOSPITAL AFTER A MILD HEART ATTACK AT THE AGE OF 46, he was handed a notebook of information on nutrition, exercise, stress reduction, and other protocols to follow to prevent another heart attack. His doctor called it his cardiac rehab packet. He also left with an appointment for the following week at the hospital's cardiac rehab center. When he showed up for his appointment, Bob met his new nutritionist, his personal trainer, and a counselor.

For 12 weeks, he had weekly appointments with each, as well as thrice-weekly workout sessions in the rehab center gym. The workout sessions included EKG monitoring and blood pressure monitoring, and an RN was on-site at all times. His new nutritionist provided him information about heart-healthy food and about shopping for and cooking this food. His counselor helped him formulate a stress-management plan that included options for group therapy, one-on-one counseling, biofeedback, massage, acupuncture, and meditative activities such as yoga, meditation, and qigong. All this happened at a large teaching hospital in a major US city.

Around the same time, Samantha left another large teaching hospital in a different major US city. She was also 46. She'd had surgery to remove a tumor from her colon, and, fortunately, the cancer was stage I. She had an excellent prognosis. When Samantha went to her last appointment with her oncologist prior to her 3-month checkup, she asked about things she could do to prevent a recurrence. Her oncologist told her not to smoke. He also gave her a number for the hospital's cancer support group. Samantha asked about any diet changes she should make, but the oncologist just reassured her that she was healthy and could go back to her "old life." Although Samantha was ecstatic about her successful treatment, and was eager to get back to normal, she found it wasn't that easy. She was anxious about her follow-up appointments and dreaded each scan. She hated feeling like there was nothing she could do to prevent her cancer from coming back, and became increasingly anxious and depressed. She ultimately went on antianxiety medication.

Two years after Samantha's and Bob's health scares, Bob has made many changes in his lifestyle. He goes to the gym regularly and stopped eating red meat. He also worked to eliminate areas of stress from his life, making a difficult decision about a stressful job. Samantha did finally quit smoking after 26 years, on her oncologist's advice. However, without guidance regarding exercise and diet, and dealing with her anxiety, she gained weight—and some other latent health concerns have become worse, such as her high blood pressure. Complications with her surgery site have made it difficult to follow an exercise regimen. She did go to a cancer support group for a few months, but seeing new friends have recurrences or die of their disease only exacerbated her anxiety.

While Bob had the impetus, guidance, and gravitas provided by the professionals at his cardiac rehab center, Samantha felt largely on her own in navigating life after cancer. Although she could have reached out to an integrative oncologist, counselor, nutritionist, or personal trainer on her own, it wasn't really something she knew much about—and, anyways, she was busy with work and family. And wasn't her prognosis positive? Her oncologist had said not to worry about lifestyle changes, so why should she?

Most oncology patients are like Samantha. They worry and wait for the other shoe to drop but are given little in the way of guidance to keep themselves physically and emotionally healthy.

We believe that if oncologists offered even the most rudimentary post-therapy program to optimize their patients' general health and help minimize the chance of cancer recurrence, it would be a great benefit. Even if there were no correlations between exercise and weight and cancer, the psychological help alone would be worth it.

Without such a program, post-treatment patients are left to wander aimlessly, worrying about their cancer coming back with nothing to help them physically, psychologically, or emotionally as this Sword of Damocles hangs over their heads. Some studies show that worry and stress can actually increase the risk of relapse.

FORMALIZING AFTER CARE

We believe the most effective way to implement our after cancer care philosophy is to build on the model now widely used after people have survived a heart attack—the same cardiac rehab that Bob was able to utilize. Rehab involves primarily supervised exercise, along with dietary counseling and stress-management guidance.

We are beginning to see some forward-thinking cancer centers establish similar "cancer rehab" programs. We feel that this needs to become a national priority, with programs placed in hospitals, cancer centers, outpatient clinics, and even health clubs. These cancer rehab centers would ideally be funded by insurance, including Medicare and Medicaid, with patients referred by their oncologists after treatment is completed. Considering that every recurrence of cancer can end up costing millions of dollars in medical treatment—not to mention the cost in human suffering for patients and their loved ones—and given new studies about the powerful effects of exercise and relaxation training on cancer survival, it seems obvious that this would be a cost-effective social and medical approach. In addition, this type of cancer rehab would have broader impacts on other lifestyle-related illnesses, such as diabetes, high blood pressure, and heart disease.

Expanding on the cardiac rehab model, cancer rehab would also include supervised exercise, relaxation training, massage, acupuncture, nutrition and cooking classes, support groups, and even guidance in nutritional supplementation. Fundamental to it would be the formula established by Moshe Frenkel, MD, director of Integrative Oncology Consultants and formerly with the MD Anderson Cancer Center: the 0, 5, 10, 30, 150 formula. This is a precise formula for good health and stands for: 0 cigarettes; 5 servings of fruits and vegetables per day; 10 minutes of silence, relaxation, or meditation per day; keeping the body mass index at less than 30 kg/m²; and 150 minutes of exercise per week.

How many cancer patients actually use this formula? According to a study published in 2008, only 4.5 percent of breast cancer patients, 5.1 percent of prostate cancer patients, and 4.6 percent of colorectal cancer patients.[1] Overall, close to 95 percent of cancer patients are not following this formula. We have a lot of work to do.

Our goal over the next 10 years is to get the medical community to embrace cancer rehab in the same way it has embraced cardiac rehab. That means oncologists would have clear next steps to provide their patients, hospitals would have designated cancer rehab centers, and insurance would pay for 12 weeks or more of cancer rehab.

In the meantime, this book provides guidelines for managing health after cancer treatment that oncologists, primary doctors, and patients themselves can follow. At a minimum, if an oncologist or primary doctor is uncomfortable making lifestyle recommendations to his patients, he can recommend this book as a start.

We are advocating a lifestyle change for patients—of the foods they eat, the attitudes they have, the level of physical activity they choose, and the environmental pollution they are exposed to. By giving cancer patients a program they can believe in and actively participate in, we are convinced they will feel better; enhance their immune system; improve their physical, psychological, and emotional well-being and overall quality of life; and minimize the chance of cancer recurrence.

We also believe that patients should have options to choose from as they make a plan for living. The choices we offer are based on scientific data and have been selected to optimize wellness. We also pay specific attention to different types of cancer and provide variations in the general program for dealing with them. We want you to feel comfortable and enjoy the pieces of this program that you integrate into your life. If they are not enjoyable, they won't be sustainable. They will become sustainable as you come to appreciate and enjoy them. Part of the program focuses on food, and you will learn that some foods promote cancer, while other foods keep it at bay. We'll explain what seems almost inconceivable: What you think or feel or fret over can actually change the very core gene expression in your body, creating an environment for either health or disease. We'll talk about managing stress and getting enough exercise, and how to fight the impact of exposure to poisons in the environment.

Ideally, we would like every oncologist to be able to say to patients at the end of treatment: "I'd like you to go to cancer rehab, which your insurance covers, and it's right over there. There's a gym and trainers, food shopping and cooking classes, progressive muscle relaxation therapy, massage therapy, and acupressure." By going to a 12-week cancer rehab program, patients would develop better habits and be far more likely to continue the health-promoting lifestyle changes long term.

Cardiac rehab is an excellent model of what cancer rehab could be. Both heart attacks and cancer are wake-up calls for premature mortality. But because doctors see heart disease as more of a lifestyle disease, it is part of mainstream medicine to modify the risk factors by exercising, changing diet, and regulating stress. We tend to see cancer as a bolt out of nowhere (as heart attacks were viewed in the 1950s and '60s). However, we now know that there are controllable factors that exacerbate the chance of cancer as well as the chance of recurrence. Unfortunately, this has not yet penetrated into the medical mind and hasn't filtered to the public mind. We hope this book will play a role in starting to change that mind-set.

While cancer rehab would be structured similarly to cardiac rehab, ideally it would evaluate each patient and then cater to an individual patient's needs. For example, a patient who can't stop crying may need a focus on counseling, while a patient who is 100 pounds overweight may need help with diet. Someone who had breast cancer might receive different nutritional advice than a person who had colon cancer. Those who have had mastectomies and lymphadenectomies need emphasis on upper-body strength training and stretching that a colon cancer patient may not need. A patient who has had a major abdominal surgery may need help strengthening the muscles that were cut during surgery.

As part of the program, progress reports would be sent to the patients' oncologists. Not only would this keep them in the loop, it would make them part of the loop—allowing them to communicate more efficiently with their patients.

STARTING YOUR OWN CANCER REHAB

You've completed chemotherapy, and your oncologist has given you the "all clear." Perhaps he's even given you this book. All the tools you need to reduce your chances of recurrence and take control of your life are here on these pages.

The first thing we recommend you do to begin your personal cancer rehab is to buy two notebooks. Label the notebooks "Nutrition" and "Exercise." Use these journals to track your daily exercise and eating habits. Be honest and detailed—these journals will help you gauge where you started and where you want to go. Be sure to bring your journals with you when meeting with your doctor or oncologist to show your progress and to remind yourself of any questions you want to bring up.

As you progress through this book, developing your own cancer rehab, your journals will be an invaluable, customized resource.

PART TWO

PHYSICAL
HEALTH

CHAPTER FOUR

EPIGENETICS

N ABOUT 1990, A FEVERISH ENDEAVOR BEGAN TO DECODE THE HUMAN GENOME TO identify the sequence of individual genes that, when taken together, make up the blueprint for the human body. The Human Genome Project was successfully completed by scientists at the National Institutes of Health, who produced a complete draft of the human genome sequence in 2003, thus putting the information in the public domain.

An explosion of scientific research and new understanding followed. Genes relating to cancer and other crippling diseases have been identified, along with many other aspects of how our bodies function.

But aspects of this impressive achievement troubled many investigators. First, the 150,000 genes hypothetically required to produce the proteins, fats, organic acids, and carbohydrates needed for life were mostly missing! The human genome actually consists of fewer than 28,000 genes—about one-fifth the number expected. This implied (which was later confirmed) that these fewer individual genes not only were capable of producing different forms of proteins, but also worked in concert with other genes in the chromosome. Thus the DNA, instead of being the governing "decision maker" of the cell, was merely a sort of blueprint filing cabinet waiting to be opened to get to the information stored within. It is not unlike the process of building a house: The builder is drawing on the essential plans held in the blueprints to guide him as to how to actually erect the home.

This surprising conclusion forced researchers to rethink their basic premise about the function of the chromosome. Half of a chromosome's makeup is the protein wrapped around the DNA. Because the DNA was the focal point of experiments conducted prior to genome sequencing, the techniques to isolate the DNA required removal of the protein. Since this discovery, we have seen a reexamination of the chromosome, including the protein wrapping. And with this, an entirely new science has evolved: epigenetics.

This approach postulates that the protein wrapping, or epigene, either responds or doesn't respond to specific proteins, amino acids, and other "information" to allow or prevent access to the DNA, which then replicates the appropriate molecules. The entire way of thinking about DNA has changed from the DNA being a sort of sacred lockbox with immutable, predestined reactions to it being more of a vending machine, supplying different products depending on the amount of money deposited and numbers pushed.

In the simplest terms, the principle of epigenetics is that genes respond to the external stimuli of food, toxins, environment, stress, exercise, and other information, and then act accordingly by either suppressing or promoting an increase of enzyme and protein production that dramatically affects the individual's wellness.

This way of thinking has led to some remarkable observations. Most startling among them is that lifestyle changes can actually regulate gene expression in clinical conditions such as hypertension, metabolic syndrome, and even cancer.

The ramifications of these findings are profound. Only 5 percent of all cancers can be traced to inherited genetic variation. This means that the rest—nearly all cancers—could be directly affected by environmental influences, such as toxin and radiation exposure, infection, nutrition and other lifestyle choices, and other outside forces, many of which can be changed! By recognizing this, we also acknowledge that there are changes we can make systemically and individually to prevent cancer or recurrence. On an individual level, this provides new possibilities for cancer patients and survivors to make positive choices to control the direction of their lives.

Everyone has cancer cells, which are simply cells that grow and divide faster than healthy cells and have their "kill switch" turned off; normally our natural killer cells and other parts of a healthy immune system eliminate them.

THE POWER OF MIND-SET

Recent mind-body research has shown that cancer survivors who consider themselves "cured" have a higher quality of life and lower rate of relapse than those who describe themselves as "in remission." It appears that our mind-set, as well as our diet and lifestyle, is very powerful.

Epigenetics, among other factors, may be triggers as to whether cells become cancerous and whether the natural killer cells work to eliminate the cancer cells as they should. Cancer remission may be described as patients having no more cancer but still having the potential for cancer. Remission is something like the proverb in which a grandfather tells his grandson that all people have two wolves raging inside them. One wolf is kindness and one is hate. The grandson asks which wolf will win, and the grandfather answers: the one you feed.

If you feed the natural killer cell—with a healthy diet, exercise, and a positive outlook—it will be better equipped to eliminate the destructive cancer cell. If you feed the cancer cell—with a diet high in inflammatory products, little exercise, and stress—the cancer cell will likely win.

INFLAMMATION AND THE LYMPH SYSTEM

Concomitant with the acceptance of epigenetic theory is an understanding of the importance of the lymphatic system. More than 30 years ago, at the Temple University School of Medicine, Dr. Lemole hypothesized based on laboratory research and clinical observation that the lymphatic system plays an important role in the creation of chronic degenerative diseases such as cancer and arteriosclerosis. Although it is the home of the immune system, the messenger for the endocrine system, the cellular waste disposal system, and the regulator of the body fluid balance (containing more fluid than the blood vessels), the lymphatic system has been grossly overlooked and understudied in medical science.

The HDL (good) cholesterol is transported through the lymph system to the liver to be recycled. The white cells, natural killer cells, and other immune cells that destroy cancer are stored in the lymph system, waiting to be recruited by messenger proteins from other parts of the body.

So how can we maximize lymphatic involvement to prevent cancer recurrence?

Lymphatic flow is increased by three to seven times by routine exercise.[1] Positive thoughts and attitudes can prevent lymphatic constriction.[2] Green tea and a vegetable-based diet high in flavonoids are also beneficial for lymphatic clearance,[3] as are practices such as massage, yoga, breathing exercises, and meditation,[4] as well as avoidance of smoking and other toxins.[5]

Another important concept arising in integrative medical research is that chronic inflammation is a critical factor in the creation of chronic degenerative diseases like cancer. Much has been written about the relationship of inflammation and cancer. Oxidative stress (free radical formation) leads to inflammation, long associated with the wide variety of chronic degenerative diseases responsible for 80 percent of health care spending today.

CANCER AND THE IMMUNE SYSTEM

Except for a small minority of tumor immunology researchers who keep chipping away, conventional oncologists until very recently have been generally skeptical about the role of the immune system in cancer treatment. The FDA approved its first advanced disease immunological therapy for prostate cancer in 2010. However, immunotherapies to promote cancer regression and maintain remission by stimulating the human immune response tend to be minimally effective in advanced cancers, where immunosuppression both from cancer and prior treatments is often profound. It makes more sense to use this approach earlier in the process, when the immune system is much more intact.

In a 2011 study conducted at University of Pennsylvania headed by Dr. Carl June, patients' T cells (immune cells) were engineered in the lab to recognize a specific receptor found in chronic lymphocytic leukemia and other B-cell malignancies; they were then grown in cultures outside of the body. Several advanced-stage chronic lymphocytic leukemia patients, who no longer responded to chemotherapy, were infused with their own reengineered T cells and obtained complete and long-lasting responses.[6] In other words, immunotherapy can prove effective.

If this can be shown to work often and in other tumor types, it may represent a fundamentally new way to harness the power and mystery of the immune system to cure cancer even in advanced stages. News of this clinical study also made many conventional oncologists sit up and take notice that immunotherapy may indeed have real promise in cancer therapy. In 2014, several new immunotherapy antibodies were approved for treatment of melanoma. Called checkpoint inhibitors, they block fundamental mechanisms by which many tumors suppress the activity of T cells, which are important components of the cellular immune system.[7] Clinical trials have also shown major activity against other solid tumor types that have never before been responsive to immunotherapies, including lung, breast, colon, and bladder cancer. Immunotherapy is finally coming of age in oncology, but it will likely be some time before these therapies are routinely applied in cancers now treated only by chemo and radiotherapy.[8]

In complementary and alternative medicine (CAM) approaches, practitioners have long believed that the immune system is primary in controlling cancer. Within the CAM community, a perhaps too-naïve assumption is that if you simply stimulate the immune system, it will kill cancer cells.

During 2 years of tumor immunology research that Dr. McKee conducted in the immunology division of the Scripps Research Institute, he was very impressed with the profound immunosuppression that tumors do indeed cause within the body, even rather small tumors.[9] Thus, in general, it makes sense to remove as much tumor from the body as possible before embarking on immune-enhancing therapies.

Inflammation is one of the body's protective mechanisms by which we isolate and dispose of harmful toxins, viruses, and bacteria that invade the body. It is also essential to healing from injuries. Inflammation is a daily part of the robust human survival mechanism, which has evolved over at least several hundred thousand years.

However, *chronic* inflammation, which is constantly present in our bodies, can cause the production of unhealthful products that can lead to cell mutation and cancer. Through this process of gene expression—or in some cases gene suppression—proteins and amino acids protecting against cancer can be shut down. Conversely, genes producing mutation and abnormal growth may be fired up. This direct link between epigenetics, inflammation, and cancer has now been documented in a number of studies, including one on colon tumors undertaken by the Johns Hopkins Kimmel Cancer Center and published in *Cancer Cell* in 2011.[10]

There is no question that it is in your best interest to minimize exposure to environments and situations that can cause chronic inflammation, which could lead to epigenetic changes within cells that can lead to cancer. It's also important to foster conditions that decrease the development of chronic inflammation in our bodies so that genes suppressing cancer are opened and genes promoting cancer are closed. Fortunately, in many cases this can be done naturally and without chemicals or medications through changes to our day-to-day lifestyles. We can reduce inflammation by paying particular attention to our lymphatic health and by incorporating lifestyle changes in our diet, stress management, and exercise.

While epigenetics is changing cancer research, so far it has not really changed cancer practice. But now that we know how it works, we can start to make these changes on our own.

CHAPTER FIVE

DIET AND NUTRITION

I N THE PAST FEW YEARS, MANY SCIENTIFIC PAPERS AND ARTICLES IN MEDICAL JOURNALS have demonstrated the relationship between obesity and cancer prevalence. Recent studies have suggested that visceral fat may act as an endocrine organ, synthesizing and releasing inflammatory chemicals called cytokines. It has also been well established that chronic inflammation facilitates cancer growth.

Guidelines for instituting whole food diets rich in fruits, vegetables, legumes, and whole grains, as well as exercise, both during and after cancer treatment, and obtaining and maintaining a healthy weight have appeared from many mainstream sources. They include the American Cancer Society and the American Society of Clinical Oncology, and are based on ever-increasing research that indicates that such interventions improve both survival and quality of life for patients during and after treatments.[1,2,3]

Obesity is second only to tobacco as a preventable cause of diseases and death in the United States. Obesity has been strongly associated with increased risk of many cancers, including colorectal, endometrial (uterus), esophageal, kidney, pancreatic, and breast (in postmenopausal women). Obesity is probably associated with an increased risk of cancer of the cervix, ovary, liver, and gallbladder, as well as multiple myeloma, non-Hodgkin's lymphoma, and aggressive forms of prostate cancer.[4] Obesity also diminishes the quality of life of cancer survivors and may worsen the prognosis of several cancers.

Yet, such information has not yet led to significant changes in behaviors of cancer patients or in the way the oncology profession counsels patients on a national and international level.[5]

Weight is related to what we eat and how much work we do with our muscles to burn energy. It is clear, given the obesity statistics for our society, that we are not eating foods that enable us to maintain a healthy weight, and we are not moving enough. Part of the problem is our culture's romance with red meat and baked goods, and the addictive nature of processed snack foods that combine fat, salt, and sugar. This is commonly known as SAD, the Standard American Diet—made up of lots of processed, fried foods, white flour, sugar, and red meat. A recently coined phrase, "Sitting is the new smoking," graphically highlights the risks associated with a sedentary lifestyle as well. (More on this in Chapter Six.)

It is not just the amounts of food we eat or their calories that affect our cancer risk, but also the chemicals found in so many foods. Often these chemicals are fat-soluble, so they concentrate in the fat cells. This means that they concentrate in breast, ovary, prostate, and lymphatic tissues, oftentimes on the lipid-rich cell membrane, disrupting hormonal balance.

The chemicals found in foods may be there because of the way they are grown or raised, because of the way they are processed, because of the way they are packaged and shipped, or because of the way we prepare them once they are in our kitchens. In Chapter Seven, we discuss in more detail the types of toxic chemicals that can be found in our foods and how to avoid them.

In the spirit of epigenetics, we can look at foods as either enhancing tumor growth or suppressing it—turning on or turning off genes that are cancer fighting or cancer promoting.

The foods that suppress tumor growth often act in quite different ways. Some suppress the tumor blood supply. Others suppress the tumor cell growth factors or contain antioxidants and enzymes that neutralize compounds required for the survival of the tumor cells. Unfortunately, cancer cells have innate mechanisms to work around many of these suppressors. That is why it's best to have a well-rounded diet, with many different types of fruits and vegetables that supply defense mechanisms to the body. Foods work in harmony, like a symphony, and it's important to have all the different players performing on the right keys at the right time. Just eating a diet of blueberries is not going to prevent cancer, no matter how much of an antioxidant they are. Our meals must consist of a panoply of foods that support the immune system, decrease inflammation, detoxify toxic chemicals, enhance apoptosis (cancer cell suicide, or the "kill switch"), block angiogenesis (new blood vessel growth in tumors), and prevent metastasis.

Great thinkers through the ages from Hippocrates to George Bernard Shaw and Thomas Edison all felt that diet profoundly influences health. Almost daily, scientific papers report the link between poor dietary choices and cancer. Regulatory governmental bodies like the National Cancer Institute routinely warn of the connection between processed meats, red meat, and high-fat and high-sugar diets and cancer of the prostate, breast, lung, and colon. Many articles in peer-reviewed journals have shown the benefit of a high-fiber plant-based diet in cancer prevention. Researchers have shown a strong correlation between obesity and many cancer types.

As we now know, new science and new information on epigenetics show that one can actually change one's gene expression by lifestyle change. Strong evidence indicates that a healthy diet prevents not only cancer but also cardiovascular, autoimmune, and other chronic degenerative diseases. Below are just a few examples of the findings that support the link between diet and cancer.

- A 14-year study of more than 100,000 men and women by American Cancer Society epidemiologists showed that nonsmokers who followed recommended lifestyle behaviors and proper diet decreased their risk of cancer by 30 percent in men and 24 percent in women. Similarly, heart disease was decreased by 48 percent in men and 50 percent in women using the same cancer prevention diet.[6]

- A study published in June 2010 looked at more than 385,000 people in Europe with an average age of 64 years and a history of drinking alcohol daily. It found that the individuals with the highest serum levels of vitamin B_6, methionine, and folate were associated with a 50 percent or greater reduction in lung cancer risk.[7] It was postulated that these nutrients were important in the metabolism of DNA in the body tissue. Amazingly, those with a higher level of B vitamins had a significantly lower risk of lung cancer whether or not they were smokers.

- A Harvard study published in 2012 showed that substituting fish, legumes, nuts, whole grains, and poultry for red meat, especially processed red meat, was associated with a significant decrease in mortality from not only heart disease but cancer.[8] Red meats are known to contain saturated fats, sodium, nitrates, and toxic hydrocarbons from the cooking process (especially grilling), all associated with increased cancer risk.

WHAT TO EAT

We recommend all our patients eat a modified Mediterranean diet or an Asian diet, both of which we call balanced diets because they are based on the idea of a balance of foods. Although we provide additional detail about the foods that are "good" and "bad" later in this chapter, here is a basic guide to a balanced diet.

1. Eat lots of vegetables and fruits. (The leafy vegetables that grow above ground are generally more nutritious than the tuberous, starchy vegetables that grow below the ground. Starchy vegetables have a high sugar and starch content.)

2. Eat whole foods, not processed foods.

3. Eat organically grown foods.

4. Limit alcohol to a small amount of red wine, consumed with meals.

5. Do not eat fried foods.

6. Eat moderate amounts of wild cold-water fish (at least weekly).

7. Eat very little red meat (use as a condiment rather than as a staple).

8. Eat small amounts of organic poultry.

9. Eat only "pastured" eggs (not from factory poultry farms).

10. Eat small amounts of organic dairy products, such as cheese, yogurt, and kefir. Avoid sugar-sweetened yogurt and kefir.

11. Eat whole grains.

12. Limit vegetable oils. Use olive oil for cooking.

13. Use herbs and spices, rather than fats or salt, to flavor foods.

14. Cook your own food.

This is essentially a Mediterranean diet modified for cancer survivors. The best vegetables and fruits—all consistent with that diet—are cabbage, broccoli, kale, Brussels sprouts, radicchio, mushrooms, tomatoes, grapes, and berries. If you are gluten sensitive, substitute quinoa, buckwheat, amaranth, hemp, chia, or flaxseeds for whole wheat pastas and breads. Given the extreme hybridizing that has led to "modern wheat," these are better and more nutritive choices even for those who are not gluten sensitive.

SHOPPING AND COOKING

Anyone can reduce his or her risk of bad health outcomes by making some basic lifestyle changes. Shopping and home cooking are two important survival skills that industry has taken over from many Americans—which has led to our increased dependence on fast food and boxed and frozen processed foods. Anyone who lives in a home where cooking goes on is way ahead of the game. One way to make positive changes in our children's future health is to teach them to cook.

Everyone should know how to select whole foods—from the supermarket or, better yet, farmers' markets—and know how to prepare them. "Whole foods" are as close to the natural form of a food as possible: a fresh fillet of fish or chicken, dried beans, fresh vegetables, and grains such as quinoa and wild rice. Today, most of us go to the supermarket and pick up frozen pizza, jars of pre-made pasta sauce, and boxes of flavored pasta mix. Our vegetables are often frozen or canned or even freeze-dried. This doesn't mean you need to bake your own bread, dismember a chicken, or press your own pasta. But knowing how to buy and make basic whole foods will be beneficial not only to your health but to the health of others in your household.

It is also far less expensive to buy and cook whole foods than to buy already cooked or processed food. Cheaper still is buying a whole chicken and cutting it up for several dinners, or buying dried beans and allowing them to soak overnight before cooking them.

All of that said, we do not want to be ideologues when it comes to diet. We doubt there is a perfect diet for all human beings. There is variation based on your ancestry, whether you live in a hot or cold place, and whether you do physical or nonphysical work. There are a number of radical diets, and there are people who thrive on each of them. Some people thrive as vegans, while others feel terrible as vegans. Whole grain bread is fine for some people, while others are sensitive to grain or to carbohydrates. If you're sensitive to dairy, you're not going to feel your best if it's part of your diet. We believe in informed trial and error. If a diet doesn't suit you, you'll drift away from it.

The fundamental survival skill is being able to intuitively recognize which foods are good for you and which are bad for you. To do this, you first need to detoxify yourself. Get off processed foods long enough for your tastebuds to recover. Many of the most healthful foods can taste bitter to a palate accustomed to added sugars and processed ingredients. Once you've been off processed foods for a few months, start taking inventory. Do you have energy after you eat, or do you feel lethargic? How does your digestive system react to a new food? Do you notice your skin breaking out after introducing a new food to your diet? This process is not unlike transitioning a baby to solid foods. Introduce a new food, wait and see your body's reaction, and then introduce another food. Your food journal will help you track foods as you introduce them into your diet. Be sure to mark down any reactions you notice.

WHEN TO EAT

Beyond knowing what to eat, you need to plan when to eat. We advise our patients to eat regular meals and snacks. This helps to regulate mood, prevent insulin spikes, and prevent overeating foods that are less healthful.

Breakfast is a particularly important meal. After the overnight fast, your body is in a specific metabolic state, and not eating breakfast can lead to insulin spikes. Insulin has been shown to be a growth factor in cancer; there are even drugs in trial phases directed at this.

Even if you're not hungry, you should eat something for breakfast. We suggest at least 7 to 10 grams of fiber and 15 to 20 grams of protein within 1 hour of waking up. An example of a breakfast that would provide this is a small bowl of high-fiber cereal and an apple. Use almond, coconut, or soy milk (although soy may be contraindicated for some cancer patients, so ask your doctor) if you are dairy sensitive. If you are not, buy organic milk from grass-fed cows. (Certain cancers, such as ovarian and breast cancer, may be stimulated by dairy, so avoid it if you've had one of these or discuss with your doctor.)

For the rest of the day, we recommend patients eat every 3 hours. Within 3 to 4 hours, your body may start to pull protein from your body structures for energy, and we don't want that. You want to use glucose and fat for energy. Your food journal will come in handy here, as it will show you when you tend to snack and will help you come up with healthful alternatives to what you may be doing now.

You can find information about fiber, carbohydrate, fat, and protein content on nutrition labels. Whole foods won't have these labels, but there are a number of Web sites that provide this information. Even easier is downloading a food-tracking app to your smartphone. Just enter the food, and it will give you the calories, sugar, carbohydrates, fats, and fiber, among other features. These apps can be very helpful when starting a food journal. Here are some of the most popular free apps:

Fooducate by Fooducate, LTD (fooducate.com)

Calorie Counter by MyFitnessPal (myfitnesspal.com)

Lose It! by FitNow (loseit.com)

Restaurant Nutrition by Foundation HealthCare Network (healthyandfitcommunities.com)

Does the following sound familiar? It's a common day-in-the-life scenario of an office worker. She starts off her day with a cup of coffee instead of breakfast and then becomes ravenous by 10 a.m., at which point she's at work with no food options other than the bowl of peanut M&Ms at the reception desk. At lunch she's still ravenous, so she adds a bag of chips to her sandwich and assumes she's set till dinner, but then gets hungry around 3. The M&Ms are all gone, so she drinks a cup of coffee, hoping that will stop the hunger pangs. By the time she gets home from work at 6, she is starving and still has to prepare dinner—so she grabs some more chips to tide her over. Of course, she's snacking as she makes dinner, so by dinner she's barely hungry and only eats half of the healthy, balanced meal she just made for her family. After doing the dishes, helping with homework, bathing the kids, and putting everyone to bed, she still has to jump back on the computer and send some e-mails she didn't get to during the day. Now it's 10 o'clock, and she's finally sitting down to relax in front of the TV . . . when she realizes she's hungry again. After all, she barely ate dinner, and the satisfaction that the chips and low-fiber snacks provided was fleeting. She remembers there's a tub of strawberry ice cream in the freezer. . . .

Unfortunately, even when we're buying the right food and cooking healthy meals for our families, our busy lives trip us up more often than we'd like to admit. And that's just the days we have time to make a healthy dinner. What about the nights when board meetings, long work hours, or a kid's soccer practice keep us from making dinner at all? Then we grab take-out or pop a frozen pizza in the oven.

Seeing what you actually eat (as opposed to what you think you eat) in your food journal can help you see where the holes are and help you plan better for filling them. If you're working long hours or have a very scheduled day, getting a good breakfast before leaving for work can help set up your entire day better. To make it easier for morning prep, you might stock your fridge with lots of individual-size (nonsugared) Greek yogurts, cut-up fruit or fruit that is easy to grab and go (such as apples, bananas, and pears), and boiled eggs. For people who hate to eat anything in the morning, smoothies are a good option. Investing in a good blender will make all the difference.

If you are a parent who makes your kids' lunches, why not use that time to also make and pack your own healthy lunch and snacks? That way when hunger pangs strike mid-morning and mid-afternoon, you'll have some healthier options to grab. Possible snacks include the same foods we listed for easy breakfasts, as well as whole grain bread or crackers with hummus or peanut butter, veggie sticks, soy or low-fat cubed cheese, and granola. Try for a combo of fiber and protein to stay full.

Instead of that cup of coffee in the afternoon, which could cause a spike and drop in your energy, a good substitute is a cup (or two or three) of green tea. Green tea has caffeine (though less than coffee) for a pick-me-up and antioxidants for added health benefits. Studies show it seems to be increasingly beneficial the more you drink. When you get home in the evening, having cut-up veggies and cold mineral water or green tea in the fridge are good options for addressing hunger while you make your healthy dinner. You won't get too full on junk while you cook and won't end up so hungry before bed that your thoughts automatically jump to ice cream. (And the best plan to avoid ice cream binges is to simply not have ice cream in the freezer!)

FOOD AND INFLAMMATION

We now know that certain foods are pro-inflammatory to our body. We also know that some cancers are directly related to chronic inflammatory exposure. In some cases, the inflammation is related to a chronic, low-grade viral or bacterial infection, which the immune system is unable to completely resolve, thus resulting in ongoing inflammation. Just a few examples of these infections include:

- Cervical cancer and the papillomavirus
- Kaposi's sarcoma and human herpesvirus 8
- Esophageal cancer and Barrett's metaplasia (related to reflux)
- Gastric MALT lymphoma, gastric cancer, and *Helicobacter pylori*
- Liver cancer and hepatitis B and C viruses
- Bladder cancer and schistosomiasis
- Ovarian cancer and pelvic inflammatory disease

There are several other chronic inflammatory syndromes not related to infections, which result in increased cancer risk, such as inflammatory bowel disease and colorectal cancers, as well as the inflammation provoked by cigarette smoke and asbestos, associated with lung cancer and mesothelioma.

The traditional Western diet—with its heavy amounts of omega-6s via vegetable oils and the use of grain-fed meats, processed meats, eggs, dairy products, white flour, and refined sugar—can be highly inflammatory. On the other hand, certain diets like the Mediterranean diet, Indian cuisine, and Asian cuisine can reduce the incidence of food-related inflammation. These diets are rich in olive oil, flaxseed oil, wild fatty fish, omega-3 eggs, curry, cilantro, ginger, and other herbs and spices.

FOODS TO AVOID

New studies point to certain foods as actually fueling cancer, or at least creating the conditions (such as chronic inflammation) that cancer thrives in. These include refined sugar, high-fructose corn syrup (a component of many processed foods), alcohol, omega-6 fats, and oxidized fats (such as produced in foods fried in vegetable oils). Foods that are rich in these substances should be avoided or restricted by anyone who wishes to practice anticancer habits. More than 50 percent of calories in the standard American diet come from sugar, trans fatty oils, and bleached flour.

The following are foods that should be avoided or strictly moderated.

Red meat

Processed meat products, including hot dogs, bacon, and processed deli meats

Hydrogenated vegetable fats, also known as trans fats

Large amounts of dairy products, including milk, cheese, and yogurt (cow's milk is a significant source of estrogen because of modern dairy herd management practices)

Processed foods

Refined/concentrated sugars

Alcohol

Red Meat

Problems associated with red meat are well known and include the amount of fat in the meat and the kinds of food given to the livestock—antibiotics, hormones, and animal parts—which affect the quality and healthfulness of the meat produced. As reported in the *Archives of Internal Medicine* in 2012, red meat consumption is directly linked to overall cancer mortality, from all cancers, as well as general morbidity.[9] It has been especially strongly linked to colon, pancreas, and endometrial cancers. Research has found that for every meal where you replace red meat with some other choice, such as fish, you lower your risk of cancer.

A Harvard review study found that even one daily serving of red meat increased the chance of premature death by 13 percent and the chance of having a heart attack or cancer by 14 percent.[10] Red meat eaters live, on average, 10 years less than those who do not eat it.

If you do eat meat, eat organic, grass-fed meat and use it as a condiment in your cooking, not as a main dish. Animals that are factory farmed and fattened with corn and other grains are also loaded with omega-6, an inflammatory entity in its own right.

Processed Meats

There is a higher rate of cancer of the stomach and esophagus in countries where the diets include large amounts of smoked foods and meats treated with nitrates and nitrites as preservatives, which become cancer-causing nitrosamines in the gut. This is especially true for hot dogs, bacon, and ham. Most bacons contain sodium nitrite and large amounts of animal fats, and should be avoided. If you insist on eating these foods occasionally, look for brands of uncured, nitrate-free meat products.

The daily ingestion of processed meats—bacon, deli chicken and turkey, hot dogs, sausage, and salami—increases your risk of having a heart attack or getting cancer by 18 percent.

Trans Fats

Trans fats have been identified as major culprits in the national obesity crisis. Trans fats are artificially made fats that increase the shelf life of foods but block normal body functions. Created in the conversion of liquid fat to solid by a process known as partial hydrogenation, trans fats are often used in processed foods—especially baked goods like doughnuts, bread, and cakes—and are found in hydrogenated vegetable oils. Trans fats have been demonstrated to contribute to many diseases, including cancer, obesity, diabetes, heart disease, and Alzheimer's.

The fact that these processed fats and oils create a great deal of inflammation may account for their link to cancer. A European study recently suggested that trans fats in the diet may increase the risk of cancer of the breast by almost 75 percent.[11] And a study of 25,000 women by the French National Institute for Health and Medical Research showed that the risk of breast cancer doubled in women with the highest level of trans fats in their blood.[12]

Currently, many foods we eat every day have an unacceptable level of trans fats. In one slice of pepperoni and cheese pizza, about one-fifth of the 490 calories come from trans fats. In addition, labeling of trans fats in processed foods can be deceptive. If a product has less than 0.5 gram of trans fats per serving, the company can legally round that to zero on the package label. You might purchase a snack that has 0.49 gram of trans fats per serving. The bag holds 10 servings, which means there is a total of 4.9 grams of trans fats. But the company that prepared and packaged this food is allowed to state on the label that there is zero gram of trans fat per serving and therefore zero gram of trans fat in all 10 servings. If you see a packaged food that states "zero gram trans fats" on the label, don't buy it and don't eat it. It's a processed food and very likely harbors these poisonous trans fats.

The National Academy of Sciences states that there is no safe level of trans fat intake and that trans fats provide no known benefit to human health. They are, in fact, metabolic poisons.

Be careful when cooking with oils. Margarines and sunflower oil are heavy in omega-6s (and margarines are rich in trans fats as well). Using them and most vegetable oils to cook with is far more dangerous than using butter. In Israel, cooking with vegetable oils and margarines has led to the Israeli paradox: A country with one of the lowest cholesterol levels when compared with Western countries has one of the highest rates of heart attacks and obesity.

We suggest you limit all vegetable oils, with the exception of coconut oil (for cooking) and unheated olive and flaxseed oil, all used sparingly. Coconut oil is a saturated fat, so it is much less susceptible to oxidation when heated. Olive oil is more heat sensitive, and if used for cooking, should be on low heat for short times. Higher heats and longer heat exposure causes oxidation of unsaturated vegetable oil but not saturated oils such as coconut oil. Oxidized fats are "unsaturated" oils (meaning they have carbon-carbon double bonds), which have been exposed to high heat and oxygen (e.g. frying). Oxygen combines with the unsaturated double bonds and creates a peroxide, which generates free radicals (oxidative stress) in the body. Many Mediterranean countries consume large amounts of olives and olive oil, but it is uncertain how much is healthy for someone who has been treated for cancer.

Dairy

When we speak of dairy products, we are talking about whole milk and milk-derived foods such as cheese, ice cream, and other processed milk products.

Dairy products are something of a conundrum. Milk has been in our diet for thousands of years and is a staple of our eating profile. However, dairy products cause concern after cancer care for several reasons, primarily because they are high in casein, a protein found in all mammalian milk products. Casein can be highly inflammatory.

Saturated fats found in meats, cream, cheese, and other dairy products have been implicated in many cancer studies. Although many of these investigations do not take into consideration the eating habits of the individuals in childhood and young adulthood, and surveys and questionnaires are often unreliable and difficult to standardize, large-scale analysis of multiple clinical trials has demonstrated a positive link between saturated animal fat intake and breast, ovarian, colon, and prostate cancer.

In *The China Study*, coauthor T. Colin Campbell, PhD, shows a correlation between powdered casein and cancer in laboratory rats, as well as an association between higher rates of cancer and the portion of the Chinese population that consumes the highest amount of dairy products. Casein is, however, found in human breast milk as well as processed dairy products, so the correlation is still being studied. Another major factor is that modern dairy practices are far different from those of our ancestors. Cows are kept continuously pregnant, which also results in high levels of bovine estrogen in modern milk and many of the products made from it. This is of particular concern to people who have had estrogen receptor positive cancers.

Cheese is an addicting concentration of salt, dairy fat, and protein. The increased consumption of salt, fat, and protein from cow's milk cheese is correlated with increased cancer incidence. Traditional cheeses made from sheep's or goat's milk contain much less of the growth-promoting factors found in cow dairy and are not produced on an industrial scale, especially in Europe. Many dairy products like ice cream and yogurt are spiked with large amounts of sugar, which only compound the possible links to inflammation and cancer.

Flavored milks should be avoided at all costs. The dairy industry has been adding aspartame, sucralose, and other artificial sweeteners to flavored milks, even those offered to children in schools. These chemicals have been associated in some studies with both formation and acceleration of tumor growth.

Besides these issues with milk in general, growth hormones (recombinant bovine growth hormone) and antibiotics, now used in most conventional dairy farms, stimulate the production of a growth hormone in humans called insulin-like growth factor 1 (IGF-1), creating a possible setup for prostate and breast cancers. Residual growth hormone is also present in standard dairy products, the effects of which on humans are not well understood.

In general, we advise that you substitute almond, rice, hemp, chia, or non-GMO soy products for dairy products as much as possible. Any dairy products in your diet should be organic, free of growth hormones, and used sparingly.

Processed Foods

Limit anything in a box. Even healthy cereals and crackers should be consumed sparingly. Michael Pollan, an American journalist and activist, famously advised readers not to eat anything with more than five ingredients or with any ingredients you can't pronounce. We love this rule of thumb and implore you to get the majority of your calories from whole foods.

It's important to recognize the pernicious nature of processed foods. Labeling of some ingredients can make the food appear to be nutritious, yet it can still be detrimental to your health. Label reading is a skill. You must consider the serving size on the label and understand what it means. Sometimes by changing the size of the labeled portions, the amount of beneficial ingredients like fiber can be overestimated or the amount of nonbeneficial sodium can be underestimated. Another way to mislabel products is to present the absolute percentage of an ingredient without the relative percentage of the ingredient in the overall product.

In the processing of foods, unhealthy substances may be added to preserve freshness, add color, or make the texture more palatable. In addition, some healthy ingredients may be removed. Avoid foods with coloring and food preservatives. Artificial sweeteners like saccharine, cyclamate, and aspartame and preservatives that produce nitrosamines are known to cause bladder and stomach cancers.

Refined Sugars

Sugar and fructose consumption is an important consideration in the prevention of cancer recurrence. Cancer cells thrive in the absence of oxygen and instead use sugar as fuel in an aerobic process called glycolysis. The high sugar levels in the blood create a rise in the insulin level, which in turn evokes the expression of hormones that encourage the growth and blood supply of cancer cells. Several studies have shown the direct correlation of elevated sugar levels and increased cancer risk. This is particularly seen in prostate, liver, esophageal, rectal, pancreatic, and breast cancers.

In the last 30 years, refined sugar has played an increasing role in the American diet. Refined sugars include white sugar, high-fructose corn syrup, molasses, corn syrup, sucrose, dextrose, sorbitol, turbinado sugar, and purified fructose, to name a few. High-fructose corn syrup is found in many processed foods and soft drinks manufactured today.

When eaten, these sugars cause a rapid rise in blood sugar, which causes the release of insulin, which in turn causes the release of IGF (insulin-like growth factor), which has been strongly associated with cancer. In a study conducted at the Harvard Medical School, women with the highest levels of IGF were seven times more likely to develop breast cancer than the group with the lowest.[13] In another study from Harvard, men with the highest IGF levels were four times more likely to develop prostate cancer than those with the lowest levels.[14] This linkage was independent of obesity.

The explosive use of fructose in our society has had a damaging effect on our health. The average American consumes 150 pounds of sugar per year, and much of it is from fructose. Although fructose does not stimulate insulin like sucrose, it does increase obesity, fat, and formaldehyde production in the liver, as well as insulin resistance, high triglycerides, and hypertension. Originally predicted as a boon to those with diabetes, fructose has not lived up to its early promise and should be consumed very cautiously.

If sugar is consumed, it's important to eat it with vegetables, fibers, and grains to blunt the insulin spike. Naturally derived sugar substitutes, such as maple syrup, honey, coconut sugar, xylitol, stevia, and erythritol, can be used sparingly. These all have a lower glycemic index, which is the level of sweetness that creates a rapid rise of insulin when ingested. Since they are natural and less refined, their absorption in the GI tract requires more energy and is slower, so they won't cause a spike in insulin as much as refined sugars do. Foods with a high glycemic index, such as white flour, should also be replaced by foods with a lower glycemic index, such as whole wheat flour and other whole grain starches. Glycemic index refers to the rate at which any carbohydrate is converted to blood sugar (glucose). Sucrose (table sugar) is given a value of 100; foods with a low glycemic index are converted very slowly into glucose, whereas those with a value of 100 (or higher) are converted rapidly and stimulate a much bigger insulin response than foods with a low glycemic index do. Equally as important as the glycemic index is the *glycemic load*, which is a measure of how much glucose is generated by a given amount of the food. For instance, although raw carrots have a relatively high glycemic index, their glycemic load is quite low, so there is not much impact on insulin. Foods such as doughnuts, baked potatoes, or white bread have both a high glycemic index *and* glycemic load, so they have a major impact on the insulin response. High insulin levels can lead to low blood sugar later on, with subsequent fatigue and craving for sweets, as well as high IGF-1 levels, which is a major growth factor for cancer cells.

Alcohol

According to the American Cancer Society, alcohol is a cause of a number of types of cancer, including mouth cancer, cancer of the pharynx and larynx, esophageal cancer, liver cancer, colorectal cancer, and breast cancer. Although it is not known whether alcohol is a factor in recurrence, it is advisable to refrain from alcohol after cancer treatment. Patients who have had breast cancer, in particular, may want to avoid alcohol as it is known to raise estrogen levels.

A 2009 study showed a link between breast cancer recurrence and alcohol, with a 34 percent increase in recurrence for women who drank three to four or more drinks per week, compared to women who had less than one drink per week.[15] One drink is equal to one serving of alcohol, meaning 12 ounces of beer, 5 ounces of wine, or 1.5 ounces of hard liquor. Two other studies of 53,000 women found a 7 to 12 percent increase in developing breast cancer for every 10-gram increase in daily alcohol intake.[16,17]

FOODS TO EAT

If you do choose to drink alcohol, you should do it in moderation. Red wine, which contains polyphenol antioxidants, may be less harmful than other forms of alcohol, which has been suggested in studies on heart disease but is not confirmed in cancer.

It's much more fun to talk about the foods that heal. For as many new studies that show what foods and contaminations possibly cause us harm, there is an equal number of studies that show us which foods are healthful and even cancer fighting!

Here are food practices that can help keep you healthy and even fight cancer or its recurrence.

1. Eat whole foods.
2. Spice it up.
3. Eat a balanced diet.
4. Eat antioxidants.

5. Prepare food properly.

6. Eat more fiber.

7. Drink lots of water.

Eat Whole Foods

Vegetables have survived over millennia by developing phytochemicals that protect them from insects, bacteria, fungi, microbes, and poor environmental conditions. These molecules, when ingested, enhance our immune system against not only these invaders but also cancer initiation. For example, green tea contains the polyphenol catechin, which prevents formation of new blood vessels by cancer cells, among other properties. According to a Harvard research study, the effect of this powerful polyphenol is enhanced when combined with soy products.[18] This is particularly true in estrogen-sensitive tumors such as breast cancer.

The healthful effects of eating fruits and vegetables are difficult to argue with, but there are some vegetables and fruits that are particularly amazing.

Cruciferous vegetables are getting a lot of play in the media of late, and for good reason. They are strong cancer-preventing foods. Cruciferous vegetables include broccoli, cabbage, cauliflower, Brussels sprouts, kale, collard, turnips, and radishes. They have very powerful cancer-suppressing amino acids and proteins called isothiocyanates, which are especially effective in breast cancer and lung cancer. They also reduce the toxicity of chemotherapy and enhance immunity response. Broccoli is especially high in sulforaphanes, chemicals found to be strongly anticancer. To preserve the chemical integrity of the proteins, they are best eaten raw or cooked lightly.

Anecdotally, daily portions of asparagus have been recommended to prevent cancer recurrence. We have had experience with one patient whose tumor markers were significantly reduced after implementation of asparagus in the diet. Asparagus is high in histones and also rich in the peptide glutathione, a first line of defense against cancer. Note, however, that glutathione production depends on the mineral selenium as a catalyst; selenium can be found in high concentrations in Brazil nuts. Two Brazil nuts daily is an effective dose.

Other vegetables like cilantro, parsley, carrots, cabbage, green and red peppers, onions, celery, tomatoes, eggplant, collard greens, and turnip greens are excellent anti-inflammatory and detoxifying foods.

The berry family, including blackberries, raspberries, and strawberries, contains anthocyanins, which are powerful antiangiogenic compounds that deprive cancer cells of blood supply. Blueberries contain specific anthocyanins that cause apoptosis. Cherries contain acids that detoxify xenoestrogens. Black raspberries have an inhibitory effect on esophageal, mouth, and colon cancers.

Recent evidence has shown that other fruits such as pomegranate and acai berry may be particularly powerful antioxidants. These berries contain a polyphenol called ellagic acid (also found in walnuts), a substance shown to be effective in normal dietary amounts. Peaches, plums, nectarines, and all stone fruits are rich in antioxidants.

In Japan, mushrooms have been known for many years to be an active anticancer food. They contain polysaccharides, including lentinan, which are powerful immune boosters. Several Japanese studies on patient survival have shown the benefit of mushroom intake in conjunction with chemotherapy.[19,20] The most famous anticancer mushrooms are shiitake, which can be found in many grocery stores, and maitake, which can be found in specialty stores.

Different fruits and vegetables contain different anticancer properties, so it is best to mix a wide variety of fruits and vegetables in your diet. A good rule to follow is "Eat a rainbow." Eating foods of all different natural colorations will help ensure that you are getting a healthy variety of nutrients. One trick is to keep a rainbow wheel chart on your refrigerator and aim to eat the whole rainbow every 2 to 3 days.

Extra-virgin olive oil (created from olives), which contains antioxidants, is another healing food.

Lignans are a group of chemical compounds found in all plants but in especially high amounts in flaxseeds and sesame seeds. Lignans have been shown to slow the progression of cancer, especially in fatty tissue of the breast, uterus, and colon. Other plants with high levels of this antioxidant are grains, including wheat, oats, barley, and especially rye; soybeans; cruciferous vegetables (such as broccoli and cauliflower); and fruits such as apricots and strawberries.

A study published in 2010 of more than 1,000 breast cancer patients found that among the postmenopausal patients, those with the highest dietary intake of lignans, versus those with the lowest, had a 70 percent reduced risk of dying of breast cancer.[21] Flax also inhibits tumor spread by metastasis and diminishes new blood vessel growth to the tumors. Dietary lignans are metabolized by intestinal bacteria into compounds called enterolactones. A 2011 study published in the *Journal of Clinical Oncology* showed that postmenopausal breast cancer patients with the highest serum levels of enterolactones had a 42 percent overall reduced risk of dying of breast cancer; for those with estrogen negative tumors, risk of death was reduced by 73 percent.[22]

Keep flaxseeds refrigerated and grind them right before eating them. We recommend a daily dosage of 1 to 2 tablespoons.

Vitamin C can prevent the synthesis of nitrite, which is converted into powerful carcinogens called nitrosamines. Foods with high levels of vitamin C include the old standby oranges but also other citrus fruits, leafy greens, berries, peppers, guavas, tomatoes, and papayas.

High-fiber foods, such as grains, beans, nuts and seeds, berries, and leafy greens, reduce the absorption of carcinogens. Sulfur-rich foods—such as cruciferous vegetables, protein-rich fish, poultry, legumes, eggs, nuts, alliums (such as onions and garlic), carotenoids (orange and yellow fruits and vegetables), and leafy greens—can promote normal cell differentiation. Grapes contain resveratrol, which helps destroy cancer cells. Lycopene, found in tomatoes, appears to have a significant effect on prostate, lung, and stomach cancer. It's also effective in the prevention of cancer and when used as an adjunct to treatment of breast and uterine cancer.

These protective compounds are found in food available to us daily. The following are examples of specific compounds and what foods they are in:

Allicin: garlic

Beta-carotene (converted to vitamin A): carrots and squash

Beta-glucans: oats, mushrooms, and onions

Carotenoids: carrots, beets, kale, sweet potatoes, and red peppers

Ellagic acid: strawberries, raspberries, and pomegranates

Fiber: all fruits and vegetables

Glucosinolate: broccoli, kale, Brussels sprouts

Isoflavones: fermented soy and alfalfa sprouts

Limonene: citrus juice and peels

Lutein: blueberries

Lycopene: tomatoes

Omega-3 fatty acids: fish, flax oil, walnuts

Polyphenols: green tea and black tea

Quercetin: apples, citrus fruits, onions, and cranberries

Selenium: Brazil nuts, garlic, and mushrooms

Sulfur: garlic, onions and leeks, shallots, and chives

When looking at the benefit of fruits and vegetables to the cancer population, scientific studies have not included the influence of pesticides and herbicide residues on the vegetables or the fluoride content of the water of the population under study. Also, they have not considered the amount of fat, the type of toxic substances that they may be exposed to during this period, or the genetic risk of the participants—or the presence of chronic inflammatory disease, which would set up the situation for cancer development. All of these contributions merit further study.

Spice It Up

Spices make your food taste wonderful and exciting, and some may have cancer-fighting elements. Adding them often has an added benefit: decreased salt consumption (because your food is tasty enough without it). Below are just a few of the amazing spices.

TURMERIC (CURCUMIN)

The Indian spice found in yellow curry, turmeric root is an exciting food ingredient that has drawn much attention in the medical world recently. Turmeric contains the curcumin molecule, which has a powerful anti-inflammatory effect. Laboratory studies show curcumin's profound inhibitory and antiangiogenic effects in lung, liver, stomach, colon, prostate, breast, ovarian, and brain cancers and leukemia. It also promotes apoptosis.

This may be the reason that the Indian population has a much lower rate of the previously mentioned cancers, in spite of higher exposure to environmental toxins.

One cautionary note: Turmeric is poorly absorbed by the digestive system unless mixed with black pepper and ginger.

BLACK PEPPER

Black pepper increases the effectiveness of antioxidants, and its use in combination with other vegetables and spices has a beneficial effect. Black pepper is particularly important when combined with the powerful anticancer spice turmeric, because it contains piperine, which can increase turmeric absorption 2,000 percent.

GINGER

Ginger has cancer-fighting chemicals and is especially helpful in combination with turmeric.

GROUND RED PEPPER

Ground red pepper is another pepper with cancer-fighting elements.

PARSLEY

More commonly a garnish than a spice, parsley has more value than just a decoration—it has cancer-fighting compounds. It also reduces cancer cell blood supply through antiangiogenic activity.

CELERY

Celery is used both as a spice and a whole vegetable, and has been shown to reduce cancer cell blood supply through antiangiogenic activity.

MINT, THYME, ROSEMARY, BASIL, AND OREGANO

These aromatic herbs are rich in fatty acids of the terpene family, which have been shown to act in a large variety of tumors, reducing cancer spread and causing cancer cell death.

CHILE PEPPER

The capsaicinoids in chile peppers decrease the inflammation of arthritis, cardiovascular disease, and thrombosis. They also lower the LDLs, but not the HDLs, in the body, directly affecting cholesterol metabolism and increasing the breakdown of cholesterol in waste.

Eat a Balanced Diet

While we recommend a modified Mediterranean or Asian diet, both of which limit animal and dairy consumption compared to the average American diet, there are other balanced diets that might be right for a particular individual. You might personally find benefits in animal proteins that outweigh their negatives. For example, retinol is the most usable form of vitamin A and is found in most animal proteins, but especially cod liver, liver, butter, eggs, and milk (beta-carotene, found in fruits and vegetables, is converted to retinol once ingested).

In general, though, patients should follow the modified Mediterranean diet, which is rich in vegetables and fruits; utilizes whole grains; limits organic red meat to maybe once or twice a month and organic poultry to no more than once a week; and includes oily, small, cold-water fish, such as salmon, mackerel, or herring, at least once a week. Use spices liberally and small amounts of olive oil for cooking.

Asian diets are also balanced diets that are rich in a variety of whole grains (usually rices and noodles), nuts, cooked vegetables, soups, green tea, and water. Fish, chicken, red meat, eggs, and soy are eaten in equal parts, but dairy and desserts are limited. Herbs and spices are used for flavor instead of salt.

As arguments for the balanced diet, look at two populations. The Seventh-day Adventists in Los Angeles County eat primarily vegetarian diets and generally abstain from alcohol; even in this polluted urban environment, they have a 54 percent lower cancer mortality than the general population. Also, a fourteenfold increase in breast cancer was experienced by one generation of Japanese women who immigrated to Hawaii and changed from the traditional Japanese diet to the standard American diet.

Eat Antioxidants

Fruits of many kinds are great sources of antioxidants. Berries such as cranberries, raspberries, strawberries, and blackberries are especially good for you. Be careful, however, in consuming these if they are not organically grown, because they can retain pesticides, even when washed very carefully. Whenever you can, obtain berries from organic producers.

The peels of grapefruits, lemons, and oranges—often used for zesting—contain substances called terpenes, which are cancer inhibitors and liver protectors; oranges and tangerines can be potentially helpful in melanoma, lung, and prostate cancers. However, be sure to obtain organically produced citrus, as fat-soluble pesticides may be present in the oils of the citrus peels of conventionally raised fruit.

Omega-3 fats are generally anti-inflammatory and reduce the risk of cancer. The primary sources of these are fish; flax, chia, and other seeds; beans; walnuts and other nuts; and oily lentils, such as dal. These oils are easily oxidized and so should be kept in the refrigerator in dark jars.

Always eat wild fish versus farmed fish, as farmed fish have fewer omega-3 fats and may have absorbed ingested hydrocarbons. Avoid larger, older fish, such as tuna and swordfish, which may have high levels of mercury, arsenic, and other environmental toxins.

Prepare Food Properly

Food preparation may be as important to healthy eating as the food itself. The most important part of food preparation is how we cook our food.

Avoid cooking with safflower, sesame, soy, corn, and canola oils, which are pro-inflammatory, especially when oxidized by heat and light. Instead, use small amounts of olive oil, rice bran oil, and coconut oil. Olive and rice bran oil are excellent for low heat cooking, while coconut oil can withstand higher temperatures.

Also avoid grilling or overcooking meats, poultry, or fish. Charring causes heterocyclic amines (HCAs) to form, and HCAs can damage your genes, raising the risk of stomach and colorectal cancer.

To avoid HCAs, do the following:

- Trim off all fat on the meat, poultry, or fish.
- Precook the meat, poultry, or fish in the microwave or oven.
- Oil the grill lightly and preheat it at a high temperature; then lower the temperature for grilling.
- After the food is done, scrub the grill well and keep it clean until the next use.

HCA formation can also be reduced by marinating food in vinegar, lemon juice, seasonings, and herbs. The bonus is that the food tastes even better!

Even when not grilling, never overcook foods as that can have the same carcinogenic consequences.

Eat More Fiber

Because of recent scientific observations and discoveries, the USDA is considering labeling fiber as a food. About 15 percent of our total caloric intake and 50 percent of the caloric intake of the colon is derived from the breakdown of soluble fiber by bacteria in the gut. About 5 pounds and 400 species of beneficial bacteria are contained in the gastrointestinal system of the average person. The amounts of bacteria in our guts have previously been grossly underestimated. It was discovered that the GI system from the mouth through the stomach—less so in the duodenum (upper small bowel), and increasingly in the ileum (distal small intestine) and jejunum (mid-small bowel)—contains bacteria living with us symbiotically, breaking down indigestible foodstuffs into short-chain fatty acids and amino acids that may harm or help the body.

The Academy of Nutrition and Dietetics recommends a minimum of 20 to 35 grams of fiber a day, yet most Americans consume half that amount. Those who eat the standard American diet consume only about 5 grams of fiber a day. Fiber can be soluble or insoluble; soluble means it is water-soluble and can be fermented with the by-products of the fermentation (short-chain fatty acids) used as energy sources or messengers to communicate with the enzymatic systems of our body.

Fiber sources have been shown to be beneficial in reducing the incidence of some types of cancer, blood cholesterol levels, obesity, diabetes, cardiovascular disease, and numerous gastrointestinal disorders, including inflammatory bowel disease, ulcerative colitis, Crohn's disease, and colon cancer. Some of the examples of soluble fiber sources are psyllium seed husks, oat bran, whole oats, rolled oats, or whole grains, such as barley. The particle size and condition of the fiber are important aspects of whether or not it can be digested by the bacteria. Softening the fiber by chewing, cooking, or other methods of breaking down the polysaccharides will be a large determinant in how much nutrition is gained from fiber ingestion.

Insoluble fiber is derived from plant foods but is not water-soluble, and escapes from the digestion and absorption at the end of the small intestine. It is then subjected to attack in the large intestine. Most soluble fibers are converted to short-chain fatty acids, such as acetic, butyric acid, or propionic acid. By contrast, the majority of insoluble fibers are composed of cellulose, which provides a surface for the bacteria to attach to and becomes a creative microclimate, a new physiochemical environment. Insoluble fiber then absorbs water, creating bulk in the stool and allowing the healthy bacteria to flourish. A significant result of this is the prevention of constipation and the creation of a more rapid transit time, which prevents toxic products from being absorbed or reabsorbed back into the bloodstream.

The foods you eat are major determinants for the prevalence of healthy bac-

A NOTE ABOUT SOY

Some discussion has taken place concerning the use of soy products for people with cancer, especially those with estrogen-sensitive tumors like breast cancer. Although there are mixed reviews on the use of soy foods, regular ingestion of moderate amounts of soy daily seems to be safe—especially with the traditional fermented soy foods such as miso, tempeh, and natto when made from organic non-GMO soybeans.

teria in the GI system. A diet low in fiber and high in sugars, processed foods, refined flour, meats, and cheese will change the environment for the healthy bacteria, allowing them to be replaced by bacteria that can cause harm to the system. You might have heard of *H. pylori,* candida, *C. diff.*, staph, and strep as bad bacteria or "pathogens," but many other beneficial bacteria can create useful breakdown products that are potentially catalysts in our body.

In the April 2013 *New England Journal of Medicine,* Cleveland Clinic investigators showed that intestinal bacteria play an important role in cardiovascular disease. Meat, cheese, milk, and other animal products, including eggs, are high in carnitine and phosphatidylcholine (lecithin). These compounds are broken down by certain bacteria in the gut and transformed into trimethylamine oxide (TMAO), which is highly inflammatory and causes arteriosclerosis. They also found that vegetarians have much lower levels of the type of bacteria that create TMAO.[23]

This illustrates just how important fiber is in our diet. We can also see the role our diet has on establishing a good environment for healthy intestinal bacteria to flourish and live symbiotically with us, helping keep our body supplied with the food, proteins, amino acids, fatty acids, and energy that we need.

FEEDING THE INDIVIDUAL

While there are some firm guidelines that anyone who is recovering from cancer should follow—such as eating a diet of mostly plant-based foods, eating organic whenever possible, and avoiding processed foods—the food that serves you best is individual. Different patients have different needs, and this may be dependent on the type of cancer you had, the treatment you went through, your current activity level, your age, your ethnic background, the climate you live in, and a host of other factors.

Cheryl, who was treated for lymphoma, made drastic changes when she was diagnosed. While going through chemotherapy, she adopted a vegetarian diet; but after finishing chemo, she was very focused on getting fit again, and her vegetarian diet did not meet her needs for being an active cyclist and hiker. In the end, she met with a nutritionist who suggested she needed more protein in her diet.

"For a long time, I just ate vegetables, grains, and I juiced and blenderized vegetables," says Cheryl. "I had some trouble with blood sugar, and we decided to add in some meat protein." She began incorporating whey shakes and other healthy foods, but also started to eat some fish, chicken, eggs, raw milk, and, rarely, red meat again—all organic and pasture-raised.

She also decided not to avoid the foods she loved and still eats some sugar and ice cream. "But I don't eat anything out of a box. I eat organic. I just pay attention in that way to everyday meals. In a way, it wasn't about cancer nutrition, it was about being fit for cycling." Her habits just happened to also be cancer-preventing.

For Jay, the right diet included juicing and lots of water, which he believes helped him tremendously during treatment and after. He still makes juicing a big part of his day.

"There were several things that helped me a lot, and one was that I started juicing vegetables. I bought a good juicer, and I drank juice almost every day. It was a lot of work, but I was able to do it because I was no longer working long hours. The juices are heavy in cruciferous vegetables—broccoli slaw and stems, cucumber, pear or apple. It's really good for anyone who is post-treatment because your stomach is just wracked. And I just love it. It gives you energy. It makes you feel strong. It's wonderful." He adds that he will sometimes use as many as 20 vegetables in one juice.

"I also drink a ton of water daily," says Jay. "A lot of the meds I took during treatment wreaked havoc on my kidneys, so I visualize rivers and energy—cleansing me, washing out all the bad guys. I meld meditational thought with intense hydrating."

Although Jay ate a moderate version of the standard American diet before he was diagnosed with cancer, since then he has embraced a balanced diet, which he believes has been essential for his health. At the same time, he still eats the food he loves, just much less of it.

"Before I had cancer, I ate a lot of meat, I ate a lot of sugar," he says. "I wasn't really overweight, but I could have lost 10 pounds. When I was first sick, I became vegan, but now I eat a very plant-strong diet. I eat a lot of fresh fish, a lot of cold-water fish because it's high in omega-3. I eat a lot of organic chicken and turkey. About a year ago, I started eating a little bit of beef. On average I have beef maybe once every 3 months. I've had a bit of pulled pork every once in a while, but I don't eat as much as I used to. If I do have a hamburger, I know the sourcing."

Jay adds, "I've learned to eat a lot of vegetables that I never really liked. I try to get a really great range of phytochemicals. I eat a lot of beans. I quit drinking milk. I drink almond milk, which tastes better to me. I try to eat chia seeds every day to help control cholesterol. I wax and wane to the extent that I avoid white flour, but I do try to avoid it. I try to eat sprouted grain instead of flour." But Jay feels strongly that his health is also related to happiness, and he avoids being so dogmatic about his diet that he doesn't enjoy the life he wasn't sure he'd be here to experience. "Last weekend I was at a barbecue, and I had a hamburger with a white bun and a cold beer. I'm just living life."

SUPPLEMENTS

An optimal post-treatment diet might look something like this: Whole foods are the base of your diet. You buy organic when possible; eat lots of vegetables, fruits, and fish; and avoid foods that are very fatty, salty, sweet, or overly processed. You do the "right" things the majority of the time, and as a result of your efforts, you are giving your body the balanced and adequate nutrition it requires for optimal health.

Ideally, this is true. We require the macronutrients of carbohydrates, fats, and proteins, as well as micronutrients like vitamins, fatty acids, minerals, and amino acids. These are all essential for health. Unfortunately, the food available to us, our medical situations, and our overall health may interfere with the natural provision of nutrition from food.

The fact is, most vegetables and fruits are grown in soil that has been depleted of much of its nutritional value. This often occurs through poor soil management, mainly as practiced by large agricultural corporations. As a result, the produce raised in some soils may not provide the nutritional support it should.

In addition, certain medications and some medical conditions can deplete your body's ability to absorb nutrients even from the wholesome food you eat. You may be eating the right types of food, but your body is not getting full benefit from that food. An example of this is the depletion of calcium, magnesium, vitamin D, vitamin B_{12}, and poor protein absorption due to extensive use of drugs like Nexium for gastric reflux. Another example is the overgrowth of candida or inflammatory bacteria in the GI system after antibiotic use. A third possibility is illnesses such as neuropathies like trigeminal neuralgia, which require increased building blocks of B_{12}, phospholipids, cholesterol, and other micronutrients to repair damaged tissue.

For these and other reasons, it is often important to supplement your nutritional intake. Supplementation is intended to correct any deficiencies in your food or your ability to properly process that food in your body.

Supplements are used to replenish the depleted micronutritional stores, repair damaged tissues, prevent common disorders, and detoxify the body. This can be especially important if you've been treated for cancer, as both the disease and the treatment can rob your body of important nutrients and create conditions in which your body poorly absorbs the nutrients in your food. In addition, the effects of many of the treatments for cancer, particularly chemotherapy, can linger in your body for many months following treatment, and detoxification may help your body get stronger faster. In the case of chemotherapy, there is no benefit to having small traces of chemotherapy in your system, so it's best to do what you can to rid the body of these toxins once treatment is complete.

SUPPLEMENTS AND CANCER

For a cancer patient, deciding whether or not to use supplements can be very difficult. So much information and advice about supplements and cancer is out in the world. Whether you are on the Internet, reading a book, or at your doctor's office, you will see information about supplements to prevent cancer, supplements to take during cancer therapy, and supplements to take to prevent recurrence. You will also see information that opposes the use of supplementation for cancer patients, particularly during treatment. Consider, too, that most orthodox oncologists and physicians oppose the use of supplementation in all of these areas.

Why is this decision so perplexing? From the doctor's standpoint, it makes sense. At first, we hear how a vitamin, mineral, protein, or phytonutrient looks extremely promising for a particular situation. Soon we hear of conflicting results and then how it may even be harmful to take these types of supplements. How can the situation change so rapidly that in one study a substance is almost miraculous, and then in the next it is purported to be dangerous?

THE CAREER PATH OF A VITAMIN PILL

So the story may unfold in the following way: Substance X is discovered in an exotic plant, then taken to the animal lab, where it is found to reduce liver cancer by 70 percent. An epidemiologic study shows that people with the highest amount of substance X in their body have the lowest cancer rates, and those with the lowest amount have the highest cancer rates. Headlines extol the virtues of substance X, and grants are funded to study prospectively the benefits of substance X over a 5-year period. This research is a randomized double-blind placebo trial, meaning the participants will be chosen randomly so they can be equally evaluated, and the observers will not know who is getting the pill with substance X or who is getting an exact replica without X (called a placebo). After 3 years, the study is stopped because it shows no benefit.

Substance X has been in the headlines three times, two showing a potential benefit and one (which is the most important in the scientific world) showing no effect.

How can this happen? Well, several possibilities exist:

- Substance X does not have any benefit in treating cancer.
- These vitamins, minerals, and phytonutrients work in harmony, as a symphony reinforcing each other's job and supplying each other with necessary ingredients to affect wellness. The test, however, picks the one substance and evaluates it as if it were a drug, not taking into account the level of other micronutrients in the population and the effect of these micronutrients on each other.
- Infrequently, companies use a synthetic micronutrient in the trial, because such a synthetic chemical is either patentable, cheaper, or less likely to be successful (serving their own interests).

Because of these factors, it can be difficult to accurately gauge the effect of a particular supplement.

When using herbs, never forget that these are medicines (albeit natural and generally far safer than pharmaceutical products). Herbs should be cautiously employed, not only because they are medicines but because they're often grown out of the country—where the application of toxic pesticides is still in practice, where the level of toxic elements such as mercury and lead is not monitored, and where the condition of the soil and climate may change the concentration of the active ingredient. That is why it's essential to use herbs purchased from a reliable source and in concert with your health provider's recommendations. With these caveats in mind, herbal medicine can be a strong force for well-being.

Nutritional supplementation can be a powerful tool that can have significant impacts on health. It is an adjunct that should be used with caution and with a reasonable understanding of the value of each supplement one takes.

In using a single-ingredient supplement, care must be taken that it does not overwhelm the ability of body cells and prevent the absorption of other nutrients. This could cause a relative deficiency of the blocked nutrients. An example is that high doses of a single B vitamin can flood the B receptors, preventing the other B vitamins from entering the cell, thus causing a relative deficiency.

TYPES OF NUTRITIONAL SUPPLEMENTS

MICRONUTRIENTS: These are elements or compounds essential for life. If they cannot be made in the body, they have to be ingested from the outside as vitamins and minerals. Other essential supplements are those proteins, amino acids, fats, and sugars necessary for life but that can be made by the body. These can be diminished, in deficiency or extreme depleting states, due to the environment or medications.

PHYTONUTRIENTS: These are the organic compounds found in fruits and vegetables that help us strengthen our immune system and ward off disease. A good example of this type of substance is turmeric, an Indian spice used in yellow curry. The turmeric root contains the powerful antioxidant curcumin, shown to be beneficial for cancer survival.

HERBS: Plants generally used for food flavoring or for their medicinal properties are designated as herbs. Almost all the parts of plants—from their green leaves to their stems, seeds, bark, roots, and fruit—can be considered as an herb when used for medicinal or culinary purposes. In many instances, these are dried or made into a tincture of alcohol.

The medicinal properties of herbs have been known for thousands of years, preserved and passed through generations and valued for their remedial benefits. These herbs are a large component of natural medicine. Indeed, fully 85 percent of our prescription drugs are still derived from compounds found in nature.

Herbs have been used in many of the cultures of the world for several thousand years. Many of the herbs found in Chinese medicine can be traced back to 100 AD and even far before. Herbs have been recorded in the Greek and Roman cultures, as well as in the rest of Europe and the Middle East, including Persia and India.

Different parts of the plant may have different effects on the body, so the leaf may be used for one malady and the root for another. Herbs may have a specific action or act as an "adaptogen," used to normalize the patient's physiology. For example, the herb *Rhodiola rosea* may be used as a stimulant in a lethargic person and as a calming potion for the hyperactive.

WHY SUPPLEMENT?

In an ideal world, the nutrients contained in all three types of supplements can be found in the whole foods we eat, and can work together symphonically with the other thousands of as-yet-undiscovered or unknown chemicals in the vegetables and fruits that help us maintain our wellness. However, as discussed earlier, many factors diminish such an ideal. Growing and harvesting methods, environmental toxins in the atmosphere, and poor dietary choices are among the problems that have often left us with less-than-optimal amounts of essential fats, vitamins, minerals, and the other necessary elements of micronutrients.

Supplements to Treat Chemotherapy Residuals

If you are continuing to have symptoms after you have finished your chemother-apy, a supplement plan and other measures may help.

FOR PERIPHERAL NEUROPATHY

- B-complex, 50 mg at breakfast and lunch
- Omega-3, 500 mg 3x daily
- Magnesium, 250 mg 2x daily
- Have your hemoglobin A1C (a blood test reflecting your average blood sugar levels) checked, and keep below 5.2

FOR CARDIOMYOPATHY

- Magnesium, 250 mg 2x daily
- Coenzyme Q10, 100 mg 2x daily
- Hawthorne berry concentrate, 500 mg daily
- L-taurine, 500 mg 2x daily

FOR "CHEMO-BRAIN" (MENTAL FOGGINESS OR MEMORY ISSUES)

- B-complex, 50 mg at breakfast and lunch
- Omega-3, 500 mg 3x daily
- Rosemary, 200 mg daily
- Vinpocetine, 20 mg 2x daily

INFLAMMATION

Although inflammation is a broad term and involves a complex interplay of a multitude of different substances throughout the body, most everyone can agree on the following facts. First, inflammation is the most significant instigator and propagator of chronic degenerative diseases, especially cancer. Any foods and supplements that decrease inflammation should be utilized, and those supplements and foods that increase inflammation should be avoided.

Second, most scientists recognize a widespread deficiency of vitamin D_3, vitamin B_{12}, and omega-3 oils in American society. So, supplement needs will start with these basic micronutrients. We will go into much more depth regarding supplements in Chapter Eight.

QUESTIONABLE SUPPLEMENT RESEARCH, DISTORTED EDITORIALS, AND MEDIA BIAS

One should look very carefully at who sponsors any research and how the studies are structured to succeed or fail, depending on the primary and secondary end points. A nonpatentable, inexpensive natural product that competes against a costly drug is certainly not desirable in the pharmaceutical industry.

One must also recognize the relationship between the media and the advertising arm of Big Pharma. Medical editors and account managers for the television, magazine, and newspaper companies are very aware of the sensitivities of these corporations. A good example of this was a study comparing the effects of the herb St. John's wort and a well-known antidepressant to control depression. The results showed that St. John's wort was equal to the medicine for mild and moderate depression, though was *as* unsuccessful as the drug for severe depression. The headlines in the newspaper stated that St. John's wort was unsuccessful in treating severe depression. No mention was made of the equal failure of the pharmaceutical or the benefit of St. John's wort in mild cases.

Along similar lines, a study was done in head and neck cancer patients receiving radiotherapy, and half of a group was given vitamin E. In the final analysis, it was found that the vitamin E group had more treatment failures and relapses. Much later, the authors discovered that the worse outcomes were entirely attributed to those patients who continued to smoke during radiotherapy—however, this is almost never mentioned when this study is cited as evidence that supplements can be harmful.

A similar finding back in the 1980s—often referred to as "the Finnish smokers study"—found that smokers who took large doses of single ingredient beta-carotene (which was also synthetic) developed more cancers than those not taking it.

Clearly smokers should not take high doses of individual antioxidants. Antioxidants always function as a network. If an individual is not taking in adequate antioxidants from his diet, and is under high oxidative stress (as from smoking and radiotherapy), large doses of single antioxidants can become pro-oxidants, since they don't have an adequate "team" to recycle them back to their nonoxidized form, and can end up doing more harm than good.

Nutrients, unlike drugs, always function within a complex web of interactions with each other. Beware research that studies nutrients with models (double-blind randomized controlled trials with few variables) that were designed to study drugs. Results are likely to not represent what happens with well-designed whole food and complex supplementation programs. Science has not yet developed good research designs to study complex systems such as this.

Another point to keep in mind is that many of the scientists who design nutritional supplement studies or who study prior studies (a type of study called "meta-analysis") are not necessarily deeply knowledgeable in the field of nutrition and often even seem to have a bias against supplementation. In 2013, Fortman et al. published a meta-analysis in the *Annals of Internal Medicine* that concluded: "Vitamins do not reduce risk of cancer or cardiovascular disease."[24]

For this meta-analysis (study of studies), about 20 different randomized controlled clinical trials of multivitamins that had been previously completed and published were chosen and studied as an aggregate. One of the primary problems with this meta-analysis is that the studies chosen for it had used many different "multivitamin" products, ranging from 3 ingredients to more than 20, so very little consistency was evident between the trials, which were lumped together.

An issue in general with meta-analysis studies is that the results depend on which clinical trials are selected to be studied and which ones are left out either inadvertently or to increase the chances of a "desired result" on the part of the meta-analysis authors. If the investigators have a bias, they can manipulate the outcome of the study by which trials they choose to include and which they exclude, and there are many ways to rationalize their reasons for inclusion and exclusion of specific prior clinical studies. They may also miss significant studies that were published in journals that weren't included in the database searched for the study.

Additionally, it seems a bit odd to be asking in a meta-analysis whether multivitamins will prevent heart disease and cancer—what they are meant to prevent is nutritional deficiencies—and there is good evidence that many people in the United States and other developed nations have less than optimal intakes of over a dozen micronutrients (vitamins and minerals) from unsupplemented diets and that supplementation with a multivitamin/mineral does indeed contribute to adequate intakes of micronutrients for a substantial proportion of the population.[25]

The conclusion of the meta-analysis by Fortman et al. was that vitamin supplementation didn't reduce the risk of cancer or cardiovascular disease. An editorial commentary in the same issue of the *Annals of Internal Medicine* was titled: "Enough is enough: Stop wasting money on vitamin and mineral supplements."[26] Here is some of this editorial's commentary, which was widely publicized in the media:

> The message is simple: Most supplements do not prevent chronic disease or death, their use is not justified, and they should be avoided. Antioxidants, folic acid, and B vitamins are harmful or ineffective for chronic disease prevention, and further large prevention trials are no longer justified. The case is closed—supplementing

the diet of well-nourished adults with (most) mineral or vitamin sup-plements has no clear benefit and may be harmful. These vita-mins should not be used for chronic disease prevention. Enough is enough.

Strong words that were widely reprinted in the press. However, when we look more closely at the phrase "well-nourished adults," we find that many Americans are, in fact, as noted above, falling well short of recommended intakes of more than a dozen vitamins and minerals.[27]

As noted previously, a major issue with meta-analysis studies as a genre is that authors are able to manipulate the outcomes of their "study of studies" simply by which studies they choose to include and which to exclude—and this applies in many areas of medicine and health research, not only to nutri-tion and supplement research. In fact, previously published clinical trials of multivitamins that were not included in the Fortman et al. meta-analysis of 2013 were two large, well-done randomized placebo-controlled clinical trials of primary prevention with multivitamin supplements—the *Su.Vi.Max* study done in France, which followed more than 13,000 adults for 7½ years, half of whom took a five-component multiantioxidant supplement and the other half a placebo, and the Harvard's Physicians' Health Study II (PHSII), which ran-domized more than 14,000 male physicians over 50 years of age to a daily multivitamin/mineral (Centrum Silver) or a lookalike placebo, and followed them for more than 10 years. In fact, both of these interventions found that major subsets of these populations had a statistically significant reduction in development of cancer. In the *Su.Vi.Max* study, a 29 percent risk reduction for all cancers was found in men but not in women. The authors hypothe-sized that this may have been due to the fact that women ate more fruits and vegetables and had higher baseline levels of certain antioxidants (particularly beta-carotene) than men.[28]

It is worth noting here the difference between primary and secondary prevention studies. Primary prevention means that an intervention is being studied to see if it has impact on a disease that no one in the study has yet been diagnosed with—such as heart disease or cancer. Secondary preven-tion studies look at a population of people who have already been diagnosed with and treated for a condition such as cancer, and an intervention is being studied to see if it can prevent a recurrence of the condition—such as a relapse of cancer or a second heart attack or stroke.

In the PHSII, among 1,312 men with a previous history of cancer (prior to entering the study), a 27 percent decrease in risk of developing cancer was demonstrated over a median follow-up time of 11.2 years.[29] Even in the total group of more than 14,000 male physicians, there was a much more modest 8 percent reduction of total cancers, which was still statisti-cally significant, likely because the study group was so large. Translating this to the entire US population, if every adult male over 50 took a standard multiple vitamin-mineral supplement, over a 15-year period there would be 135,000 fewer cases of cancer in men. Thus, we see within the PHSII study both a primary prevention trial and a subset of the physicians who essentially made up a secondary prevention trial within the larger study—the group of more than 1,300 physicians who had previously been diagnosed with and treated for cancer—and in this population, this modest intervention with a multiple vitamin-mineral, had a much stronger cancer preventive effect than in the larger population who had not previously had cancer.

Despite the positive outcome of the PHSII study, an invited editorial published in the same issue of *JAMA* cast doubt on the findings.[30] Drs. Bach and Lewis opined:

> The PHSII study was a well-done, large-scale, blinded, randomized clinical trial with objective verification of cancer outcomes. (But) . . . the biological plausibility of the study hypothesis—that a multivitamin would be protective in a well-nourished population—is limited. This matters, because the chance that the study finding of a protective effect is true is intrinsically related (via Bayes theorem) to the plausibility of the hypothesis. . . . [B]efore drawing a definitive conclusion from this study that daily multivitamins reduce the risk of cancer in men, physicians and other readers must be convinced that the observed treatment effect is real and thus is likely to be reproduced in future experience rather than a random event that is unlikely to recur. The marginal statistical significance* and perplexing and somewhat counterintuitive nature of the study findings make drawing any firm conclusion premature. Thus, it may be inappropriate to recommend that men take multivitamins to prevent cancer.

Plausibility depends a great deal on what one knows and how deeply one cares to ponder the question. On the surface, it may seem implausible to academic medical doctors that vitamins and mineral supplements could prevent cancer in well-nourished people (and the physicians in the PHSII study ate better than average diets and exercised more than the average American population). Biochemically, the function of vitamins and minerals are as coenzymes, meaning that they are necessary for enzymes to function properly. Enzymes are the biological catalysts that allow every biochemical reaction in human cells to take place at body temperature. This includes enzymes that repair DNA and that allow mitochondria (the

---

*The statistics for the entire group indicated that there was a 4 out of 100 probability that the results could occur by chance (known as a p value of .04), and for the group of physicians with a prior history of cancer, it was 2 in 100 probability that the results occurred by chance (p value of .02).

energy-producing parts of our cells) to function. There is good evidence that as we get older and accumulate more environmental toxins in our bodies (which interfere with enzyme function), we require higher levels of specific vitamins and minerals for optimal enzyme function and hence for cellular repair.[31]

Clearly, it depends which studies are included in a meta-analysis as to whether multivitamins appear to be worthless (and perhaps dangerous) or whether they save lives. It also depends on how the individual studies that are meta-analyzed were designed, which nutrients, in what doses, and in what forms were used in the study. Because nutrients act in networks, studies that use larger numbers of nutrients in natural forms and in modest doses are more likely to be positive than studies that use only a few nutrients, especially when synthetically produced and given in relatively high dosages.

More to the point, people who have been diagnosed with a life-threatening cancer and have been successfully treated for it are much more likely than the general population to emerge from such treatment with more significant deficiencies of important nutrients. And this population, the intended audience for this book, has not yet been the subject of large-scale nutritional studies. Let's hope that can be rectified in the not-too-distant future.

WHERE IN OUR BODY DOES IT ALL GO?

It's worthwhile to note where the micronutrients are absorbed in our digestive tract, since many drugs, operations, infections, and localized conditions change the absorption of specific areas.

- The stomach absorbs water and minerals like zinc and iodide.
- The duodenum (upper small bowel) absorbs minerals such as calcium, magnesium, copper, selenium, iron, and phosphorus; the B vitamins riboflavin, niacin, and biotin; electrolytes; and the fat-soluble vitamins A, D, E, and K.
- The jejunum (mid-small bowel) absorbs minerals such as chromium, manganese, molybdenum, phosphorus, magnesium; the fat-soluble vitamins A, D, E, and K; and vitamin C, biotin, pantothenate, niacin, thiamin, riboflavin, and some amino acids.
- The ileum (distal small intestine) absorbs vitamins A, C, D, and K and folate, vitamin B_{12}; the mineral magnesium; and bile salts and bile acids.

VITAMIN D

Of special interest, almost requiring a chapter of its own, are the benefits of vitamin D. Vitamin D is not actually a vitamin but a prohormone that is created in the skin by the effects of ultraviolet rays from the sun on cholesterol. It is stored in the liver as vitamin 25-hydroxycholecalciferol, and transformed to its active form of 1,25 dihydroxycalciferol in the peripheral tissues.

Vitamin D receptors are found in almost 2,000 of our genes—out of 26,000. These receptors are located in more than 13 systems, including the cardiovascular, immune, endocrine, gastrointestinal, genitourinary, musculoskeletal, pulmonary, and neurologic. More than 200 vitamin D receptors are located in cardiovascular tissue, including the endothelium, the smooth muscle cells of the vessels, and the cardiac muscle cell itself. They are also found in the parathyroid, thyroid, and pancreas.

Vitamin D shuts down renin, a protein essential to the production of hypertension. We now know that renin can cause left ventricular hypertrophy without hypertension, induce inflammation and oxidative stress, and create constriction of smooth muscle. Levels of renin have recently been found a good prognosticator for cardiovascular disease, even when there are no other such risk factors present.

Cedric Garland, DrPH, of the University of California, San Diego, Moores Cancer Center, in the February 21, 2013, *Journal of Anticancer Research*, states that by taking between 4,000 and 8,000 IU a day of vitamin D, one may be able to prevent or contain cancer, multiple sclerosis, and type 1 diabetes.[32] He recommends that to prevent cancer, a blood level range of 40 to 60 ng/mL should be sought. Unfortunately, less than 10 percent of the US population has this level of vitamin D. Preventing cancer recurrence requires even a higher blood level, a range of 60 to 80 ng/mL.

Dr. Garland reports on a new theory of cancer formation called "micro Darwinism." Under this theory, the initiating event prior to cancer is the disruption of intracellular junctions. These are cilia-like connections between cells that allow them to communicate with each other, and to modulate and interrelate cells for tissue function. When the cells are tightly connected, they can more readily talk to each other. With the disintegration of the intracellular junction, the cells become autonomous, and the more rapidly proliferating cells can mutate and become malignant.

Vitamin D is the hormone that creates this tight intracellular bond, and lack of it allows the cells to become dysfunctional and autonomous. This process is described with the acronym DINOMIT: disjunction, initiation, natural selection, overgrowth, metastasis, involution, and transition. Dr. Garland believes that vitamin D will prevent, cure, or control cancer growth in any of these stages. This theory opens an exciting new era in the treatment and prevention of cancer.

CHAPTER SIX

EXERCISE

THE SECOND ELEMENT OF THE TRIAD TO POSTCANCER SUCCESS IS EXERCISE. OF course, any book about health improvement will recommend an exercise program because of its obvious benefits. Exercise lowers weight, blood pressure, and blood sugar levels; increases bloodflow and endorphins; helps control osteoporosis; and relieves anxiety and depression.

We know that obesity is related to cancer, and there are hard reasons for cancer patients to actively work to keep their weight down to prevent recurrence. It now appears that the relationship between exercise and cancer goes beyond that: Exercise itself is directly linked to cancer prevention.

Exercise lowers inflammation markers, and there are strong correlations between exercise and mental health, which could relate to cancer recurrence.

According to Moshe Frenkel, MD, founder of the Integrative Oncology Clinic at the MD Anderson Cancer Center, walking every day for half an hour, seven times a week, reduces the mortality of breast cancer survivors by 50 percent.[1] In addition, a study published in the *Journal of the American Medical Association* reported that women who actively walk saw a 45 percent reduction in breast cancer recurrence.[2] This is a greater improvement in the risk of recurrence than that seen with the antiestrogen therapies like tamoxifen.

A prospective cohort study of lifetime physical activity and survival in women with breast cancer followed 1,231 women diagnosed with breast cancer between 1995 and 1997 for a minimum of 8.3 years. Both moderate- and vigorous-intensity recreational physical activity decreased the risk of breast cancer death between 26 and 44 percent. Moderate-intensity recreational walking (defined as about 100 steps in 1 minute) decreased the risk of a recurrence or progression of a new primary cancer by an average of 44 percent.[3]

Another study done on patients with prostate cancer found something very similar. Between 1990 and 2008, 2,705 men diagnosed with nonmetastatic prostate cancer were observed. Men who walked 90 minutes or more per week—about 30 minutes three times a week—at a normal to very brisk pace reduced their risk of mortality by 46 percent compared with men who walked shorter durations at an easy walking pace. When they increased this exercise to greater than 3 hours per week of vigorous activity, they lowered their risk of death from prostate cancer by 60 percent compared to men who did less than 1 hour a week of vigorous activity.[4]

A report from the United Kingdom's oldest and most respected charitable patient-support organization, Macmillan Cancer Support, says that cancer patients should exercise at moderate intensity for at least 2½ hours every week. Regular exercise can both reduce the risk of dying from cancer and minimize the side effects of treatment.[5]

Exercise is clearly strong medicine against cancer. But despite the fact that it is an easy, free, and nontoxic recommendation that rivals the effectiveness of existing protocols, few oncologists prescribe it.

Ciarán Devane, former chief executive of Macmillan Cancer Support, says, "Cancer patients would be shocked if they knew just how much of a benefit physical activity could have on their recovery and long-term health, in some cases reducing their chances of having to go through the grueling ordeal of treatment all over again. It doesn't need to be anything too strenuous—doing the gardening, going for a brisk walk, and swimming all count."

Such advice is a major reversal from a time not that long ago when patients were encouraged not to exercise. "The advice that I would have previously given to one of my patients would have been to 'take it easy,' says Jane Maher, MD, Macmillan Cancer Support's chief medical officer. "This has now changed significantly because of the recognition that if physical exercise were a drug, it would be hitting the headlines."[6]

According to the center, research shows that their recommended levels of exercise—6 hours of moderate physical activity per week—can reduce the risk of breast cancer recurrence by 40 percent. The risk of dying from prostate cancer can be reduced by up to 30 percent. Bowel cancer patients can cut their risk of dying from their disease by almost 50 percent.

Jennifer Ligibel, MD, of Harvard Medical School reported in the 2007 *Journal of Clinical Oncology* that exercise intervention was associated with a significant decrease in insulin levels and hip circumference in breast cancer survivors.[7] This is an important finding because a strong association exists between cancer and obesity, insulin, and sugar levels. In a recent editorial of the *Journal of Clinical Oncology,* Pamela Goodwin, MD, of the Mount Sinai Hospital in Toronto stated: "If you look at the effect of insulin, the women in the highest quartile of insulin levels in the studies that have been done all yield the same result. They have a triple risk of death."[8]

We know that sugar suppresses the immune system and that insulin and obesity increase inflammation, which then sets up an environment for cancer spread. So it would seem beneficial to minimize these parameters in the post-therapy period. Exercise helps with insulin resistance and obesity in two ways. When you exercise, you burn more calories than you would if you were sedentary. A 190-pound man burns about 80 calories an hour at rest, such as when watching TV or reading. An hour spent jogging at the light pace of 12 minutes per mile would burn about 600 calories. In addition, exercise boosts your metabolism not just for the hour you exercise but for the entire day after you exercise. This metabolism boost occurs at a cellular level through the resulting increase in muscle mass (the amount of which depends on the type of exercise).

So what does that mean for losing weight (another component of preventing cancer recurrence)? If you engage in an exercise that burns 250 calories in an hour and also reduce your caloric intake by another 250 calories that day, you will lose about 1 pound in a week. One pound of muscle burns about 2.5 times as many calories as 1 pound of fat, just to maintain life. The average woman carries about 30 percent of her weight as body fat, but as a result of daily exercise, she can increase muscle mass and burn fat. So even if she does not lose any net weight, she will trade body fat for new muscle, which then will burn more than twice the calories that the fat did—while she does nothing but breathe!

EXERCISE FOR CANCER PATIENTS

Because of the short- and long-term complications that can arise in cancer therapy, many survivors—for reasons both physical and emotional—become sedentary. Surgery recovery and chemotherapy and radiation side effects may inhibit exercise in the short term, while fatigue and depression can contribute to longer-term avoidance of exercise.

While this is understandable, it also increases the risk of cancer recurrence. And excessive rest, which was the earlier advice for patients going through treatment, may result in loss of function, strength, and range of motion for a person with a chronic illness. Fortunately, once patients develop a regular exercise program, they usually find that the exercise not only gets easier but also helps alleviate the fatigue and depression that kept them from participating.

Some researchers and providers recognize the hurdles to starting an exercise regimen and are aware that merely providing this information to patients is not enough. Patients need to have a directed regimen prescribed by their doctor or a medically affiliated program.

This is why cardiac rehab programs work so well and why we recommend a comprehensive, prescribed cancer rehab program.

Without a cancer rehab program in place, and without clear prescriptions for exercise from your oncologist, it is up to you to create your own prescription. We highly recommend that, if you can afford it, you sign up with a local gym and work with a personal trainer to establish your exercise regimen. Some health insurance companies will provide discounts on gym memberships and even pay for a few hours with a personal trainer, so contact your insurance representative to ask about these possibilities. You may also be able to find no-cost or low-cost directed exercise classes and programs through local community centers, senior centers, or even a local hospital. Look for a trainer with some experience and/or certification in chronic disease or cancer. The American Council on Exercise and the American College of Sports Medicine both have specialized training available to their experienced trainers.

A NEW LIFE TO LIVE

Cancer survivors have essentially been given a new life. A change in normal life habits can positively or negatively impact how that "second life" is lived.

If you were sedentary before cancer, or became sedentary as a result of your illness and treatment, you may need to make a fundamental shift in how you approach exercise. People often look at fitness as an additional burden in an already chaotic schedule. Maybe you're thinking, "I don't have the time." But everyone has the time. You just need to prioritize your health and commit to increasing your activity level.

There are many small ways in which you can increase your exercise throughout the day. We highly recommend purchasing a wearable exercise tracker, which will show you your activity during the day, and can help you set goals and track the progress you are making. Aim to walk at least 5,000 steps per day. As you begin your exercise regimen, track your progress in your fitness journal. You'll be surprised by the progress you make in just a few months! Some ways to increase your activity are:

- Take the stairs instead of the elevator.
- Park at the outer edge of the parking lot at the mall or grocery store (when it's safe).
- Get on and off the bus at the second stop from your home or work.
- Walk to lunch instead of driving.

- Park farther away from your office.
- Do the housework and gardening, instead of hiring a housekeeper to clean or a neighborhood kid to mow. Consider these activities part of your weekly regimen. You'll save money and get exercise!

ATTITUDE MATTERS

Instead of looking at exercise as a chore and additional activity that you must squeeze into your day, try to look at it as simply a part of your day—every day. Your daily walk, run, swim, bicycle ride, or yoga class should be as much a part of your routine as eating dinner. We eat dinner every night, but some nights dinner is a gourmet meal while other nights it's just soup and salad.

This same concept applies to exercise. Some days, you'll go to the gym or a class and have a great hour-long workout. On other days, you may just have time for a brisk walk. Both are beneficial and important. If you go into an exercise program with the mind-set that it has to be a long, gut-busting, sweat-filled workout every time, you're setting yourself up to dread it. You're also setting yourself up for an exercise regimen that will be very short lived, which makes it less likely that you will restart a new program down the road. If people have failed to follow through on a fitness program once, they often avoid trying again. So give yourself a break.

The fact is, you will not always be able to follow through with your workout plan, but that doesn't mean you won't tomorrow or next week. You may have the best of intentions to go to the gym or for a 10-mile bike ride, but then work runs late, your child comes down with the flu, or you need to get home for a host of

A PERFECT STORM

As our cancer treatments improve, more people are surviving longer, and more people are being cured of this dreaded illness. More than 60 percent of people diagnosed with cancer between 1999 and 2006 were still alive 5 years later. In 1977, that survival statistic was only 40 percent. That's a more than 50 percent improvement in just 3 decades!

That means we have more people who are diagnosed with cancer earlier as screening studies are more widely used, more people who are cured, and more people who are living with cancer. With baby boomers now entering their retirement years, this means we will have a population "bump" of cancer survivors. Resources must be found to focus attention on this tremendous influx of patients into the world of cancer survivorship. Exercise/fitness is one cost-efficient and highly effective way to manage the health of the many current and future cancer survivors.

reasons. In those instances, instead of considering your workout a failure, try to fit in something quick, like a short walk or playing soccer in the yard with your child. Then refocus for the next day or even the next week. Even after weeks off, you can always get back on track.

As Yogi Berra said so profoundly, "Ninety percent of [the] game is half mental."

BENEFITS OF EXERCISE

Evidence of the benefits of exercise for cancer patients has been mounting for the past 15 to 20 years. In 1996, the American Cancer Society added "regular physical activity" to the list of measures included in their cancer prevention guidelines, finally bringing to an end the "get more rest" mentality that pervaded the oncology community for so many years. The role of exercise is rapidly emerging as one of the foremost areas of cancer research, with recently proven benefits like higher quality of life, improved mood, less cancer-related fatigue, better pain and nausea control, and, perhaps most importantly, a lower risk of recurrence.

We know that estrogen is the driving force behind many breast cancers and that fat tissue harbors estrogen. As such, a recent study demonstrated that obesity may contribute to the risk of breast cancer recurrence. Exercise seems to benefit people from the standpoints of primary prevention (preventing cancer from ever occurring), secondary prevention (preventing a recurrence), improving quality of life and tolerance during treatment, and improving overall health and survival in patients who have metastatic cancer and are living with it every day.

In 1997, the American Institute for Cancer Research (AICR) concluded that as many as 30 to 40 percent of all cancers could be prevented if everyone ate a healthful diet, avoided becoming obese, and participated in a regular exercise program. The international panel of experts recommended the equivalent of a brisk walk 1 hour per day, along with 1 hour of more vigorous exercise per week for those who performed sedentary jobs. However, we know that the vast majority of the population does not come anywhere near to achieving these guidelines.

In 2011, the AICR released a surprising analysis. It estimated that some 50,000 cases of breast cancer and 43,000 cases of colon cancer occurred as a direct result of physical inactivity. Specifically, it condemned prolonged periods of sitting, dubbing this new affliction "Sitting Disease." In this analysis, the AICR cut in half its daily exercise recommendations—from 60 minutes per day to a daily 30-minute brisk walk. An even more startling finding was that even for those of us who are physically active, prolonged sitting is a significant detriment to our health. At the very least, we should be standing and taking a quick walk or doing a few minutes of exercise every hour or two. We should also try to stand as much as possible during the day. As a cancer risk factor, sitting now rivals smoking!

MORE SCIENCE IS NEEDED

In laboratory studies, investigators have injected mice with cancer-causing substances and then divided them into groups—those that exercise and those that don't. Based on these studies, it seems that exercise on its own may actually slow the growth of cancer cells. The mechanisms by which exercise contributes to this outcome are likely numerous, but one explanation is that exercise enhances the natural defensive activity of some of the most vital cells in the immune system.

A recent Nurses' Health Study of more than 3,000 cancer survivors showed that higher levels of activity after a diagnosis of breast cancer resulted in a 25 to 40 percent reduction in the risk of breast cancer recurrence and risk of death from breast cancer.[9] These benefits extended to women who did as little as 1 to 3 hours of moderately intense exercise per week, with greater benefit to those who did more. Similar benefits have been demonstrated in colon cancer survivors.

EXERCISE CAUTION

Getting a diagnosis of cancer is frightening, but with proper guidance, some motivation, a bit of insight into how your body works—along with an understanding of your disease and its treatment—and a healthy dose of common sense, you can improve your odds for avoiding recurrence and optimizing survival. Exercise, which can improve your daily physical functioning and overall quality of life, can be one of many pieces that allow you to reclaim your life.

All of that said, it is important that you discuss an exercise plan with your doctor and, if possible, get the help of a physical trainer to individualize the exercise program to match your particular limitations, strengths, needs, and goals. Your primary doctor can perform an exercise assessment, which is valuable no matter what type of exercise you are doing. We generally consider five aspects of assessment: aerobic capacity, muscular strength, flexibility, neuromuscular adaptation, and functional ability. Each of these then needs to be tailored to the specific patient.

Your physician or physical trainer can measure the following basic parameters:

1. Resting heart rate
2. Resting blood pressure
3. Serum cholesterol
4. HDL cholesterol (also known as good cholesterol)
5. Percentage of body fat

6. Maximum VO$_2$
7. Sit and reach flexibility test
8. Hand grip dynamometer

From these basics, you can set sensible fitness goals. Patients with cancer are also advised to take into account some general precautions when exercising.

- Always talk to all of your oncology caregivers prior to beginning any new physical activity. This includes, where applicable, your surgical oncologist, radiation oncologist, and medical oncologist. They are all different specialists who perform different functions. They may be able to advise you on specific limitations based on their treatments.

- If you go to a personal trainer, try to find one who has some experience with patients being treated for cancer and other chronic diseases. The American Council on Exercise and the American College of Sports Medicine both have additional certifications in these areas.

- If you received chemotherapy treatment, ask your oncologist to explain your blood counts to you. Neutrophils are white blood cells that fight bacterial infections; they should be above 1,500 to prevent infection and to exercise safely. Platelets are cells involved in clotting blood; they should be above 50,000 to prevent bleeding. Red blood cells carry oxygen to your organs and tissues. Hemoglobin is a measure of your red blood cells. When it's low, you are anemic and often tired. Unless the count is severely low—below 8.0—it should not deter you from exercising.

- Never exercise with a fever, as this may worsen an incipient infection.

- Certain chemotherapy drugs, such as vincristine or Taxol, can lead to peripheral neuropathy—an irritation of nerves causing pain, numbness, or tingling of the arms and legs. Neuropathy can cause difficulty with balance. If you have neuropathy, talk to a trainer about seated exercise and exercises where there is no risk of falling. Also talk to your trainer about exercises that can help alleviate the symptoms of neuropathy.

- Other chemotherapeutics, such as Adriamycin or Herceptin, can contribute to heart damage, so if you feel worsening shortness of breath or develop chest pain or palpitations while exercising, stop and contact your physician. If you were on any of these chemotherapy drugs, talk to your doctor about their effects before starting an exercise program.

- Cancer can generate blood clots. If you have had one, you may be on blood thinners, which increases risk of bleeding and makes exercise risky. Check regularly with your oncologist to make sure your blood is not overly thinned.

- If you still have a port—a catheter in one of your veins—be careful about exposure to water and avoid rigorous movement of muscles surrounding that catheter's location.

- If you had surgery, this may limit—or at least make more difficult—certain exercise motions. For example, some breast cancer patients have had a section of their abdominal muscles removed to reconstruct their breast, which makes abdominal strengthening difficult but all the more vital, so take things slowly. Other patients may have had multiple lymph nodes removed from their arm, which decreases the range of motion in that arm.

- If you received radiation therapy, make sure the skin around the area is not torn or cracked. Some exercises will cause the skin to stretch, leading to more damage or discomfort and possible infection.

- Always stay well hydrated during exercise by drinking clear liquids. This is vital to maintaining adequate kidney function and electrolyte balance. Ask your oncologist about your recent potassium, magnesium, and calcium levels. They can all affect exercise tolerance. Plain water is great, and plain coconut water is another recommendation because of its levels of potassium and magnesium. Aim for drinking 8 to 10 glasses of water each day. Your doctor can quickly tell through some blood work and a physical exam if you might be dehydrated. Minimize alcohol and caffeine, both of which can lead to dehydration.

CARDIOVASCULAR EXERCISE

Cardiovascular exercise has been intensively studied in cancer patients both during and after treatment, including how it may affect recurrence. Its benefits are as many and as varied as the types of exercises that you can do. Cardiovascular exercise:

- Strengthens respiration muscles, which improves airflow in and out of the lungs
- Strengthens the heart muscle, which makes the heart more efficient with each beat
- Lowers your heart rate
- Improves circulation
- Reduces blood pressure
- Increases endorphin levels (the "feel-good" chemicals in the brain)
- Lowers body fat
- Increases general muscle mass

AEROBIC VERSUS ANAEROBIC EXERCISE

The term *cardiovascular exercise* is often used interchangeably with *aerobic exercise,* though they are not necessarily the same. Aerobic exercise refers to physical activity of relatively low intensity. This type of exercise does not result in the formation of lactic acid, which leads to burning muscles, sore muscles, and sometimes—if there's too much of it in the body—nausea and vomiting. Anaerobic activity is characterized by short bursts of intense exercise, during which the muscles run out of oxygen quickly and lactic acid builds up fast. This is why you can't sprint for an hour. During aerobic exercise like brisk walking, both sugar and fat from within your body can be utilized as energy sources, though the relative contributions of each depend on the intensity of exercise.

Although lower-intensity exercise burns proportionately more fat than high intensity, the overall number of calories burned is substantially higher with higher-intensity workouts. High-intensity exercise also revs up your calorie burning for the next 24 hours, while low-intensity workouts do not. All of which is to say that immediately following your treatment, you may need to take it easy on yourself, but you can still get meaningful benefit from any lower-intensity activities. Later, when you are able, you can mix in some activities that require more effort but provide an even greater reward.

- Decreases the risk of diabetes and other chronic lifestyle-related conditions
- Lowers stress levels
- Improves mental health through sound physical conditioning

RATING YOUR WORKOUT

When exercising, it's important to gauge your exercise intensity accurately. The Rate of Perceived Exertion (RPE) scale helps you estimate how intense your activity level is at any given time, just by thinking about how you're feeling. This method requires no equipment and has been demonstrated to correlate well with target heart rate, which is another method of measuring intensity.

The RPE chart loosely follows these levels:

0–1: You feel no exertion or very, very light exertion. It is any passive sedentary activity, including watching TV or reading.

2–3: Light to moderately light activity. You could do it for a sustained period and maintain a conversation. It is easy to breathe.

4–6: Moderate activity. You can sustain the activity for an hour or more. You can have short conversations, but you are breathing heavily.

7–8: Vigorous activity. You are breathing very heavily and can only speak a sentence or so. You cannot sustain the activity for long periods.

9: Very hard activity: You have difficulty breathing and talking, and cannot maintain the activity for more than short periods.

10: Max effort activity. You can barely breathe, and you can't talk. You can only maintain the activity for very short durations.

We advise you to aim for an RPE level between 3 and 6 for most activities—starting even slower, if necessary. Begin your workouts at a comfortable level, about the 3 range on the scale, for a duration of at least 10 minutes and as long as 45 minutes. Try to do the 3–6 activity level workouts at least every other day.

TYPES OF CARDIO

Entire volumes have been written on the different types of cardiovascular exercises, but we'd like to spotlight a few that are easy to do and that most people find enjoyable. Always remember the first rule of exercise: If it's not enjoyable, it's not sustainable.

Running and Walking

Running and walking are the most common of all cardiovascular exercises. When you begin exercising—especially when starting during cancer treatment or immediately after—it's a good idea to monitor your walking. Because you may not realize how many miles you actually cover in a day, this will be a good gauge. You can purchase a relatively inexpensive pedometer, which simply detects your body movement, counts each step you take, and then calculates the total number of feet (and subsequently miles) you've covered over a given time period. We generally suggest you aim for at least 5,000 steps per day.

Walking is something that you can start even before completing therapy because it is low impact. When you walk, one foot is always on the ground; when you run, both feet are airborne at the top of your stride, and then you land on one foot, causing a greater shock to the joints with each step (which is why it's called high impact). This is one reason that running can lead to more hip and knee problems than walking can, especially if not done correctly.

The relevance of impact can be even greater for those patients who have had treatment that resulted in diminished bone density and are now at higher risk for fractures. This includes, among others, antiestrogen therapies for breast cancer, hormonal therapy for prostate cancer, and certain chemotherapy agents that accelerated the onset of menopause. If you have a question about this—and if you've been advised against running—ask your doctor for a bone density scan (aka a DEXA scan) as a baseline.

If you are not able to run, walking briskly is a great low-impact option and a great way to reduce stress. Walking may also be a better form of exercise to do with a partner, as the lower intensity allows you to carry on a conversation. Studies have shown that brisk walking 30 minutes a day, 6 days a week is a highly effective way to prevent cancer recurrence.

Biking

Biking is another great low-impact exercise, whether you use a stationary or conventional bicycle. Both come in two main varieties: the recumbent and the upright (standard). In the recumbent bike, the weight is distributed more broadly across the back and buttocks, and therefore it leads to less hunching of the back and more of a focus on the legs. Conversely, the standard upright bicycle is more of a challenge; it forces the rider to sit up straight, resulting in a harder workout for the erector muscles of the spine. As more of your muscles are recruited to keep your body upright, it also tends to be a tougher workout.

You should be wary of any residual nerve damage (neuropathy) you may have sustained with your chemotherapy because this can lead to balance dysfunction and subsequent injury. It can take up to a year for your nerves to fully recover from drugs like paclitaxel (Taxol) or vincristine, and some patients' nerves never recover. If you have any concerns about balance, you may want to stick with a stationary bike until you feel more stable.

As you advance in your bike training, you may wish to join a bike team or find a bike buddy for longer rides. Most areas offer organized bike rides on a regular basis. Participating in a long ride can be an excellent long-term goal.

For those who prefer to ride stationary bikes, there are also ways to increase the intensity of your workout as you develop your strength, stamina, and skills. Spin classes have become very popular and are widely available through gyms and Spin training centers. These are directed stationary bike classes in which an instructor leads participants on a simulated "ride," utilizing the resistance on the bike to increase and decrease intensity throughout.

Swimming

Almost every community has an indoor pool within a few miles. Make use of it! Swimming is another low-impact exercise and has many benefits. It's a great activity for cancer survivors who are suffering from balance problems due to their illness or treatment, and is excellent for obese or previously sedentary patients slowly easing into an exercise regimen. (And if you can't swim, take the opportunity to learn now; it's a survival skill that everyone should have.)

Swimming can be as light or as intense as you want it to be, based on the speed at which you swim. Many swimmers prefer to do longer, slower workouts, but you can also do sprint workouts, utilizing the timers at the side of public pools. Most lifeguards will enthusiastically give you pointers on doing timed workouts and, as you progress, may even be able to provide you with set workouts.

Swimming is also a very meditative activity, and many swimmers find that doing laps is a way to clear their minds. If you are looking for social connections through your sport, look into local master's level swim teams. Master's swim clubs are open to swimmers at all levels and to anyone over the age of 18.

If you have less experience in the pool, or are looking for a low-impact workout that is not just doing laps, excellent pool activities are water Zumba or water aerobics—or even just walking in the water, which provides a low-impact, high-resistance exercise.

RESISTANCE TRAINING

Resistance training is often the least understood area of exercise. It is typically associated with lifting impossibly heavy weights to achieve grossly oversized muscles. But resistance training should not be confused with powerlifting or bodybuilding, just as cardiovascular training should not be confused with Ironman-type triathlons. These are extreme examples of activities that are usually done by normal folks. Most of the equipment in modern gyms today—other than treadmills, stationary bikes, and elliptical trainers—is there to support some specific form of resistance exercise. Make no mistake: Resistance training provides multiple and significant benefits for patients who have gone through cancer therapy.

By definition, resistance training is any type of exercise in which effort is performed against a specific opposing force that generates resistance and leads to contraction of muscles. The American Sports Medicine Institute defines the goal of resistance training as "to gradually and progressively overload the musculature system so it gets stronger." This type of exercise not only improves muscle strength but also strengthens the tendons (which connect muscle to muscle) and ligaments (which connect muscle to bone) around the joints. This leads to improved balance and posture and, for many patients, a quicker return to full functional capacity. Chemotherapy itself, along with the limited activity that often follows treatment, can lead to muscle atrophy—the loss of muscle mass—fairly quickly. Prostate cancer and breast cancer patients, in particular, also receive hormonal or antihormonal therapies, which tend to further diminish muscle mass and bone density. Resistance exercises are the best remedy for this drop in muscle and bone mass.

Exercise guidelines tend to stress the importance of "increasing metabolism." While this is a complex process, much of it actually revolves around decreasing body fat while increasing muscle. We know that when the ratio of fat to muscle decreases, you will burn more calories at rest due to the higher caloric needs of maintaining muscle versus fat tissues.

This leads to the other important, if somewhat intangible, benefit of resistance training, which should not be underestimated. Physical appearance and the psychological impact of looking fit are vital to emotional well-being for most of us, but particularly for patients who have undergone often-harrowing regimens of chemotherapy, radiation, and surgery. It is resistance exercises that accomplish the definition and tone many of us seek. This style of workout can be an integral part of a return to body normalcy.

Dr. Mehta prefers that his patients use free weights, rather than machines. These include barbells and dumbbells (with dumbbells preferred for most exercises), which come in a wide range of weights to match your lifting capacity. Free weights work more muscles at the same time than machines do. Individual machines are designed to target specific individual muscles, which may not be particularly useful when doing exercises for rehabilitation. The more muscles you are working during resistance training, the better. Free weight exercises often mimic everyday motions, so they result in what's called functional fitness—strength that translates to real life, not just the gym.

If you are not familiar with handling free weights, make sure you get proper guidance from a trained professional before venturing into the weight room because improper form can easily cause an injury. Most gyms will provide one or two free or reduced-cost sessions with a physical trainer with your membership.

One advantage to weight machines is that your form is determined by the way the machine is designed to move. You don't have to think about it—you just push and pull. The drawback is that if you have a specific issue with one arm or leg from surgery, for example, the limited range of motion preset by the machine may be a tough test for a weakened limb, and there's little opportunity for other muscles to help you out.

In some cases, simple exercise bands may be your best bet. They provide resistance without the risk of injury of free weights or the restrictions of weight machines. A combination of all these approaches may be optimum; a good trainer will help you make these important decisions.

STRETCHING

In many Eastern traditions, mental and physical flexibility is said to be the key to a balanced and happy life. It is our ability to adapt to the difficult situations we are put in that can determine the degree of satisfaction we have with our lives. Not much is more stressful and demanding than a cancer diagnosis. Often, without realizing it, new cancer patients make profound adjustments to the way they approach living their lives. Both emotional and spiritual flexibility are essential.

All exercise involves some degree of stretching, but we want you to learn safe and effective stretching techniques with the specific goal of gaining overall physical flexibility. To accomplish this, we recommend you seek out the assistance of a trained professional who understands your specific medical needs as well as proper stretching techniques that apply to everybody.

Once again, whether you accomplish this by doing yoga, Pilates, or simple floor mat activities, stretching is a great place to start getting used to the "feel" of moving your body correctly.

While Pilates may be more expensive, yoga classes are routinely offered through gyms and community centers for minimal cost. Joining a yoga class twice a week is a way to combine exercise, stretching, and meditation.

Balance can be a special challenge for cancer patients. Side effects of the various treatments, residual effects of the cancer itself, and overall debility and fatigue can put you at risk for a fall. Fortunately, exercise itself—including dancing and especially yoga stretching and tai chi—has been found to help improve balance, even in older persons or those with neurological challenges. We advise that in addition to the rest of your workout, you do 15 or 20 minutes of stretching per day. This will help your body warm up and cool down from other exercise. It also increases the lymphatic flow in your body and is often meditative. Plus, it feels good.

If you have issues with balance, you can start in a chair. In general, err on the side of being cautious until you have fully recovered. Start slowly, but you should find improvement in just a few sessions.

MOTIVATION

Sometimes just hearing that exercise can increase your health or make you feel better isn't enough to get started. If you fall into this category, consider some ways to motivate yourself.

START SMALL: Go for a walk around the block and then increase your walk by a block every day. Maybe the first 30 walks are only 5 minutes each. Regardless, you are doing something, and eventually you will find that adding length and a distance—minutes at a time—is extremely rewarding.

GET A DOG: Adopt a dog or make more time for an existing pet. Dogs need to be walked, and they will make daily walks far more enjoyable for you. And once you get started, it's hard to resist those pleading brown eyes.

FIND AN EXERCISE BUDDY: Solicit a friend to be your exercise buddy

Cheryl's Story: Back to Biking

After Cheryl finished her treatment for lymphoma, she found herself increasingly drawn to doing the activity she once loved: biking. "I loved bike riding, and I started doing that until I built up my strength. I had very little muscle tone, so it was like starting all over again. But I just loved riding, and I was addicted to it. I felt so free. It was also something my husband and I could do together after what had been such a solo journey."

Cheryl continued, "Little by little, I lost weight and gained strength. It was just uphill from there. We started biking longer and longer distances. We really focused on that. We went on organized bike rides and joined a biking club. It certainly has helped me mentally. I use activity to provide a sense of accomplishment. Looking at what my body can do. It's kind of an affirmation."

and set a standing date. Knowing someone else is waiting for you is a huge motivation to get up and out.

JOIN A CLASS: Paying for a class just may be enough to get you there! Before you know it, you'll be having fun and making new friends who you'll look forward to seeing.

REDISCOVER A PASSION: Did you love dancing, playing baseball, or surfing when you were a kid? Well, guess what? You can reacquaint yourself with these activities no matter how old you are—even into your eighties and nineties! There are adult and senior dance classes, softball teams, Hula-Hoop classes, and surfing groups, as well as adult-league kickball and dodgeball teams. You'll be having so much fun, you won't even realize you're exercising!

SOLICIT YOUR FRIENDS OR FAMILY: Ask your family or a group of friends to commit to a weekly hike, bike ride, walk, swim, or other physical activity. Doing so will help strengthen bonds and provide health benefits for all of you.

LOVE WHAT YOU DO: Remember, exercise is like dinner. There is your soup-and-salad day: a half-hour walk and some stretching; your lasagna day: an hour at the gym or a good, long run or swim; and your oysters-and-caviar day: surfing in the ocean, backcountry cross-country skiing, or a destination bike ride. Anything is better than nothing, so don't hold yourself to unrealistic expectations—fit in what you can!

CHAPTER SEVEN

AVOIDING TOXINS

RIDDING YOUR LIFE OF TOXINS CAN BE AN IMPORTANT PART OF YOUR AFTER cancer care. There is no doubt that the toxins in our food and our environment contribute to cancer. There are the well-known and obvious connections—such as cigarettes and lung and mouth cancer, or asbestos and mesothelioma—but also many less-known toxins that definitively or possibly cause cancer.

When we discuss toxic substances, we are talking about those substances that are ingested or inhaled or that we otherwise come in contact with that can cause degenerative diseases to develop or intensify. These toxic agents can affect the nervous system along with many other bodily functions, introducing or aggravating many degenerative diseases, including several types of cancers.

Diseases can develop or become worse when an initiating factor intrudes from outside of the body or if a toxic substance is produced from within. Toxins that come from the outside include gases such as carbon monoxide, liquids such as alcohol, and heavy metals like mercury. Internal toxicities can develop from certain neurotransmitters such as glutamate, an excitatory amino acid that, in excess, creates neurologic damage; metabolism products like homocysteine, an amino acid that, when produced by the body in excess, generates inflammation; or trimethylamine, an oxidative by-product of metabolism that in excess likewise leads to inflammation. All of these, at high levels, can cause toxicity and cell death.

One of the most vigorous controversies in cancer research is how important the influence of environmental and ingested toxins are on the development of human malignancies. The materials we incorporate into our body's makeup come from not only what we eat but also from what we take in by breathing and what is absorbed through the largest organ of our body, the skin. An ongoing debate rages over which chemicals are responsible—and what their level of culpability actually is—for causing different types of cancer. We're all agreed that cigarette smoke and asbestos do cause cancer, but what about the pesticide on our apple or the fertilizer on our lawn? And if they do cause cancer at some amount, what's the level of safety, if there is any?

The Environmental Protection Agency (EPA) can compound the confusion. Only a small fraction of the 80,000 chemicals we are exposed to actually get tested for carcinogenicity, and although it's well intentioned, the EPA's Integrated Risk Information System maintains a complex and perplexing rating system that doesn't clearly help people identify what substances to avoid. The system divides chemicals into five groups: from the most harmful ones in group A—those chemicals that are clearly carcinogens for humans—to the least dangerous in group E—those not likely to be carcinogenic to humans. Between these extremes are groups B (likely to be carcinogenic), C (evidence suggests carcinogenic potential), and D (inadequate information exists to assess carcinogenic potential).

This mass of information only serves to put the cancer survivor in a deeper quandary as to which substances to avoid in trying to maintain a cancer-free life. To add to the confusion, many of the substances on the list often go by several different names, so salt might be listed as sodium chloride, or methanol might be listed as methyl alcohol, making it difficult to find a particular substance in the alphabetical listing that may not always use its most common name.

Also, other organizations, such as the American Cancer Society, National Cancer Institute, and National Institute for Occupational Safety and Health, may from time to time take positions on specific chemical exposures, which can confound even experts. Hundreds of chemicals, elements, and exposure levels are listed by the International Agency for Research on Cancer and the National Toxicology Program. They are divided into known human carcinogens and probable carcinogens. Reviewing these lists is not very helpful either because—here as well—the offending chemical may be labeled with another name.

Our individual exposure or sensitivity to the substance cannot be quantified, and reading the caveat by these organizations does not instill great confidence. At the head of the list, the American Cancer Society warns: "Looking at the list can tell you whether or not something may increase your risk of cancer, but it is important to try to get an idea of how much it might increase your risk. It is also important to know what your risk is to begin with. Many factors can enter into this, including age, gender, family history, and lifestyle factors, such as tobacco and alcohol use, weight, diet, physical activity level, etc. The type and extent of exposure to a substance may also play a role. You should consider the actual amount of increased risk when deciding if you should limit or avoid exposure."

To a person without any guidance from a health program or professional about what substances to avoid, this is a daunting admonition. We suggest that the best way to approach this problem is to avoid those chemicals suggested as possibly carcinogenic, even if there is no firm proof. If the evidence comes from the laboratory or from epidemiologic studies that have not yet been fully proven, it is best to err on the side of caution and stay away from these products, to maximize your chances for staying healthy.

For a current list of known and probable carcinogens, go to the American Cancer Society's Web site, cancer.org, and click on "Learn About Cancer" and "What Causes Cancer?" and "Other Carcinogens," and then scroll through the options.

TOXINS IN THE ENVIRONMENT

In 2010, the President's Cancer Panel warned of grievous harm from chemicals and other hazards, and cited a growing body of evidence linking environmental exposure to toxins to cancer. These warnings were accompanied by a statement that cancers caused by environmental exposure were "grossly underestimated." It advised the government to strengthen research and regulation, and cautioned individuals to limit exposure to threats like pesticides, industrial chemicals, medical x-rays, vehicle exhaust, plastic food containers, and overexposure to sunlight.

Of the many tens of thousands of potentially carcinogenic chemicals now in regular use in the United States, only a few hundred have been tested for safety. The panel stated that our government's regulatory approach is "reactionary rather than precautionary." Instead of taking preventive measures in cases where uncertainty exists, government inaction prevails unless there is actual proof of harm.

Many environmental researchers estimate that the carcinogens in our environment are responsible for about 50 percent of all cancers in the United States. However, the American Cancer Society estimates that only about 6 percent of cancers in this country are related to environmental causes. Their position is that environmental causes may be overestimated and confounded due to the population's exposure to so many chemicals, the lack of specific patient information, and the potential risk from medical-imaging radiation.

No definite link has been established between many of the chemicals proven to be carcinogenic to laboratory test animals and the actual development of cancer in humans. Despite this, it is advisable to avoid any chemical that is shown to have carcinogenic potential. However, you should recognize that carcinogenicity may not be related exclusively to the simple presence of any given chemical substance, but also to the amount (dosage) and duration of exposure and to the susceptibility of the individual to that chemical.

There are many more sources of possibly carcinogenic toxins that we encounter on a regular basis, both as the more typically perceived industrial waste and in forms as seemingly benign as how we cook our meat for dinner.

HOW TO AVOID TOXINS

Unfortunately, there are so many toxins in our environment and in our homes that it's almost impossible to avoid all of them. You can, however, limit your toxin exposure by becoming familiar with the names of toxins that should be avoided and by reading labels to avoid them when possible.

So what is there to be done to avoid toxins in your immediate environment as well as the wider environment?

THE ENVIRONMENT IN YOUR HOME

To mitigate some of the effects of pollution entering your home, follow the same protocols that many people with allergies follow, including these precautions.

Use a HEPA air filter, which traps fine particles of dust in the air. Dust surfaces and windowsills (by wiping down surfaces with a cloth, rather than just using a duster to move dust around), and mop, sweep, and vacuum floors frequently.

Remove shoes inside your home. This cuts down on the amount of sweeping and mopping you'll have to do, too!

Wash your hands after digging in your garden or digging in dirt. Make sure children wash their hands when they come inside after playing. The soil around many homes has large amounts of lead, especially if you have an older home. If you are concerned about your home in particular, you can have your soil tested for lead contamination.

Crack your windows. It's important to keep air circulating to ventilate your home.

Wash pets at least every few weeks. Their fur can trap contaminants.

Wash linens weekly.

Do the Detox

In addition to the microscopic contaminants that enter your home from the environment, there are many potentially toxic household products that you can avoid with a little thought. Detoxifying your home can be a freeing experience, and it will force you to go through all those cleaning supplies and lidless food storage containers once and for all!

GET RID OF YOUR EXISTING REUSABLE PLASTIC CONTAINERS AND UTENSILS. Replace them with BPA- and BPH-free plastic or containers made of ceramic or glass.

GET RID OF ALL CLEANING SUPPLIES MADE WITH INGREDIENTS THAT MIGHT BE CARCINOGENIC. Common toxic ingredients in household cleaners include chlorine bleach, ammonia, lye, diethanolamine (DEA) and triethanolamine (TEA), alkylphenol ethoxylates, butyl cellosolve, phosphates, petroleum, and chemical fragrances. Of course, it's not that easy to interpret the ingredients on a product bottle, so the Organic Consumers Association recommends this trick. Instead of looking at individual ingredients, look for the terms *Danger, Poison, Warning,* or *Caution.* Products with the words *Danger* or *Poison* are the most toxic. Products with the word *Warning* are moderately hazardous. And products noting *Caution* are slightly toxic.

Replace them with products that display none of these words. Most cleaning can be done with some basic, nontoxic supplies, including vinegar, liquid castile soap, and baking soda. You can also find cleaners free of toxins by shopping at a natural foods store. Ask a store clerk for guidance in picking the best product for your needs. Recent to the market are mops that use boiling water to clean and disinfect surfaces, avoiding toxic ingredients altogether.

GET RID OF NONSTICK POTS AND PANS, ESPECIALLY IF THEY ARE SCRATCHED OR DAMAGED. Nonstick pans contain perfluorinated chemicals or PFCs, which can be released—even if the pot or pan is brand-new—when heated to 500 degrees or higher. Perfluorinated chemicals have been shown in studies to likely be carcinogenic and cause a host of other health problems. Replace them with new stainless steel or cast-iron pots and pans.

CONSIDER GETTING RID OF WALL-TO-WALL CARPETS AND REPLACING THEM WITH HARDWOOD FLOORS AND AREA RUGS. Wall-to-wall carpets can release chemicals, or off-gas, for many years after purchase. If you're not in a position to get rid of your carpet, however, you can mitigate the effects of off-gassing by providing good ventilation in the rooms where you have carpets. Open windows and doors and turn on the fan whenever possible.

If possible, get rid of standard mattresses, which can also off-gas, and replace them with mattresses made of organic materials.

DO NOT USE VINYL SHOWER CURTAINS, WHICH CAN RELEASE CHEMICALS. Replace them with curtains made of EVA or PEVA plastic, nylon, cotton, or polyester. If you're not sure whether a curtain is vinyl, look for the number 3 or the letters PVC on the packaging. Another tell-tale sign of a PVC curtain is the distinctive new curtain smell.

GET RID OF PESTICIDES. Replace them with mouse or rat traps, and keep counters and floors clean of anything sweet or sticky to avoid ants. If you need something stronger, there are a few products on the market that have lower toxins.

GET RID OF FURNITURE TREATED WITH TRADITIONAL STAIN-RESISTANT PRODUCTS. These products have been shown to break down into PFCs. Instead, buy a couch made of fabric that is easy to clean, such as leather or hemp, and consider using a slipcover and pillows with covers so they can be slipped off and cleaned.

Personal Products and Toxins

SUNSCREEN: Peeling or blistering sunburns are associated with melanoma, the deadliest form of skin cancer. However, not all sunscreens protect against the most damaging rays, UVA, and some sunscreens may even be linked to cancer themselves.

According to the Environmental Working Group (EWG) and other experts, you should avoid sunscreens that only protect against UVB and contain oxybenzone and retinyl palmitate. Oxybenzone is a hormone disruptor that may be linked to cancer. Retinyl palmitate may have links to lesions and tumors. Also avoid spray, powder, and towelette suncreens—all three contain particulates that could be inhaled.

Instead, use a sunscreen that protects against UVA and UVB and is made with zinc oxide or titanium dioxide. These are mineral sunscreens, which are not absorbed into the skin in the same way chemical sunscreens are.

Sunscreen is something of a conundrum because while it is very important to protect the skin from serious sunburns, it is equally important for humans to have access to vitamin D on a daily basis, which decreases the risk of all cancers and many other diseases. Many doctors suggest using sunscreen for prolonged periods in the sun (like a midday trip to the beach or park) and relying on clothes to cover skin the rest of the time. Wearing a hat and long sleeves when out and about will likely provide you the best protection against sunburn while still allowing access to the benefits of the sun's rays on a daily basis.

COSMETICS: Some of the possibly cancer-causing agents found in cosmetics include petroleum, PEG compounds, siloxanes, parabens, phthalates, DEA-related ingredients, BHA, and BHT. Many of these are industrial chemicals with effects that range from being hormone disruptors to having heavy metal contaminants. Avoid cosmetics with fragrance and, when in doubt, stick to cosmetics you purchase from a natural foods store that you trust.

SHAMPOO/CONDITIONER AND BODY WASH: Sodium laureth sulfate, cocamide DEA, and glycol disteareate are different names for a foaming product made from coconut oil. Sounds innocuous, but according to the EWG, it's not. It's gone through an ethoxylation process that results in cancer-causing

1,4-dioxane. Instead, look for its safer cousin, also made from coconut oil, called sodium lauryl sulfate.

There are many nontoxic shampoos and conditioners available through natural foods stores. Also look for shampoo and body wash bottles that are BPA- and phthalate-free. This is especially important for baby shampoos and body washes.

PETROLEUM JELLY: Derived from a by-product of oil refining, petroleum jelly is used for everything from lip balm to diaper cream. Although it's derived from carcinogenic products, it's triple-refined and considered noncarcinogenic. However, many people who are detoxing their medicine cabinets opt to swap it out for one of the many nonpetroleum jellies on the market, most of which work just as well.

FEMININE PRODUCTS: Tampons and menstrual pads are generally made of bleached cotton or from cotton sprayed with chemicals. Both the chlorine used for the bleach and the pesticides used on the cotton may be carcinogenic. Instead, use unbleached, organic cotton pads and tampons found at natural foods stores. Avoid using plastic applicators, which may be made using phthalates.

LOTIONS: Avoid lotions made with fragrance, petroleum products, or parabens, a possible hormone disruptor. Instead use a fragrance-free, paraben-free lotion, easily available at natural foods stores, or a natural oil, such as olive oil or coconut oil.

TOOTHPASTE: Triclosan is an antibacterial that may lurk in some toothpastes and is under review by the FDA. It's been banned in some states and should be avoided. If you are avoiding commercial toothpastes, look for a natural toothpaste that is ADA-approved and includes fluoride.

ANTIPERSPIRANT/DEODORANT: Although there is no definitive link between antiperspirant and cancer, antiperspirants do often contain parabens and aluminum, which have some estrogen-like qualities. There are deodorants without parabens or aluminum available at natural foods stores.

DRY CLEANING: Conventional dry cleaning uses chemicals such as estrogenic nonylphenol and nonylphenol ethoxylates (NPEs), which are potentially hormone disruptors. Perchloroethylene (also called tetrachloroethylene or PERC) is classified as "likely carcinogenic." Avoid these dry-cleaning products by buying clothes that do not require dry cleaning or by using a dry cleaner who utilizes nontoxic alternatives (although be aware that there are levels of nontoxicity in the industry, and you should research individual dry cleaners before assuming "organic" or "natural" cleaners are what they claim to be). If you do use a conventional dry cleaner, always air out clothes for at least 4 hours before wearing them.

Toxins from Electronics

Electromagnetic fields (EMFs) are a new area of concern. An electromagnetic field is the physical field created by an electronic device. The question as to whether EMFs are harmful, particularly those around microwaves and cell phones, continues to be disputed, but there is growing evidence and concern stemming from strong scientific data. Two Swedish studies, published together in 2014, showed an association between brain tumors and cell phones.[1]

To be on the safe side, we suggest limiting your exposure to these potentially harmful energies. Cell phones should be shut off when not in use, should be carried away from the body, and should always be used in the speakerphone mode or with wireless earphones (not Bluetooth next to your ear). Practice prudent avoidance in general, by doing the following:

- Locate your microwave oven away from areas where people congregate—in a hallway or pantry, if possible.
- Do not use your lap as a "desk" for your laptop computer.
- Do not sit directly under or beside a compact fluorescent light bulb.
- Be aware that electrical appliances and wires emit EMFs, which for the most part drop off in intensity within about 12 inches, making it not too difficult to avoid exposure.

Other Environmental Toxins

Radon is a naturally occurring radioactive gas found in the cellars of both older and recently built stone homes. It is a known carcinogen, thought to be second only to smoking in causing lung cancer. Hire a licensed professional to inspect your home for radon if your home has not been inspected previously. Radon is often concentrated in the cellar or attic, and a simple ventilation system can usually rectify the problem.

Dioxins, which have been called the most lethal compounds ever created by man, are related to the PCBs once used in plastic but banned in the United States since 1979. Dioxins cause cancer, liver disease, and hormonal disruption of the reproductive systems, retarding normal development. However, Rolf Halden, PhD, with the Department of Environmental Health Sciences and the Center for Water and Health at the Johns Hopkins Bloomberg School of Public Health, states unequivocally that there are no dioxins in plastics themselves, but that dioxins are created by the incineration of plastics. Hospital waste products contain large quantities of polyvinyl chloride and other dioxin precursors like aromatic organic chemicals. When these are incinerated, they release large amounts of dioxin. Most industrial incinerators have state-of-the-art emission controls that minimize this pollution.

There are other activities that release dioxins as well. Backyard burning of trash can release dioxin into the air. The toxin rises up and attaches to small particles in the atmosphere, which are eventually precipitated into our waters and land. The dioxin is subsequently concentrated and stored in the fatty tissue of animals of all types. People who eat fat-rich fish or meat then become the unknowing recipients of this toxic chemical.

TOXINS IN YOUR FOOD

In addition to the environmental toxins outside and inside our homes, we are also exposed to toxins through the things we ingest. Even the most healthful of foods—fruits and vegetables—may be exposing us to high levels of toxins through the use of pesticides in their growth.

Fatty meat products can contain organic chlorine contaminants. Imported vegetables can be tainted with DDT and arsenic, both of which are banned from use as pesticides in the United States but are still used in China, Argentina, and Chile—countries we import food from. These are known cancer-causing agents with a disturbing staying power. DDT has been banned here since 1972, but tests of women's breast tissues continue to show evidence of the presence of DDT.

Excessive amounts of phosphates in our diet may activate genetic pathways that stimulate the development of lung cancer. These additives, used to improve food texture and soften water, can be found in processed pork products, cheeses, pastries, and almost all sodas, including colas and sparkling sweet drinks. Phosphates are particularly used in frozen meals, including pizza and fish sticks, and in food prepared with evaporated milk, including processed ice cream.

Naturally occurring carcinogens are even found in some food plants, not to mention the residue of pesticides still on produce even after it reaches the store. Tannins—found in red wine, tea, coffee, and cocoa—have been shown to cause liver tumors in lab animals and may be linked to esophageal cancers in humans. Another category of toxins includes those synthesized as a product or by-product of the human body. Alcohol, tobacco, excessive radiation, ultraviolet exposure from sunlight, and sexually transmitted diseases all are examples of such naturally occurring carcinogenic exposures.

Additionally, there are the toxins that are inhaled, absorbed, or ingested and which are often found in nature, including mercury, lead, and arsenic. Mercury is a prevalent toxin in the modern world, with 50 percent of all mercury in the environment released from coal burned to generate electricity. Mercury in coal smoke escapes into the atmosphere, where it is "washed out" of the air by rain. With time, it is carried into our streams, rivers, and oceans. There, fish incorporate this toxin into their tissue, and it is very difficult for them to eliminate it from their bodies. As the larger fish eat smaller fish, the mercury continues to build up in the larger fish through a process called bioaccumulation.

The result of this toxic food chain is the concentration of dangerously high amounts of mercury in older, larger fish such as swordfish, tuna, sturgeon, and shark. You should avoid all of these at the grocery store and at your favorite restaurant. Instead, choose smaller cold-water fish such as herring, salmon, smelt, and sardines, as well as sole and sanddabs, because they have had less time to accumulate large amounts of mercury into their tissue. (And always buy wild rather than farmed fish.)

Foods stored or packaged in plastics made with bisphenol A, or BPA, have been linked to breast and prostate cancer, among other health problems. Because of this, there are growing concerns about the use of BPAs in food storage. It is a known hormone disruptor but is also potentially carcinogenic. In the President's Cancer Panel Annual Report for 2008–2009, LaSalle Leffall Jr. and Margaret Kripke, two members of the panel, wrote: "With nearly 80,000 chemicals on the market in the United States, many of which are used by millions of Americans in their daily lives and are un- or understudied and largely unregulated, exposure to potential environmental carcinogens is widespread. One such ubiquitous chemical, bisphenol A (BPA), is still found in many consumer products and remains unregulated in the United States, despite the growing link between BPA and several diseases, including various cancers."[2]

It is used in the production of plastic bottles and the linings of tin cans. The chemicals can leach into the contents of the container over time, especially if the containers are kept in a heated or sunlit room. To be safe, avoid food and beverages from tin cans and plastic bottles, and always store water and foods in glass, ceramic, or stainless steel containers.

Sources of carcinogenic risk have also been found in food preparation itself. Frying or otherwise overheating starchy carbohydrates, such as when making french fries and potato chips, generates a known carcinogen called acrylamide. Its effects and potential risks to human health continue to be studied. Barbecuing meat on an open fire creates polycyclic hydrocarbons like those found in cigarette smoke. At least 20 chemicals that are by-products of frying and broiling food can increase the risk of prostate, pancreatic, breast, and colon cancers.

GO ORGANIC

In order to avoid ingesting these toxins, we suggest everyone, but especially those who have had cancer, avoid eating conventionally grown produce and opt for organic-grown produce instead. However, because price and availability may make this challenging, we suggest at least avoiding the produce with the highest traces of pesticides.

Although an apple a day is purported to keep the doctor away, this may not be true, depending on many factors in the apple's life. Every year the nonprofit advocacy organization EWG releases a list of the 12 most pesticide-laden fruits and vegetables on the market. Unfortunately, the mythic apple turns up again and again because of the heavy use of pesticides in its agriculture.

Every year since 2000, EWG researchers have studied nearly four dozen popular fruits and vegetables chosen on the basis of pesticide-load reports from the USDA and Food and Drug Administration. The database includes 60,700 samples taken over a 10-year period. It's important to note that all of the testing was conducted on fruits and vegetables that had been washed and/or peeled—the typical precautions taken by American consumers.

Some information is not included in the basic list. For example, while apples were ranked as the most contaminated overall, imported nectarines had a shocking 100 percent rate of positive pesticide test results, more than any other product. Bell peppers and grapes were contaminated with 15 different pesticides in a single sample—the highest overall diversity of contamination.

The EWG labels the 12 most contaminated products the Dirty Dozen. These fruits and vegetables are so contaminated with pesticides that you should not eat them when they are grown conventionally. On the positive side, there is an opposite end of the spectrum in what the EWG calls the Clean 15. These are the 15 least contaminated fruits and vegetables. They can be safely eaten even when conventionally grown and are good options when organically grown produce is not available.

THE DIRTY DOZEN

Apples	Nectarines	Potatoes
Celery	Grapes (imported)	Blueberries
Strawberries		Lettuce
Peaches	Sweet bell peppers	Kale
Spinach		

THE CLEAN 15

Onions	Asparagus	Sweet potatoes
Sweet corn	Mangoes	Grapefruit
Pineapples	Eggplant	Watermelon
Avocado	Kiwi	Mushrooms
Cabbage	Cantaloupe (domestic)	
Sweet peas		

The Dirty Dozen include some of the most healthful fruits and vegetables available, with life-preserving nutrients, so you shouldn't eliminate them from your diet. The solution is to generally eat organically grown vegetables and fruits, to limit one's exposure to pesticides overall.

It is more important to buy the Dirty Dozen in organic form than to buy the Clean 15 in organic form. All 15 of these products are relatively free of pesticides even when conventionally grown.

In general, however, we advise that you buy and consume organic produce whenever you can. If you cannot obtain organically grown versions of these fruits and vegetables, you do still have some options to include them in your diet. Peppers, squash, and cucumbers are sold covered with pesticide-impregnated wax. To eliminate pesticides from these vegetables, scrub or peel off this wax.

Toxins and Meat

The use of artificial growth hormones is becoming an increasing concern when it comes to our health and the food we eat. Beef cattle, dairy cows, and sheep are treated with artificial hormones to promote growth, and studies have shown an increased risk of breast, prostate, and colorectal cancer associated with higher levels of IGF-1 (insulin-like growth factor 1). The hormone rBGH (recombinant bovine growth hormone, also known as recombinant bovine somatotropin or rBST) is often used in dairy cows and causes increased IGF-1 levels in the milk of those cows. The European Union has banned the use of these growth hormones due to their possible health effects (including cancer). And while the United States banned the use of the hormones in pork products, they are still commonly used in beef and dairy products. Increasing numbers of dairy producers are phasing out the use of growth hormones in their products, so look for the rBST- or rBGH-free notation on the label.

Conventionally grown meat is also a concern because of the use of prophylactic antibiotics, which is necessary due to the crowded conditions in which factory-farmed cattle and chicken are grown. They are also fed an inadequate grain diet, derived from grains that have generally been treated heavily with pesticides that concentrate in the animals and pass to the person who eventually eats them. Author Michael Pollan does an excellent job of walking through the ramifications of our factory-farming lifestyle in his book *The Omnivore's Dilemma*.

We recommend that you avoid eating red meat and pork altogether and eat only organic chicken and wild fish once or twice per week. If you choose to eat meat, buy and eat only organic beef and pork. Even better, buy your meat directly from a small farmer whose practices you can see for yourself or from a small butcher who is familiar with the farms where the meat is sourced. It is true that organic and local meats will cost you more. However, by limiting the amount of meat you eat and eating mostly plant-based foods, you may well save on your weekly grocery bill.

Toxins and Water

It is best to filter the water coming into your home or workplace to remove many such potentially harmful elements, as well as any bacteria or residual pharmaceutical medications that may have contaminated your water supply. You can use either carbon filters that are attached to the tap or in a pitcher, or a reverse osmosis filter.

Avoid water bottled in plastic containers, especially if they may have been exposed to heat and light, and do not reuse single-use plastic bottles as they can leach contaminants. Filtering your own water is a far better option than bottled water, both for your health and the health of the planet.

QUICK CHECK

Below is a quick list of ways to reduce the toxins in your environment.

- Filter your tap water and then store it in stainless steel, glass, or ceramic containers to avoid exposure to BPA or other plastic components.
- Avoid produce grown with chemical fertilizers or pesticides, and wash all produce thoroughly before eating.
- Buy meat, chicken, fish, and dairy that is free of hormones and antibiotics.
- Buy organic vegetables and fruit.
- Avoid processed, charred, or well-done meat.
- Do not use plastic containers to heat food in your microwave.
- Reduce exposure to cell phones.
- Go organic in caring for your home and garden.
- Check your home's radon level.
- Use nontoxic personal products.
- Use BPA-free or glass storage containers.
- Throw out nonstick cookware.
- Do not use conventional dry cleaners, and avoid wall-to-wall carpeting and stain-proof furniture.

CHAPTER EIGHT

CANCER PROTOCOLS

THE RECOMMENDATIONS WE'VE OUTLINED UP TO THIS POINT ARE APPLICABLE AND beneficial to any patient with a cancer diagnosis. In this chapter, however, we will summarize the available evidence regarding lifestyle modifications and their specific impact on some of the most common cancers.

Breast cancer	Bladder cancer	Lymphoma
Colon cancer	Endometrial cancer	Melanoma
Lung cancer		Renal cancer
Prostate cancer	Leukemia	Thyroid cancer

Although we have mentioned the word *cancer* throughout this book as some monolithic entity, it is in fact a myriad of different diseases wreaking havoc on various parts of the body, with vastly different growth patterns and biologic stimuli. Lending further support to the theory that each cancer has its own unique set of molecular and biologic underpinnings is the fact that while certain medications work wonders for some cancers, they may do absolutely nothing for others. Along those lines, we should also give credence to the notion that there are certain nutritional and supplemental approaches that may work specifically for certain cancers; perhaps surprisingly, a reasonable body of scientific literature now supports this.

We must also remember that even within each type of cancer, many different subtypes may behave quite differently from one another. For example, we know that breast cancer is often fueled by estrogen (the primary female hormone) and prostate cancer by testosterone (the male hormone), respectively. However, some breast and prostate cancers have figured out how to grow in an environment completely independent of hormones.

BREAST CANCER
Breast Cancer Basics

- Nearly 230,000 new cases of breast cancer, most of which were in women, were diagnosed in 2012, with a total of nearly 40,000 deaths from the disease.[1]
- Aside from skin cancer, it is the most commonly diagnosed cancer and the second leading cause of cancer death among women.
- Both the occurrence and death due to breast cancer have declined somewhat in recent years, largely due to a decline in hormone replacement therapy (HRT) use among postmenopausal women.
- Breast cancer is significantly influenced by dietary and lifestyle factors, in part evidenced by the nearly threefold higher occurrence in developed countries compared to underdeveloped ones.[2]

Causes/Contributing Factors

A number of risk factors are known to be associated with breast cancer occurrence, and the risk factors for younger women are not necessarily the same for women over 40.

Among the most well-established risk factors include:

- A history of cancer in your family, particularly a first-degree relative
- Dense breast tissue

Risk factors for younger women also include:

- Not having a child until after age 35
- Having a prior breast biopsy[3]

Other known risk factors include:

- Alcohol intake
- Smoking
- Higher amounts of dietary fat

- Obesity in postmenopausal women
- Early menarche, late menopause
- Night-shift work

Relevant Diagnostic Testing

- **MAMMOGRAPHY:** Screening by mammography is recommended by a number of cancer organizations. The U.S. Preventive Services Task Force recommends individualized, informed decision making about when to start mammography.
- **PHYSICAL EXAMS, IMAGING PROCEDURES, LABORATORY TESTS, PATHOLOGY REPORTS, AND SURGICAL REPORTS** provide information to determine the stage of a cancer.
- **GENOMIC EVALUATION:** Genomic evaluation of your tumor may be recommended, as a number of genetic mutations have been associated with prognosis (outlook) and help to predict how beneficial different treatments may be.
- **VITAMIN D LEVEL:** Vitamin D levels have been found to be predictive of breast cancer risk and higher-grade tumors.[4,5]

CANCER STAGING

Staging is the process of finding out how much cancer there is in a person's body and where it's located. It's how the doctor learns the stage of a person's cancer and allows them to develop a treatment plan specific to that situation. The higher that stage, the greater the burden of cancer that exists in that patient.

Most cancers are staged into four or five groups (stages 0, I, II, III, and IV) with the T, N, M system. T describes size and characteristics of the primary tumor, N describes lymph node involvement, and M describes metastases. Most cancer staging systems use stage IV to indicate the presence of metastases.

BREAST CANCER STAGING SYSTEM

- **Stage 0 (TIS, N0, M0):** This is *ductal carcinoma in situ* (DCIS), but it is not cancer or precancer. Its presence, however, is a marker for increased future breast cancer risk. Many consider DCIS the earliest form of breast cancer. In DCIS, cancer cells are still within a duct and have not invaded deeper into the surrounding fatty breast tissue. *Lobular carcinoma in situ* is sometimes also classified as stage 0 breast cancer. Paget disease of the nipple (without an underlying tumor mass) is also stage 0. In all cases, the cancer has not spread to the lymph nodes or to distant sites.
- **Stage IA (T1, N0, M0):** The tumor is 2 cm or less across (T1) and has not spread to lymph nodes (N0) or distant sites (M0).

- **Stage IB (T0 or T1, N1MI, M0):** The tumor is 2 cm or less across or is not found (T0 or T1), with micrometastases in one to three axillary lymph nodes. The cancer in the lymph nodes is greater than 0.2 mm across and/or more than 200 cells but is not larger than 2 mm (N1mi). The cancer has not spread to distant sites (M0).

- **Stage IIA:** One of the following applies:
  - » **T0 or T1, N1 (but not N1MI), M0:** The tumor is 2 cm or less across or is not found (T1 or T0) and either:
    - It has spread to one to three axillary lymph nodes, with the cancer in the lymph nodes larger than 2 mm across (N1a); or
    - Tiny amounts of cancer are found in the internal mammary lymph nodes on a sentinel lymph node biopsy (N1b); or
    - It has spread to one to three lymph nodes under the arm and to the internal mammary lymph nodes, found on a sentinel lymph node biopsy (N1c).

    OR

    - **T2, N0, M0:** The tumor is larger than 2 cm but less than 5 cm across (T2) but hasn't spread to the lymph nodes (N0).
    - The cancer hasn't spread to distant sites (M0).

- **Stage IIB:** One of the following applies:
  - » **T2, N1, M0:** The tumor is larger than 2 cm but less than 5 cm across (T2). It has spread to one to three axillary lymph nodes and/or tiny amounts of cancer are found in the internal mammary lymph nodes on a sentinel lymph node biopsy (N1). The cancer hasn't spread to distant sites (M0).

    OR

  - » **T3, N0, M0:** The tumor is larger than 5 cm across but does not grow into the chest wall or skin and has not spread to lymph nodes (T3, N0). The cancer hasn't spread to distant sites (M0).

- **Stage IIIA:** One of the following applies:
  - » **T0 to T2, N2, M0:** The tumor is not more than 5 cm across or cannot be found (T0 to T2). It has spread to four to nine axillary lymph nodes, or it has enlarged the internal mammary lymph nodes (N2). The cancer hasn't spread to distant sites (M0).

    OR

  - » **T3, N1 or N2, M0:** The tumor is larger than 5 cm across but does not grow into the chest wall or skin (T3). It has spread to one to nine axillary nodes or to the internal mammary nodes (N1 or N2). The cancer hasn't spread to distant sites (M0).

- **Stage IIIB (T4, N0 to N2, M0):** The tumor has grown into the chest wall or skin (T4), and one of the following applies:
  » It has not spread to the lymph nodes (N0).
  » It has spread to one to three axillary lymph nodes, and/or tiny amounts of cancer are found in the internal mammary lymph nodes on a sentinel lymph node biopsy (N1).
  » It has spread to four to nine axillary lymph nodes, or it has enlarged the internal mammary lymph nodes (N2).
  » The cancer hasn't spread to distant sites (M0).
  Inflammatory breast cancer is classified as T4d and is at least stage IIIB. If it has spread to many nearby lymph nodes (N3), it could be stage IIIC; if it has spread to distant lymph nodes or organs (M1), it would be stage IV.
- **Stage IIIC (any T, N3, M0):** The tumor is any size (or can't be found), and one of the following applies:
  » Cancer has spread to 10 or more axillary lymph nodes (N3).
  » Cancer has spread to the lymph nodes under the clavicle, or collarbone (N3).
  » Cancer has spread to the lymph nodes above the clavicle (N3).
  » Cancer involves axillary lymph nodes and has enlarged the internal mammary lymph nodes (N3).
  » Cancer has spread to four or more axillary lymph nodes, and tiny amounts of cancer are found in the internal mammary lymph nodes on a sentinel lymph node biopsy (N3).
  » The cancer hasn't spread to distant sites (M0).
- **Stage IV (any T, any N, M1):** The cancer can be any size (any T) and may or may not have spread to nearby lymph nodes (any N). It has spread to distant organs or to lymph nodes far from the breast (M1). The most common sites of spread are the bone, liver, brain, or lung.

Breast Cancer Supplement Program

Multiple nutritional supplements have been associated with reduced cancer occurrence and/or cancer progression. The list below contains those with the greatest evidence base and benefit, though it is not necessary that they all be included.

VITAMIN D
SUGGESTED DOSE: May require 5,000 IU per day or more, depending on blood levels

Vitamin D levels are associated with both the risk of breast cancer and the risk of dying from it. The suggested dose is sufficient to raise 25-OH vitamin D levels to >40 ng/mL and optimally between 50 and 80 ng/mL.[6]

OMEGA-3 FATTY ACIDS

SUGGESTED DOSE: 2–3 g combined EPA and DHA per day, with at least 1–2 g of a GLA source

Omega-3 fatty acids, DHA and EPA, have been shown to exert numerous antiproliferative effects on breast cancer cells, as well as reduce inflammation and fatigue among breast cancer survivors.[7] DHA and EPA have also demonstrated protective effects when combined with several chemotherapeutic agents.[8] Additionally, GLA, another omega-3, helps to maintain balance in the fatty acids and enhances the anti-inflammatory effect.[9, 10]

ISOTHIOCYANATES AND DIM (3,3'-DIINDOLYLMETHANE)

SUGGESTED DOSE: DIM 250 mg, isothiocyanates 600 mcg per day

Isothiocyanates, which are abundant in cruciferous vegetables like broccoli, cauliflower, and cabbage, have shown antitumor activity. DIM (3,3'-Diindolylmethane), a metabolite of indole-3-carbinol, one of the isothiocyanates, inhibits cancer cell proliferation in estrogen-receptor positive and negative cells. DIM also modulates estrogen metabolism, as reflected by a change in urinary estrogen metabolite profiles to those associated with lower cancer risk among cancer survivors.[11, 12, 13]

SCUTELLARIA BARBATA

SUGGESTED DOSE: 1–2 g per day

Scutellaria barbata is an herb that grows in Korea and southern China. An extract of this plant has been shown to be safe in a clinical trial of women with advanced breast cancer; it inhibits cell proliferation and induces cancer cell death.[14, 15]

CURCUMIN

SUGGESTED DOSE: 1–2 g per day of Meriva or Longvida curcumin

The active extract from the spice turmeric, curcumin displays an ability to inhibit many tumor cell types and also may sensitize cancer cells to other therapies.[16] Recently it was combined with docetaxel, a commonly used chemotherapy medication, in patients with advanced and metastatic breast cancer with encouraging results.[17] Doses range depending on the type of curcumin, yet Meriva and Longvida have been shown to be much more efficiently absorbed forms.[18, 19]

GREEN TEA EXTRACT

SUGGESTED DOSE: 1 g EGCG and mixed catechins per day

Catechins, antioxidants that are found in green tea, particularly EGCG (epigallocatechin-3-gallate), are known to have numerous antimetastatic and antiproliferative properties. Also, clinical trials suggest EGCG may enhance other therapies.[20, 21]

RESVERATROL
SUGGESTED DOSE: 100–200 mg per day

Found in red wine and grapes, this antioxidant has been shown to influence the methylation of genes in women at high breast cancer risk, and to reduce the toxicity of radiation therapy.[22, 23]

MILK THISTLE
SUGGESTED DOSE: At least 500 mg silymarin per day

Silymarin and silibinin from milk thistle have antiproliferative and antimetastatic properties, and may enhance the effectiveness of other therapies.[24, 25]

QUERCETIN
SUGGESTED DOSE: 200–400 mg three times per day

This antioxidant has multiple mechanisms by which it inhibits breast cancer proliferation and induces apoptosis (programmed cell death), and alters the metabolism of estrogen to less toxic compounds.[26, 27] It may be particularly beneficial for HER2/neu-positive cancer.[28]

GRAPE SEED EXTRACT AND/OR PYCNOGENOL
SUGGESTED DOSE: 100–200 mg per day

Grape seed extract has been shown to inhibit breast cell carcinogenesis in response to several common toxins, and to inhibit the enzyme aromatase, a factor in hormone-sensitive cancers.[29, 30]

MELATONIN
SUGGESTED DOSE: At least 3 mg at night, preferably time-released

Intake of supplemental melatonin, a hormone, has improved survival in a number of cancers and may enhance conventional therapy effectiveness.[31] In clinical trials, up to 20 mg has been used.

VITAMIN E
SUGGESTED DOSE: 200–400 IU per day of mixed tocopherols and tocotrienols

Various components of vitamin E have shown anticancer properties. Although alpha-tocopherol is often used in clinical trials, when given alone it may deplete other important components of vitamin E.[32, 33]

VITAMIN K$_2$
SUGGESTED DOSE: 100 mcg vitamin K$_2$ (MK-7)

Vitamin K$_2$ (MK-7) has the longest half-life, meaning it is the most stable, of all forms of vitamin K. Shown to improve bone and cardiovascular health, higher intakes of this form have also been associated with reduced cancer incidence and death, and may improve effectiveness of other therapies.[34, 35, 36]

Dietary Action Plan

EMPHASIZE

- Brightly colored fresh vegetables, leafy greens, and fresh fruits; choose organic if possible
- Cruciferous vegetables, such as broccoli, cauliflower, and cabbage
- Whole foods (foods that are as close to their natural form as possible)
- Low sugar/low glycemic diet; glycemic index and glycemic load are measures of the effect on blood glucose level after a food containing carbohydrates is consumed
- Omega-3 fatty acids, found in cold-water fish such as sardines, wild-caught salmon, cod, mackerel, and tuna
- High fiber, from whole grains, beans, vegetables, and fruits
- Healthy fats, from avocados, nuts, seeds, olive oil, coconut oil, and cold-water fish
- For animal protein, choose lean poultry and fish over red meat, and aim to view meat as a condiment rather than a staple. Try to choose grass-fed and organic meats and eggs whenever possible. Eat no fish larger than a salmon to minimize environmental contaminants, including mercury.

AVOID

- Processed and grilled meats; try to limit intake of red meat
- Fast foods, fried foods, baked goods, and packaged, processed foods
- Sugar, sweeteners, and artificial sweeteners
- Vegetable oils, shortening, margarine, and anything with hydrogenated or partially hydrogenated oils

Top 5 Lifestyle Interventions

1. Maintain a healthy weight.[37]
2. Most studies suggest physical activity lowers breast cancer mortality.[38]
3. Avoid alcohol and smoking.
4. Consume a vegetable-rich, Mediterranean-style diet, emphasizing whole foods and cruciferous vegetables (such as broccoli, cauliflower, kale, and Brussels sprouts).[39]

5. Practice mindfulness-based stress reduction, like breathing techniques, yoga, Pilates, and meditation.[40]

Important Nutrient/Drug Interactions

Given that many nutritional interventions have the potential to both increase the effectiveness of conventional treatments and possibly interfere with their effects, combined use should always be supervised. For example, DHEA, an adrenal hormone that can be metabolized into many other hormones including estrogen, may also interfere with the effectiveness of chemotherapy, particularly for estrogen receptor positive cancers.[41] Doses higher than 50 mcg of vitamin K_2 (MK-7) may interfere with some anticoagulant medications.[42]

COLON CANCER
Colorectal Cancer Basics

- Nearly 150,000 people were diagnosed with colorectal cancer in the United States in 2008, the most recent year we have data for, with roughly 50,000 deaths attributed to this disease.[43]

- It is the second leading cause of cancer death among cancers that affect both men and women, although it is thought to be largely preventable, with rates tenfold higher reported in Western countries.[44]

- One study of nearly 50,000 men found that more than 70 percent of colorectal cancer incidence could be prevented by diet, physical activity, and specific health behaviors such as refraining from smoking.[45]

- Nearly all colorectal cancers are adenocarcinomas, with the great majority arising from an adenomatous polyp.[46] Recently, six lifestyle factors were found to cumulatively increase the risk for adenomas: cigarette smoking, obesity, aspirin use, high intake of red meat, low intake of fiber, and low intake of calcium. This provides strong evidence that lifestyle modification is important for the prevention of colorectal polyps, especially advanced and multiple adenomas, which are established precursors of colorectal cancer.[47]

Causes/Contributing Factors

- Colorectal cancer occurs more commonly in those over age 50, men, and individuals of African American descent, and those with a family history of colorectal cancer or a personal history of polyps, inflammatory bowel disease, or low socioeconomic status.[48]

- Smoking increases the risk for colorectal cancer for as long as 25 years after quitting, although having a normal body mass index (BMI) and having high fruit consumption mitigate this risk to a small degree.[49]

- Other dietary factors associated with risk include consumption of animal foods, particularly a high intake of red and processed meat and a low intake of fiber and calcium.[50]

- Obesity increases the risk of colorectal cancer.

- Alcohol and an elevated BMI are also risk factors, while physical activity has a dose-dependent benefit for reducing risk.[51, 52, 53]

Relevant Diagnostic Testing

- A number of screening tests for colorectal cancer are available and require a physician's guidance to determine the most appropriate. A colonoscopy, for example, is the most likely to find polyps or cancer, but there is a small risk of complications such as bowel tears or infection.

- Several tumor markers may be used to monitor progress or guide treatment decisions, including carcinoembryonic antigen (CEA) and tissue polypeptide antigen (TPA).

- Low vitamin D levels have been associated with the risk of developing colorectal cancer, as well as both overall and colorectal cancer specific mortality.[54, 55]

CANCER STAGING

Staging is the process of finding out how much cancer there is in a person's body and where it's located. It's how the doctor learns the stage of a person's cancer.

Most cancers are staged into four or five groups (stages 0, I, II, III, and IV) with the T, N, M system. T describes size and characteristics of the primary tumor, N describes lymph node involvement, and M describes metastases. Most cancer staging systems use stage IV to indicate the presence of metastases.

COLORECTAL CANCER STAGING SYSTEM

- **Stage 0 (TIS, N0, M0):** The cancer is in the earliest stage. It has not grown beyond the inner layer (mucosa) of the colon or rectum. This stage is also known as carcinoma in situ or intramucosal carcinoma.

- **Stage I (T1-T2, N0, M0):** The cancer has grown through the muscularis mucosa into the submucosa (T1), or it may also have grown into the muscularis propria (T2). It has not spread to nearby lymph nodes or distant sites.

- **Stage IIA (T3, N0, M0):** The cancer has grown into the outermost layers of the colon or rectum but has not gone through them (T3). It has not reached nearby organs. It has not yet spread to the nearby lymph nodes or distant sites.

• **Stage IIB (T4A, N0, M0):** The cancer has grown through the wall of the colon or rectum but has not grown into other nearby tissues or organs (T4a). It has not yet spread to the nearby lymph nodes or distant sites.

• **Stage IIC (T4B, N0, M0):** The cancer has grown through the wall of the colon or rectum and is attached to or has grown into other nearby tissues or organs (T4b). It has not yet spread to the nearby lymph nodes or distant sites.

• **Stage IIIA:** One of the following applies:

   » **T1-T2, N1, M0:** The cancer has grown through the mucosa into the submucosa (T1), and it may also have grown into the muscularis propria (T2). It has spread to one to three nearby lymph nodes (N1a/N1b) or into areas of fat near the lymph nodes but not the nodes themselves (N1c). It has not spread to distant sites.

   OR:

   » **T1, N2A, M0:** The cancer has grown through the mucosa into the submucosa (T1). It has spread to four to six nearby lymph nodes (N2a). It has not spread to distant sites.

• **Stage IIIB:** One of the following applies:

   » **T3-T4A, N1, M0:** The cancer has grown into the outermost layers of the colon or rectum (T3) or through the visceral peritoneum (T4a), but has not reached nearby organs. It has spread to one to three nearby lymph nodes (N1a/N1b) or into areas of fat near the lymph nodes but not the nodes themselves (N1c). It has not spread to distant sites.

   OR

   » **T2-T3, N2A, M0:** The cancer has grown into the muscularis propria (T2) or into the outermost layers of the colon or rectum (T3). It has spread to four to six nearby lymph nodes (N2a). It has not spread to distant sites.

   OR

   » **T1-T2, N2B, M0:** The cancer has grown through the mucosa into the submucosa (T1), or it may also have grown into the muscularis propria (T2). It has spread to seven or more nearby lymph nodes (N2b). It has not spread to distant sites.

• **Stage IIIC:** One of the following applies:

   » **T4A, N2A, M0:** The cancer has grown through the wall of the colon or rectum (including the visceral peritoneum) but has not reached nearby organs (T4a). It has spread to four to six nearby lymph nodes (N2a). It has not spread to distant sites.

   » **T3-T4A, N2B, M0:** The cancer has grown into the outermost layers of the colon or rectum (T3) or through the visceral peritoneum (T4a) but has not reached nearby organs. It has spread to seven or more nearby lymph nodes (N2b). It has not spread to distant sites.

» **T4B, N1-N2, M0**: The cancer has grown through the wall of the colon or rectum, and is attached to or has grown into other nearby tissues or organs (T4b). It has spread to at least one nearby lymph node or into areas of fat near the lymph nodes (N1 or N2). It has not spread to distant sites.

• **Stage IVA (ANY T, ANY N, M1A)**: The cancer may or may not have grown through the wall of the colon or rectum, and it may or may not have spread to nearby lymph nodes. It has spread to one distant organ (such as the liver or lung) or set of lymph nodes (M1a).

• **Stage IVB (ANY T, ANY N, M1B)**: The cancer may or may not have grown through the wall of the colon or rectum, and it may or may not have spread to nearby lymph nodes. It has spread to more than one distant organ (such as the liver or lung) or set of lymph nodes, or it has spread to distant parts of the peritoneum, or the lining of the abdominal cavity (M1b).

Colorectal Cancer Supplement Program

Multiple nutritional supplements have been associated with reduced cancer incidence and/or cancer progression. The list below contains those with the greatest evidence base and benefit, though it is not necessary that they all be included.

VITAMIN D
SUGGESTED DOSE: May require 5,000 IU per day or more, depending on blood levels

Vitamin D levels have been associated with both the incidence of colorectal cancer as well as overall mortality. The suggested dose is sufficient to raise 25-OH vitamin D levels to >40 ng/mL and optimally between 50 and 80 ng/mL.[56]

CURCUMIN
SUGGESTED DOSE: 1–2 g per day of Meriva or Longvida curcumin

Extracted from the spice turmeric, curcumin has been shown to arrest cancer cell growth, induce programmed cell death (apoptosis), and increase the efficacy of chemotherapy for treatment-resistant colorectal cancer cells.[57] While trials of curcumin suggest at least 4 g per day may be more beneficial than lower doses,[58] Meriva and Longvida curcumin have been shown to be much more efficiently absorbed forms.[59, 60]

GREEN TEA EXTRACT
SUGGESTED DOSE: 1 g EGCG and mixed catechins per day

EGCG (epigallocatechin-3-gallate) from green tea has multiple anticancer mechanisms of action, is associated with a reduced incidence of colorectal cancer, and has been shown to reduce the incidence of adenoma formation in patients who have had them previously removed.[61, 62]

RESVERATROL
SUGGESTED DOSE: 500–1,000 mg per day

This antioxidant interferes with all stages of cancer development, and its low bioavailability may make it more suitable for colorectal cancer.[63] When given to patients with colorectal cancer at a dose of 500 to 1,000 mg per day, it reduced tumor proliferation.[64]

GRAPE SEED EXTRACT AND/OR PYCNOGENOL
SUGGESTED DOSE: 100–200 mg per day

Grape seed extract inhibits the growth of cancer cells through several mechanisms and may have synergistic benefit when used with resveratrol.[65, 66]

PROBIOTICS
SUGGESTED DOSE: 1 capsule two times per day, at least 25 billion CFU/capsule

While probiotic therapy for colorectal cancer treatment is not well established, microbiota are thought to influence multiple pathways by which cancer develops and progresses. Additionally, presurgery supplementation has been shown to improve outcomes and reduce treatment side effects.[67]

OMEGA-3 FATTY ACIDS
SUGGESTED DOSE: 1–2 g combined EPA and DHA per day, with at least 1–2 g of a GLA source

The omega-3 fatty acids DHA and EPA have broad health benefits, such as reducing the oxidative stress and inflammation thought to influence colorectal cancer progression and recurrence.[68] Current evidence suggests several grams of these fatty acids improve nutritional status and potentially the effectiveness of other cancer therapies.[69] Additionally, GLA, another omega-3, helps to maintain balance in the fatty acids and enhances the anti-inflammatory effect.[70, 71]

DIM (3,3′-DIINDOLYLMETHANE)
SUGGESTED DOSE: 250 mg per day

Extracted from cruciferous vegetables such as broccoli, cauliflower, and cabbage, DIM has been shown to target several mechanisms by which colorectal cancer cells are resistant to apoptosis (programmed cell death).[72, 73]

QUERCETIN
SUGGESTED DOSE: 200–400 mg three times per day

Dietary consumption of this flavonoid is associated with a reduced risk of colorectal cancer, as well as in vitro induction of apoptosis in colorectal cancer cells and improved efficacy of 5-fluorouracil, the most commonly used chemo-therapy for colorectal cancer.[74, 75]

MELATONIN
SUGGESTED DOSE: At least 3 mg at night, preferably time-released

Intake of supplemental melatonin, a hormone, has improved survival in a number of cancers and may enhance conventional therapy effectiveness.[76] In clinical trials, up to 20 mg has been used.

VITAMIN E
SUGGESTED DOSE: 200–400 IU per day of mixed tocopherols and tocotrienols

Various components of vitamin E have shown anticancer properties. Although alpha-tocopherol is often used in clinical trials, when given alone it may deplete other important components of vitamin E.[77, 78]

VITAMIN K$_2$
SUGGESTED DOSE: 100 mcg vitamin K$_2$ (MK-7)

Vitamin K$_2$ (MK-7) has the longest half-life, meaning it is the most stable, of all forms of vitamin K. Shown to improve bone and cardiovascular health, higher intakes of this form have also been associated with reduced cancer incidence and death, and may improve effectiveness of other therapies.[79, 80, 81]

Dietary Action Plan

An optimal diet would be rich in whole plant-based foods and rich in fiber and antioxidants, while also having a low glycemic index. Glycemic index and glycemic load are measures of the effect on blood glucose level after a food containing carbohydrates is consumed. A high glycemic index has been associated with a greater risk of recurrence and mortality among colorectal cancer patients.[82] A Western dietary pattern—including high intakes of meat, fat, refined grains, and sugar—has been associated with more than a threefold risk of recurrence and/or death among patients with stage III colorectal cancer, even those receiving chemotherapy.[83]

EMPHASIZE

- Brightly colored fresh vegetables, leafy greens, and fresh fruits (choose organic if possible)
- Cruciferous vegetables, such as broccoli, cauliflower, and cabbage
- Whole foods (foods that are as close to their natural form as possible)
- Low sugar/low glycemic diet
- Omega-3 fatty acids, found in cold-water fish such as sardines, wild-caught salmon, cod, mackerel, and tuna
- High fiber, from whole grains, beans, vegetables, and fruits

- Healthy fats, from avocados, nuts, seeds, olive oil, coconut oil, and cold-water fish
- For animal protein, choose lean poultry and fish over red meat, and aim to view meat as a condiment rather than a staple. Try to choose grass-fed and organic meats and eggs whenever possible. Eat no fish larger than a salmon to minimize environmental contaminants, including mercury.

AVOID

- Processed and grilled meats; try to limit intake of red meat
- Fast foods, fried foods, baked goods, and packaged, processed foods
- Sugar, sweeteners, and artificial sweeteners
- Vegetable oils, shortening, margarine, and anything with hydrogenated or partially hydrogenated oils

Top 5 Lifestyle Interventions

1. Be physically active every day. Even light-intensity exercise has benefit.[84]
2. Limit alcohol intake and do not smoke.
3. Reduce animal-based and high glycemic index foods.
4. Emphasize plant-based whole foods, rich in micronutrients, cruciferous vegetables, omega-3 fatty acids, fiber, and calcium.
5. Maintain a healthy weight.

Important Nutrient/Drug Interactions

Many nutritional interventions have the potential to both increase the efficacy of conventional treatments and possibly interfere with their effects, thus combined use should always be supervised. For example, calcium supplementation may improve chemotherapy effectiveness, but also increase its toxicity.[85] Doses higher than 50 mcg of vitamin K_2 (MK-7) may interfere with some anticoagulant medications.[86]

LUNG CANCER
Lung Cancer Basics

- Lung and bronchus cancer is the leading cause of cancer death in the United States, with more than 225,000 new diagnoses in 2012 and an estimated

87,750 and 72,590 deaths predicted to occur yearly in men and women, respectively. This is nearly as many cancer deaths from prostate, breast, and colon cancer combined.

- Eighty-five percent of all cases are non-small cell lung cancer, with most patients diagnosed after the disease has advanced.
- Lung cancer has a mortality rate that has changed very little, getting slightly worse over the last 40 years.[87]
- In the United States 85 to 90 percent of all cases are due to tobacco smoking, making this a very preventable condition.

Causes/Contributing Factors

- Smoking increases the risk for lung cancer by a factor of tenfold to thirtyfold compared to "never-smokers."
- Secondhand smoke is also thought to contribute to nearly 20 percent of lung cancer cases among nonsmokers, raising lung cancer risk approximately 30 percent versus those with no exposure.[88] Smoking also has an additive effect in patients with other environmental exposures, such as radon or asbestos.
- Because smoking is responsible for such a large percentage of lung cancer cases, the fact that nonsmoking causes of lung cancer are still one of the top 10 causes of cancer mortality is often ignored.[89] This includes occupational exposure to known lung carcinogens, such as asbestos, arsenic, nickel, and radon, as well as environmental air pollution, such as that caused by fossil fuel combustion.

Relevant Diagnostic Testing

- **SCREENING LOW-DOSE CT SCANS:** These may be of benefit for those at high risk, such as older individuals with a long history of smoking.
- **IMAGING, INCLUDING CT, MRI, AND POSITRON EMISSION TOMOGRAPHY:** These are likely to be used to monitor treatment efficacy and detect recurrence.[90]
- **VITAMIN D LEVELS:** Vitamin D levels have been associated with both risk of developing lung cancer and survival among lung cancer patients.[91]
- **C-REACTIVE PROTEIN LEVELS:** Elevated C-reactive protein levels have been associated with a greater risk of early death and may help guide appropriate anti-inflammatory treatments.[92]

CANCER STAGING

Staging is the process of finding out how much cancer there is in a person's body and where it's located. It's how the doctor learns the stage of a person's cancer.

Most cancers are staged into four or five groups (stages 0, I, II, III, and IV) with the T, N, M system. T describes size and characteristics of the primary tumor, N describes lymph node involvement, and M describes metastases. Most cancer staging systems use stage IV to indicate the presence of metastases.

LUNG CANCER STAGING SYSTEM

• **Occult (hidden) cancer (TX, N0, M0):** Cancer cells are seen in a sample of sputum or other lung fluids, but the cancer isn't found with other tests, so its location can't be determined.

• **Stage 0 (TIS, N0, M0):** The cancer is found only in the top layers of cells lining the air passages. It has not invaded deeper into other lung tissues and has not spread to lymph nodes or distant sites.

• **Stage IA (T1A/T1B, N0, M0):** The cancer is no larger than 3 cm across, has not reached the membranes that surround the lungs, and does not affect the main branches of the bronchi. It has not spread to lymph nodes or distant sites.

• **Stage IB (T2A, N0, M0):** The cancer has one or more of the following features:

» The main tumor is larger than 3 cm across but not larger than 5 cm.

» The tumor has grown into a main bronchus but is not within 2 cm of the carina (and it is not larger than 5 cm).

» The tumor has grown into the visceral pleura (the membranes surrounding the lungs) and is not larger than 5 cm.

» The tumor is partially clogging the airways (and is not larger than 5 cm).

» The cancer has not spread to lymph nodes or distant sites.

• **Stage IIA:** Three main combinations of categories make up this stage.

» **T1A/T1B, N1, M0:** The cancer is no larger than 3 cm across, has not grown into the membranes that surround the lungs, and does not affect the main branches of the bronchi. It has spread to lymph nodes within the lung and/or around the area where the bronchus enters the lung (hilar lymph nodes). These lymph nodes are on the same side as the cancer. It has not spread to distant sites.

OR

» **T2A, N1, M0:** The cancer has one or more of the following features:

- The main tumor is larger than 3 cm across but not larger than 5 cm.
- The tumor has grown into a main bronchus but is not within 2 cm of the carina (and it is not larger than 5 cm).
- The tumor has grown into the visceral pleura (the membranes surrounding the lungs) and is not larger than 5 cm.
- The tumor is partially clogging the airways (and is not larger than 5 cm).
- The cancer has also spread to the lymph nodes within the lung and/or around the area where the bronchus enters the lung (hilar lymph nodes). These lymph nodes are on the same side as the cancer. It has not spread to distant sites.

OR

» **T2B, N0, M0**: The cancer has one or more of the following features:
- The main tumor is larger than 5 cm across but not larger than 7 cm.
- The tumor has grown into a main bronchus but is not within 2 cm of the carina (and it is between 5 and 7 cm across).
- The tumor has grown into the visceral pleura (the membranes surrounding the lungs) and is between 5 and 7 cm across.
- The tumor is partially clogging the airways (and is between 5 and 7 cm across).
- The cancer has not spread to lymph nodes or distant sites.

- **Stage IIB**: Two combinations of categories make up this stage.
  » **T2B, N1, M0**: The cancer has one or more of the following features:
  - The main tumor is larger than 5 cm across but not larger than 7 cm.
  - The tumor has grown into a main bronchus but is not within 2 cm of the carina (and it is between 5 and 7 cm across).
  - The tumor has grown into the visceral pleura (the membranes surrounding the lungs) and is between 5 and 7 cm across.
  - The cancer is partially clogging the airways (and is between 5 and 7 cm across).
  - It has also spread to lymph nodes within the lung and/or around the area where the bronchus enters the lung (hilar lymph nodes). These lymph nodes are on the same side as the cancer. It has not spread to distant sites.

OR

» **T3, N0, M0**: The main tumor has one or more of the following features:

- It is larger than 7 cm across.
- It has grown into the chest wall, the breathing muscle that separates the chest from the abdomen (diaphragm), the membranes surrounding the space between the lungs (mediastinal pleura), or membranes of the sac surrounding the heart (parietal pericardium).
- It invades a main bronchus and is closer than 2 cm to the carina, but it does not involve the carina itself.
- It has grown into the airways enough to cause an entire lung to collapse or to cause pneumonia in the entire lung.
- Two or more separate tumor nodules are present in the same lobe of a lung.
- The cancer has not spread to lymph nodes or distant sites.

- **Stage IIIA:** Three main combinations of categories make up this stage.
  - » **T1-T3, N2, M0:** The main tumor can be any size. It has not grown into the space between the lungs (mediastinum), the heart, the large blood vessels near the heart (such as the aorta), the windpipe (trachea), the tube connecting the throat to the stomach (esophagus), the backbone, or the carina. It has not spread to different lobes of the same lung.
  - » The cancer has spread to lymph nodes around the carina (the point where the windpipe splits into the left and right bronchi) or in the space between the lungs (mediastinum). These lymph nodes are on the same side as the main lung tumor. The cancer has not spread to distant sites.

  OR

  - » **T3, N1, M0:** The cancer has one or more of the following features:
    - It is larger than 7 cm across.
    - It has grown into the chest wall, the breathing muscle that separates the chest from the abdomen (diaphragm), the membranes surrounding the space between the lungs (mediastinal pleura), or membranes of the sac surrounding the heart (parietal pericardium).
    - It invades a main bronchus and is closer than 2 cm to the carina, but it does not involve the carina itself.
    - Two or more separate tumor nodules are present in the same lobe of a lung.
    - It has grown into the airways enough to cause an entire lung to collapse or to cause pneumonia in the entire lung.

- It has also spread to lymph nodes within the lung and/or around the area where the bronchus enters the lung (hilar lymph nodes). These lymph nodes are on the same side as the cancer. It has not spread to distant sites.

OR

» **T4, N0 OR N1, M0:** The cancer has one or more of the following features:
  - A tumor of any size has grown into the space between the lungs (mediastinum), the heart, the large blood vessels near the heart (such as the aorta), the windpipe (trachea), the tube connecting the throat to the stomach (esophagus), the backbone, or the carina.
  - Two or more separate tumor nodules are present in different lobes of the same lung.
  - It may or may not have spread to lymph nodes within the lung and/or around the area where the bronchus enters the lung (hilar lymph nodes). Any affected lymph nodes are on the same side as the cancer. It has not spread to distant sites.

- **Stage IIIB:** Two combinations of categories make up this stage.
  » **Any T, N3, M0:** The cancer can be of any size. It may or may not have grown into nearby structures or caused pneumonia or lung collapse. It has spread to lymph nodes near the collarbone on either side, and/or has spread to hilar or mediastinal lymph nodes on the side opposite the primary tumor. The cancer has not spread to distant sites.

OR

» **T4, N2, M0:** The cancer has one or more of the following features:
  - A tumor of any size has grown into the space between the lungs (mediastinum), the heart, the large blood vessels near the heart (such as the aorta), the windpipe (trachea), the tube connecting the throat to the stomach (esophagus), the backbone, or the carina.
  - Two or more separate tumor nodules are present in different lobes of the same lung.
  - The cancer has also spread to lymph nodes around the carina (the point where the windpipe splits into the left and right bronchi) or in the space between the lungs (mediastinum). Affected lymph nodes are on the same side as the main lung tumor. It has not spread to distant sites.

- **Stage IV:** Two combinations of categories make up this stage.
  » **Any T, Any N, M1A:** The cancer can be any size and may or may not

have grown into nearby structures or reached nearby lymph nodes. In addition, any of the following is true:

- The cancer has spread to the other lung.
- Cancer cells are found in the fluid around the lung (called a malignant pleural effusion).
- Cancer cells are found in the fluid around the heart (called a malignant pericardial effusion).

OR

» **Any T, Any N, M1B:** The cancer can be any size and may or may not have grown into nearby structures or reached nearby lymph nodes. It has spread to distant lymph nodes or to other organs such as the liver, bones, or brain.

Lung Cancer Supplement Program

Multiple nutritional supplements have been associated with reduced cancer occurrence and/or cancer progression. The list below contains those with the greatest evidence base and benefit, though it is not necessary that they all be included.

VITAMIN D

SUGGESTED DOSE: May require 5,000 IU per day or more, depending on blood levels

Lower levels of vitamin D have been associated with an increased risk for developing lung cancer as well as lung cancer death. The suggested dose is sufficient to raise 25-OH vitamin D levels to >40 ng/mL and optimally between 50 and 80 ng/mL. [93]

OMEGA-3 FATTY ACIDS

SUGGESTED DOSE: 2–3 g combined EPA and DHA per day, with at least 1–2 g of a GLA source

Clinical trials with the omega-3 fatty acids EPA and DHA have shown improved nutritional status, better functional status, reduced inflammation, and improved effectiveness of chemotherapeutic agents.[94, 95, 96] Additionally, GLA, another omega-3 found in evening primrose oil, helps to maintain balance in the fatty acids and enhances the anti-inflammatory effect.[97, 98]

ALPHA LIPOIC ACID

SUGGESTED DOSE: 300 mg, one to two times per day

Shown to protect healthy cells from oxidative stress and induce apoptosis (programmed cell death) in cancer cells, and when combined with N-acetylcysteine was found to restore function to the immune cells of cancer patients.[99, 100]

ISOTHIOCYANATES

SUGGESTED DOSE: 600 mcg per day

Isothiocyanates occur in many commonly consumed cruciferous vegetables (such as broccoli, cauliflower, and kale) and have numerous anticancer properties. They have recently been shown to reduce the drug resistance of some lung cancer cells.[101, 102]

GREEN TEA EXTRACT

SUGGESTED DOSE: 1 g EGCG and mixed catechins per day

Catechins, antioxidants that are found in green tea, particularly EGCG (epigallocatechin-3-gallate), have been shown to have numerous anticancer effects and may enhance chemotherapy effectiveness.[103] The suggested dose has been used with benefit in clinical trials.

CURCUMIN

SUGGESTED DOSE: 1–2 g per day of Meriva or Longvida curcumin

The pharmacologically active component of the spice turmeric, curcumin inhibits tumor growth by multiple mechanisms and has shown synergistic function with several chemotherapeutic agents.[104] While trials often use doses of at least 1 g per day, Meriva and Longvida curcumin have been shown to be much more efficiently absorbed forms.[105, 106]

RESVERATROL

SUGGESTED DOSE: 100–200 mg per day

Found in red wine and grapes, this antioxidant inhibits the invasion and metastasis of lung cancer cells.[107]

QUERCETIN

SUGGESTED DOSE: 200–400 mg three times per day

A high intake of this antioxidant has been associated with a reduced risk of developing lung cancer, as it appears to influence several antiproliferative pathways.[108, 109]

MELATONIN

SUGGESTED DOSE: At least 3 mg at night, preferably time-released

Intake of supplemental melatonin, a hormone, has improved survival in a number of cancers and may enhance conventional therapy effectiveness.[110, 111] In clinical trials, 20 mg is most commonly used.

VITAMIN E

SUGGESTED DOSE: 200–400 IU per day of mixed tocopherols and tocotrienols

Various components of vitamin E have shown anticancer properties.

Although alpha-tocopherol is often used in clinical trials, when given alone it may deplete other important components of vitamin E.[112, 113]

VITAMIN K$_2$
SUGGESTED DOSE: 100 mcg vitamin K$_2$ (MK-7) per day

Vitamin K$_2$ (MK-7) has the longest half-life, meaning it is the most stable, of all forms of vitamin K. Shown to improve bone and cardiovascular health, higher intakes of this form have also been associated with reduced cancer incidence and death, and may improve effectiveness of other therapies.[114, 115, 116]

Dietary Action Plan

A diet rich in specific foods, such as apples, peaches, strawberries, sweet potatoes and yams, carrots, and cruciferous vegetables (broccoli, cauliflower, kale), has been associated with the lowest risk for lung cancer development.[117] Flavonoid-rich foods, such as brightly colored vegetables and fruits, green tea, and even dark chocolate, have also shown a protective influence.[118]

EMPHASIZE

- Brightly colored fresh vegetables, leafy greens, and fresh fruits (choose organic if possible)
- Cruciferous vegetables, such as broccoli, cauliflower, and cabbage
- Whole foods (foods that are as close to their natural form as possible)
- Low sugar/low glycemic diet; glycemic index and glycemic load are measures of the effect on blood glucose level after a food containing carbohydrates is consumed
- Omega-3 fatty acids, found in cold-water fish such as sardines, wild-caught salmon, cod, mackerel, and tuna
- High fiber, from whole grains, beans, vegetables, and fruits
- Healthy fats, from avocados, nuts, seeds, olive oil, coconut oil, and cold-water fish
- For animal protein, choose lean poultry and fish over red meat, and aim to view meat as a condiment rather than a staple. Try to choose grass-fed and organic meats and eggs whenever possible. Eat no fish larger than a salmon to minimize environmental contaminants, including mercury.

AVOID

- Processed and grilled meats; try to limit intake of red meat
- Fast foods, fried foods, baked goods, and packaged, processed foods

- Sugar, sweeteners, and artificial sweeteners
- Vegetable oils, shortening, margarine, and anything with hydrogenated or partially hydrogenated oils

Top 5 Lifestyle Interventions

1. Avoid smoking and secondhand smoke.
2. Eat a plant-rich diet, with diverse fruits and vegetables, emphasizing cruciferous vegetables, colorful fruits and veggies, and flavonoid-rich foods (dark chocolate, tea).
3. Avoid animal-based foods, particularly meats and foods high in nitrites, such as salami and processed meats.
4. Be physically active—this has been shown to be associated with a better quality of life among lung cancer patients.[119]
5. Avoid exposure to environmental toxins such as air pollution, radon, and wood smoke.

Important Nutrient/Drug Interactions

Many nutritional interventions have the potential to both increase the efficacy of conventional treatments and possibly interfere with their effects, thus combined use should always be supervised. Although dietary intake of vitamin A and carotenoids has been associated with a reduced risk of lung cancer, supplementation with beta-carotene has been shown to increase the risk among smokers and should be avoided as a single supplemented nutrient.[120] Some antioxidants, such as N-acetylcysteine, may theoretically impact the effectiveness of specific chemotherapeutic agents. Doses higher than 50 mcg of vitamin K_2 (MK-7) may interfere with some anticoagulant medications.[121]

PROSTATE CANCER
Prostate Cancer Basics

- Other than skin cancer, prostate cancer is the most commonly diagnosed cancer in the United States, with nearly 250,000 men expected to be diagnosed with it in 2012.[122]
- Prostate cancer incidence is highly influenced by lifestyle and environmental factors, with a nearly sixtyfold higher incidence in Japanese and Chinese men living in the United States than living in their native countries.[123]

- In the United States, it affects 16 percent of men, and 3 percent will die from it, representing the second leading cause of cancer death.

- Despite this frequent occurrence, most men who have prostate cancer are roughly six times more likely to die from another cause than from prostate cancer itself. In other words, they will die with prostate cancer rather than from prostate cancer. This apparent "overdiagnosis" of prostate cancer has challenged previous recommendations for widespread screening,[124] and also lends itself to the use of lifestyle and nutritional interventions, either used alone or combined with more aggressive treatments when warranted.

Causes/Contributing Factors

A number of risk factors have been identified for prostate cancer, the most important of which are:

- Having a positive family history
- Being over age 60
- Being African American

A number of environmental, dietary, and lifestyle factors have been found to influence prostate cancer risk:

- **HIGHER INTAKE OF REFINED CALORIES, FAT, AND ANIMAL-BASED FOODS** has been associated with a significant increase in risk for prostate cancer, while a plant-based diet rich in cruciferous vegetables, soy, micronutrients, and omega-3 fatty acids is associated with a reduced risk.

- **OBESITY** influences multiple hormonal pathways and inflammatory chemicals thought to be involved in prostate cancer progression and development.[125]

- **HIGHER EXPOSURE TO CADMIUM** has been associated with an increase in risk, while a higher intake of zinc and selenium may have a protective role.[126, 127, 128]

Relevant Diagnostic Testing

- **PSA (prostate-specific antigen)**: Several large studies have found minimal to no benefit for PSA screening, with a significant impact on quality of life as a result of screening and subsequent treatment.[129, 130] Using PSA to monitor therapy effectiveness and progression, however, is widely accepted.[131]

- **BIOPSY**: A biopsy is required for diagnosis, from which the pathologist who looks at the specimen will assign what's called a Gleason score. The Gleason score may help to guide appropriate treatments.

- **VITAMIN D LEVELS:** Higher levels of vitamin D are associated with a 57 percent reduction in risk of death from prostate cancer.[132, 133]

CANCER STAGING

Staging is the process of finding out how much cancer there is in a person's body and where it's located. It's how the doctor learns the stage of a person's cancer.

Most cancers are staged into four or five groups (stages 0, I, II, III, and IV) with the T, N, M system. T describes size and characteristics of the primary tumor, N describes lymph node involvement, and M describes metastases. Most cancer staging systems use stage IV to indicate the presence of metastases. In prostate cancer staging, the Gleason score (an estimation of how normal or abnormal the cancer cells look under the microscope compared to normal prostate cells) and the PSA (prostate-specific antigen) are used in the staging system as well as the size and location of the tumor, lymph nodes, and metastases.

PROSTATE CANCER STAGING SYSTEM

- **Stage I:** One of the following applies:
  - » **T1, N0, M0, Gleason score 6 or less, PSA less than 10:** The doctor can't feel the tumor or see it with an imaging test such as a transrectal ultrasound—it was either found during a transurethral resection or was diagnosed by needle biopsy done for a high PSA (T1). The cancer is still within the prostate and has not spread to nearby lymph nodes (N0) or elsewhere in the body (M0). The Gleason score is 6 or less, and the PSA level is less than 10.

    OR

  - » **T2A, N0, M0, Gleason score 6 or less, PSA less than 10:** The tumor can be felt by digital rectal exam or seen with imaging such as a transrectal ultrasound and is in one-half or less of only one side (left or right) of the prostate (T2a). The cancer is still within the prostate and has not spread to nearby lymph nodes (N0) or elsewhere in the body (M0). The Gleason score is 6 or less, and the PSA level is less than 10.

- **Stage IIA:** One of the following applies:
  - » **T1, N0, M0, Gleason score of 7, PSA less than 20:** The doctor can't feel the tumor or see it with imaging such as a transrectal ultrasound—it was either found during a transurethral resection or was diagnosed by needle biopsy done for a high PSA level (T1). The cancer has not spread to nearby lymph nodes (N0) or elsewhere in the body (M0). The tumor has a Gleason score of 7, and the PSA level is less than 20.

    OR

» **T1, N0, M0, Gleason score of 6 or less, PSA at least 10 but less than 20:** The doctor can't feel the tumor or see it with imaging such as a transrectal ultrasound—it was either found during a transurethral resection or was diagnosed by needle biopsy done for a high PSA (T1). The cancer has not spread to nearby lymph nodes (N0) or elsewhere in the body (M0). The tumor has a Gleason score of 6 or less, and the PSA level is at least 10 but less than 20.

OR

» **T2A or T2B, N0, M0, Gleason score of 7 or less, PSA less than 20:** The tumor can be felt by digital rectal exam or seen with imaging such as a transrectal ultrasound and is in only one side of the prostate (T2a or T2b). The cancer has not spread to nearby lymph nodes (N0) or elsewhere in the body (M0). It has a Gleason score of 7 or less, and the PSA level is less than 20.

- **Stage IIB:** One of the following applies:
  » **T2C, N0, M0, Any Gleason score, any PSA:** The tumor can be felt by digital rectal exam or seen with imaging such as a transrectal ultrasound and is in both sides of the prostate (T2c). The cancer has not spread to nearby lymph nodes (N0) or elsewhere in the body (M0). The tumor can have any Gleason score, and the PSA can be any value.

  OR

  » **T1 or T2, N0, M0, any Gleason score, PSA of 20 or more:** The cancer has not yet spread outside the prostate. It may (or may not) be felt by digital rectal exam or seen with imaging such as a transrectal ultrasound (T1 or T2). The cancer has not spread to nearby lymph nodes (N0) or elsewhere in the body (M0). The tumor can have any Gleason score, and the PSA level is at least 20.

  OR

  » **T1 or T2, N0, M0, Gleason score of 8 or higher, any PSA:** The cancer has not yet spread outside the prostate. It may (or may not) be felt by digital rectal exam or seen with imaging such as a transrectal ultrasound (T1 or T2). The cancer has not spread to nearby lymph nodes (N0) or elsewhere in the body (M0). The Gleason score is 8 or higher, and the PSA can be any value.

- **Stage III (T3, N0, M0, any Gleason score, any PSA):** The cancer has grown outside the prostate and may have spread to the seminal vesicles (T3), but it has not spread to nearby lymph nodes (N0) or elsewhere in the body (M0). The tumor can have any Gleason score, and the PSA can be any value.

- **Stage IV:** One of the following applies:

» **T4, N0, M0, any Gleason score, any PSA**: The cancer has grown into tissues next to the prostate (other than the seminal vesicles), such as the urethral sphincter (muscle that helps control urination), rectum, bladder, and/or the wall of the pelvis (T4). The cancer has not spread to nearby lymph nodes (N0) or elsewhere in the body (M0). The tumor can have any Gleason score, and the PSA can be any value.

OR

» **Any T, N1, M0, any Gleason score, any PSA**: The tumor may or may not be growing into tissues near the prostate (any T). The cancer has spread to nearby lymph nodes (N1) but has not spread elsewhere in the body (M0). The tumor can have any Gleason score, and the PSA can be any value.

OR

» **Any T, any N, M1, any Gleason score, any PSA**: The cancer may or may not be growing into tissues near the prostate (any T) and may or may not have spread to nearby lymph nodes (any N). It has spread to other, more distant sites in the body (M1). The tumor can have any Gleason score, and the PSA can be any value.

Prostate Cancer Supplement Program

Multiple nutritional supplements have been associated with reduced cancer occurrence and/or cancer progression. The list below contains those with the greatest evidence base and benefit, though it is not necessary that they all be included.

VITAMIN D

SUGGESTED DOSE: May require 5,000 IU per day or more, depending on blood levels

As mentioned above, low vitamin D blood levels are associated with a higher risk of dying from prostate cancer. In a trial of men given 4,000 IU per day for 1 year, vitamin D levels increased from 33 ng/mL to 66 ng/mL, and more than half had a decrease in the number of positive needle biopsies or the Gleason score on pathology. Higher Gleason scores represent a more aggressive type of prostate cancer.[134] The suggested dose is sufficient to raise 25-OH vitamin D levels to >40 ng/mL.[135] Many integrative cancer experts feel that 40 ng/mL is a minimum safe amount, and levels as high as 80 ng/mL are safe. Research has not yet established if levels significantly higher than 40 ng/mL provide extra protection.

LYCOPENE

SUGGESTED DOSE: 30 mg per day

This tomato-based antioxidant has been shown to inhibit cell proliferation via several pathways.[136, 137, 138] Eating a portion of pasta sauce containing 30 mg of lycopene per day increased evidence of cancer cell death in pathology specimens from patients who had subsequent prostatectomy.[139]

GREEN TEA EXTRACT

SUGGESTED DOSE: 1 g EGCG and mixed catechins per day

Catechins, antioxidants that are found in green tea, particularly EGCG (epigallocatechin-3-gallate), have been shown to increase prostate cancer cell death by at least two mechanisms.[140] The suggested dose has been used with benefit in clinical trials.[141, 142]

CURCUMIN

SUGGESTED DOSE: 1–2 g per day of Meriva or Longvida curcumin

The pharmacologically active component of the spice turmeric, curcumin inhibits tumor growth by multiple mechanisms.[143] While trials often use doses of at least 1 g per day, Meriva and Longvida curcumin have been shown to be much more efficiently absorbed forms.[144, 145]

RESVERATROL

SUGGESTED DOSE: 100–200 mg per day

Found in red wine and grapes, this antioxidant has inhibited prostate cancer cell growth and metastasis.[146] It also appears to improve the effectiveness of radiotherapy.[147]

OMEGA-3 FATTY ACIDS

SUGGESTED DOSE: 2–3 g combined EPA and DHA per day, with at least 1–2 g of a GLA source

Omega-3 fatty acids have been shown to reduce the risk of prostate cancer, and higher intakes have been associated with greater survival.[148] Several grams of DHA and EPA have been used in clinical trials.[149] Additionally, GLA, another omega-3 found in evening primrose oil, helps to maintain balance in the fatty acids and enhances the anti-inflammatory effect.[150, 151]

MILK THISTLE EXTRACT (SILYMARIN)

SUGGESTED DOSE: 500 mg, two times per day

Silymarin and silibinin from milk thistle have antiproliferative and antimetastatic properties. A variety of dosing regimens have been used, and at least the suggested dose is likely needed.[152, 153]

DIM (3,3'-DIINDOLYLMETHANE)

SUGGESTED DOSE: 250 mg per day

A number of extracts from cruciferous vegetables (such as broccoli, cauliflower, and cabbage), particularly diindolylmethane (DIM), may explain the benefit of these vegetables on cancer progression, as it has been shown to inhibit multiple mechanisms of cancer growth.[154, 155]

QUERCETIN

SUGGESTED DOSE: 200–400 mg three times per day

This antioxidant found primarily in onions has been shown to inhibit invasion and metastasis of prostate cancer cells.[156]

GRAPE SEED EXTRACT AND/OR PYCNOGENOL

SUGGESTED DOSE: 100–200 mg per day

In a large cohort of more than 35,000 men, use of a grape seed extract supplement was associated with a 41 percent reduced risk of prostate cancer.[157] It is thought to influence hormonal and inflammatory pathways.[158]

MELATONIN

SUGGESTED DOSE: At least 3 mg at night, preferably time-released

Intake of supplemental melatonin, a hormone, has improved survival in a number of cancers, and may enhance conventional therapy effectiveness.[159] In clinical trials, 20 mg is most commonly used.

VITAMIN E

SUGGESTED DOSE: 200–400 IU per day of mixed tocopherols and tocotrienols

Various components of vitamin E have shown anticancer properties. Although alpha-tocopherol is often used in clinical trials, when given alone it may deplete other important components of vitamin E.[160, 161]

VITAMIN K_2

SUGGESTED DOSE: 100 mcg vitamin K_2 (MK-7) per day

Vitamin K_2 (MK-7) has the longest half-life, meaning it is the most stable, of all forms of vitamin K. Shown to improve bone and cardiovascular health, higher intakes of this form have also been associated with reduced cancer incidence and fatality, and may improve effectiveness of other therapies.[162, 163, 164]

Dietary Action Plan

Plant-based whole foods rich in omega-3 fatty acids should be the mainstay of the diet. Avoiding refined carbohydrates, including sugar-sweetened beverages, and animal-based foods affects not only the risk of prostate cancer but its progression.[165, 166] Whole milk, for example, has been associated not only with a heightened risk for prostate cancer, but also with a more than twofold increase in prostate cancer mortality.[167]

EMPHASIZE

- Brightly colored fresh vegetables, leafy greens, and fresh fruits (choose organic if possible)
- Cruciferous vegetables, such as broccoli, cauliflower, and cabbage

- Whole foods (foods that are as close to their natural form as possible)
- Low sugar/low glycemic diet; glycemic index and glycemic load are measures of the effect on blood glucose level after a food containing carbohydrates is consumed
- Omega-3 fatty acids, found in cold-water fish such as sardines, wild-caught salmon, cod, mackerel, and tuna
- High fiber, from whole grains, beans, vegetables, and fruits
- Healthy fats, from avocados, nuts, seeds, olive oil, coconut oil, and cold-water fish
- For animal protein, choose lean poultry and fish over red meat, and aim to view meat as a condiment rather than a staple. Try to choose grass-fed and organic meats and eggs whenever possible. Eat no fish larger than a salmon to minimize environmental contaminants, including mercury.

AVOID
- Processed and grilled meats; try to limit intake of red meat
- Fast foods, fried foods, baked goods, and packaged, processed foods
- Sugar, sweeteners, and artificial sweeteners
- Vegetable oils, shortening, margarine and anything with hydrogenated or partially hydrogenated oils

Top 5 Lifestyle Interventions

1. Be physically active, every day. Even light-intensity exercise has benefit.[168]
2. Limit alcohol intake.
3. Reduce animal-based and high-fat food consumption, and avoid cooking at high temperatures.[169, 170]
4. Emphasize plant-based whole foods, especially cruciferous vegetables (such as broccoli, cauliflower, and cabbage), and omega-3 fatty acids.[171]
5. Maintain a healthy weight.

Important Nutrient/Drug Interactions

Given that many nutritional interventions have the potential to both increase the effectiveness of conventional treatments and possibly interfere with their effects, combined use should always be supervised. For example, resveratrol appears to sensitize tumors to the effects of chemotherapy, suggesting an important therapeutic benefit.[172] Androgen deprivation therapies are known to increase the risk for cardiometabolic conditions, such as diabetes, and nutritional interventions may help mitigate these adverse effects.[173] Doses higher than 50 mcg of vitamin K_2 (MK-7) may interfere with some anticoagulant medications.[174]

BLADDER CANCER
Bladder Cancer Basics

- Nearly 70,000 individuals in the United States will be diagnosed with bladder cancer in 2011, the fifth most common cancer, and almost 15,000 will die of the disease.[175]
- Eighty percent of bladder cancer diagnoses occur in those over 60, with a three times higher occurrence in men than women. Although it is more prevalent in Caucasians, delayed diagnosis leads to worse prognosis in African Americans individuals.[176]
- It occurs at a rate roughly three times higher in the United States than in Asian countries.[177]
- Seventy percent of cases are non-muscle invasive lesions, which recur frequently but do not often affect mortality, and 30 percent are muscle invasive, which tend to be progressive and have poor survival.[178]
- Because most people with bladder cancer have recurrences and survive long-term, lifelong monitoring is required.

Causes/Contributing Factors

- Smoking is the largest contributor to bladder cancer occurrence, responsible for half of all cases, with an increase in risk that persists as long as 20 years after quitting.[179]
- Urothelial carcinoma of the bladder is thought to be significantly influenced by environmental factors, particularly cigarette smoking, which accounts for roughly 50 percent of all cases.[180]
- Other environmental and occupational toxins have also demonstrated risk, including toxins found commonly in industrial and agricultural settings.
- One subtype is linked to the infectious agent *Schistosoma haematobium*, though this is mainly limited to Africa and the Middle East.
- Dietary factors include a higher processed meat intake, while vitamin B_{12} appears to have a protective effect.[181]
- A recent study found that higher intakes of alpha-linolenic acid content, derived from plant foods, were associated with a 74 percent lower risk of developing bladder cancer.[182]

Relevant Diagnostic Testing

- **CYSTOSCOPY**: a procedure to see inside the bladder and urethra
- **BIOPSY**: a sampling of cells collected for further testing
- **IMAGING**: allows the doctor to examine the structures of the urinary tract
- **URINE CYTOLOGY**: the examination of urine cells under a microscope
- **VITAMIN D LEVEL**: Low vitamin D levels have been associated with increased risk for bladder cancer. The ratio of 25-OH vitamin D to D binding protein may be the most predictive.[183, 184]

CANCER STAGING

Staging is the process of finding out how much cancer there is in a person's body and where it's located. It's how the doctor learns the stage of a person's cancer.

Most cancers are staged into four or five groups (stages 0, I, II, III, and IV) with the T, N, M system. T describes size and characteristics of the primary tumor, N describes lymph node involvement, and M describes metastases. Most cancer staging systems use stage IV to indicate the presence of metastases.

BLADDER CANCER STAGING SYSTEM

- **Stage 0A (TA, N0, M0)**: The cancer is a noninvasive papillary carcinoma (Ta). It has grown toward the hollow center of the bladder but has not grown into the connective tissue or muscle of the bladder wall. It has not spread to lymph nodes (N0) or distant sites (M0).
- **Stage 0IS (TIS, N0, M0)**: The cancer is a flat, noninvasive carcinoma (Tis), also known as flat carcinoma in situ. The cancer is growing in the inner lining layer of the bladder only. It has neither grown inward toward the hollow part of the bladder nor invaded the connective tissue or muscle of the bladder wall. It has not spread to lymph nodes (N0) or distant sites (M0).
- **Stage I (T1, N0, M0)**: The cancer has grown into the layer of connective tissue under the lining layer of the bladder but has not reached the layer of muscle in the bladder wall (T1). The cancer has not spread to lymph nodes (N0) or to distant sites (M0).
- **Stage II (T2A or T2B, N0, M0)**: The cancer has grown into the thick muscle layer of the bladder wall, but it has not passed completely through the muscle to reach the layer of fatty tissue that surrounds the bladder (T2). The cancer has not spread to lymph nodes (N0) or to distant sites (M0).
- **Stage III (T3A, T3B, or T4A, N0, M0)**: The cancer has grown into the layer of fatty tissue that surrounds the bladder (T3a or T3b). It might have spread into the prostate, uterus, or vagina, but it is not growing into the pelvic or abdominal wall

(T4a). The cancer has not spread to lymph nodes (N0) or to distant sites (M0).

- **Stage IV**: One of the following applies:
  - » **T4B, N0, M0**: The cancer has grown through the bladder wall and into the pelvic or abdominal wall (T4b). The cancer has not spread to lymph nodes (N0) or to distant sites (M0).

  OR

  - » **Any T, N1 TO N3, M0**: The cancer has spread to nearby lymph nodes (N1-N3) but not to distant sites (M0).

  OR

  - » **Any T, any N, M1**: The cancer has spread to distant lymph nodes or to sites such as the bones, liver, or lungs (M1).

Bladder Cancer Supplement Program

Multiple nutritional supplements have been associated with reduced cancer incidence and/or cancer progression. The list below contains those with the greatest evidence base and benefit, though it is not necessary that they all be included.

VITAMIN D

SUGGESTED DOSE: May require 5,000 IU per day or more, depending on blood levels

Low vitamin D levels have been associated with a greater occurrence and risk of dying from bladder cancer. The suggested dose is sufficient to raise 25-OH vitamin D levels to >40 ng/mL and optimally between 50 and 80 ng/mL.[185]

ISOTHIOCYANATES

SUGGESTED DOSE: 600 mcg per day

Isothiocyanates occur in many commonly consumed cruciferous vegetables (such as broccoli, cauliflower, and kale) and exhibit significant anticancer activities. Available data suggest that they are particularly promising for bladder cancer prevention and/or treatment.[186]

GREEN TEA EXTRACT

SUGGESTED DOSE: 1 g EGCG and mixed catechins per day

Catechins, antioxidants found in green tea, particularly EGCG, have been shown to inhibit bladder cancer cell invasion and spreading (metastasis).[187, 188]

VITAMIN E AND MIXED TOCOPHEROLS

SUGGESTED DOSE: 400 IU per day of mixed tocopherols and tocotrienols

A small trial of vitamin E for patients with low-grade bladder cancer significantly reduced cancer recurrence in both smokers and nonsmokers.[189] A previous study found that long-term vitamin E supplementation was associated with a 40 percent reduction in bladder cancer mortality, and some evidence suggests it may enhance the effectiveness of some chemotherapy.[190, 191] Although 400 IU alpha tocopherol is often used, mixed tocopherols and tocotrienols are likely to have greater benefit.

N-ACETYLCYSTEINE
SUGGESTED DOSE: 600 mg, two to three times per day

This antioxidant has been shown to inhibit several processes in bladder cancer cells, including adhesion, invasion, and migration.[192]

CURCUMIN
SUGGESTED DOSE: 1–2 g per day of Meriva or Longvida curcumin

Derived from the spice turmeric, curcumin has multiple mechanisms of anticancer action. Additionally, it may enhance the effects of Bacillus Calmette-Guerin (BCG), the most commonly used agent for treating superficial bladder cancer.[193, 194] Doses range depending on type of curcumin, but Meriva and Longvida have been shown to be much more efficiently absorbed forms.[195, 196]

MILK THISTLE
SUGGESTED DOSE: At least 500 mg silymarin per day

Silymarin and silibinin from milk thistle have antiproliferative and antimetastatic properties, and have increased apoptosis (programmed cell death) in bladder cancer cells.[197, 198]

DIM (3,3′-DIINDOLYLMETHANE)
SUGGESTED DOSE: 250 mg per day

Diindolylmethane (DIM), extracted from cruciferous vegetables, such as broccoli, cauliflower, and cabbage, has been shown to induce apoptosis (programmed cell death) and reduce the invasiveness of bladder cancer cells, and may improve chemotherapeutic effectiveness against more resistant cells.[199]

QUERCETIN
SUGGESTED DOSE: 200–400 mg three times per day

The antioxidants in quercetin have been shown to inhibit the growth of cancer cells and protect bladder cancer cells from carcinogenic toxins.[200, 201]

MELATONIN
SUGGESTED DOSE: At least 3 mg at night, preferably time-released

Intake of supplemental melatonin, a hormone, has improved survival in a number of cancers, and may enhance conventional therapy effectiveness.[202] In clinical trials, up to 20 mg has been used.

VITAMIN K$_2$
SUGGESTED DOSE: 100 mcg vitamin K$_2$ (MK-7)

Vitamin K$_2$ (MK-7) has the longest half-life, meaning it is the most stable, of all forms of vitamin K. Shown to improve bone and cardiovascular health, higher intakes of this form have also been associated with reduced cancer occurrence and death, and may improve effectiveness of other therapies.[203, 204, 205]

Dietary Action Plan

EMPHASIZE

- Brightly colored fresh vegetables, leafy greens, and fresh fruits (choose organic if possible)
- Cruciferous vegetables, such as broccoli (especially raw), cauliflower, and cabbage
- Foods high in alpha-linolenic acid, such as flaxseeds, pumpkin seeds, walnuts, Brussels sprouts and soybeans, among others
- Whole foods (foods that are as close to their natural form as possible)
- Low sugar/low glycemic diet; glycemic index and glycemic load are measures of the effect on blood glucose level after a food containing carbohydrates is consumed
- Omega-3 fatty acids, found in cold-water fish such as sardines, wild-caught salmon, cod, mackerel, and tuna
- High fiber, from whole grains, beans, vegetables, and fruits
- Healthy fats, from avocados, nuts, seeds, olive oil, coconut oil, and cold-water fish
- For animal protein, choose lean poultry and fish over red meat, and aim to view meat as a condiment rather than a staple. Try to choose grass-fed and organic meats and eggs whenever possible. Eat no fish larger than a salmon to minimize environmental contaminants, including mercury.

AVOID

- Processed and grilled meats; try to limit intake of red meat
- Fast foods, fried foods, baked goods, and packaged, processed foods
- Sugar, sweeteners, and artificial sweeteners
- Vegetable oils, shortening, margarine, and anything with hydrogenated or partially hydrogenated oils

Top 5 Lifestyle Interventions

1. Avoid smoking and secondhand smoke.
2. Increase cruciferous (cauliflower, kale, Brussels sprouts, and

especially broccoli), root, and leafy vegetable consumption, and foods rich in alpha-linolenic acid (flaxseeds, pumpkin seeds, walnuts, soybeans, and, again, Brussels sprouts).[206]

3. Be physically active, every day. Even light-intensity exercise has benefit.[207]

4. Avoid exposure to occupational and environmental toxins.

5. Make sure drinking water is free of arsenic.

Important Nutrient/Drug Interactions

Many nutritional interventions have the potential to both increase the effectiveness of conventional treatments and possibly interfere with their effects, thus combined use should always be supervised. N-acetylcysteine, for example, may be contraindicated with some types of chemotherapy, while curcumin may increase the efficacy of BCG, the most common treatment for bladder cancer. Beta-carotene has been shown to increase the risk of bladder cancer and should be avoided.[208] Doses higher than 50 mcg of vitamin K_2 (MK-7) may interfere with some anticoagulant medications.[209]

ENDOMETRIAL CANCER
Endometrial Cancer Basics

- About 2.7 percent of women will be diagnosed with endometrial cancer at some point during their lifetime, based on the SEER 2009–2011 data.[210]
- Endometrial cancer is the most common malignancy of women in developed countries, and its incidence is 10 times higher there than in developing countries.
- Of women with endometrial cancer, 81.1 percent have a 5-year survival rate.[211]
- Endometrial cancer is heavily influenced by estrogen exposure, therefore it is found in higher amounts in women with early menarche, no children, and late menopause.

Causes/Contributing Factors

A number of risk factors are known to be associated with endometrial cancer occurrence, with different risk factors among different age groups. Endometrial cancer occurs much more frequently in postmenopausal women.[212]

Among the most well-established risk factors include:

- A history of cancer in the family, particularly a first-degree relative.
- Tamoxifen use for breast cancer. Women with breast cancer who take the

hormone therapy drug tamoxifen have a twofold to threefold higher risk of developing endometrial cancer (though the increased risk is still low, at 3 percent).

- Starting menses prior to age 12 and having no pregnancies significantly increases the risk.
- Hereditary nonpolyposis colorectal cancer (HNPCC) is a syndrome that increases the risk of endometrial cancer. HNPCC occurs because of a gene mutation from parents to their offspring.

Risk factors for older women:

- Taking hormones after menopause that contain estrogen but not progesterone increases the risk of endometrial cancer. Unopposed estrogen is associated with increased risk of endometrial hyperplasia at all doses, and durations of therapy between 1 and 3 years.[213]

Other known risk factors include:

- Alcohol intake
- Higher amounts of dietary fat
- Elevated blood sugar. Overweight women with an elevated blood glucose had a 260 percent increase in risk for female reproductive cancers, while overweight women with a normal glucose had only a 70 percent increase in risk, as compared with healthy weight women.[214]
- High percentage of body fat

Relevant Diagnostic Testing

- **SYMPTOMS**: There is not one lab test to diagnose endometrial cancer. Rather it is most often suspected from an initial physical exam and history. It is estimated that 90 percent of women with endometrial cancer experience changes in their menses, abnormal vaginal bleeding, or postmenopausal vaginal bleeding, and 10 percent present as a nonbloody discharge. Later stages of the cancer may show up as pain in the pelvis, feeling a mass in the abdomen or pelvis, and losing weight without trying.
- **IMAGING AND TISSUE STUDIES**: Noninvasive methods include ultrasounds of the pelvic region and endometrial cytology (cell study). Invasive methods include dilation and curettage (D&C), endometrial biopsy, and hysteroscopy with biopsy of the endometrium (uterine lining).

CANCER STAGING

Staging is the process of finding out how much cancer there is in a person's body and where it's located. CT or MRI is often used to monitor and stage.

ENDOMETRIAL CANCER STAGING SYSTEM

• **Stage 0**: The abnormal cells are found only on the innermost lining of the uterus or carcinoma in situ.

• **Stage I**: The tumor has grown through the inner lining of the uterus to the endometrium. It may also have invaded the myometrium.

• **Stage II**: The tumor has invaded the cervix.

• **Stage III**: The tumor has grown through the uterus to reach nearby tissues, most often the vagina or lymph nodes.

• **Stage IV**: The tumor has invaded the bladder or intestine. Or cancer cells have spread to parts of the body far from the uterus, most commonly the liver or lungs.

Endometrial Cancer Supplement Program

Multiple nutritional supplements have been associated with reduced cancer occurrence and/or cancer progression. The list below contains those with the greatest evidence base and benefit, though it is not necessary that they all be included.

VITAMIN D

SUGGESTED DOSE: May require 5,000 IU per day or more, depending on blood levels

Vitamin D levels are associated with the risk of most hormone cancers, including endometrial cancers. Studies on human cells demonstrate that vitamin D protects against endometrial cancer progression.[215, 216] Individuals with a history of lymphoma should also monitor 1,25 dihydroxy-vitamin D levels, as rapid conversion to this active form has been observed. The suggested dose is sufficient to raise 25-OH vitamin D levels to >40 ng/mL and optimally between 50 and 80 ng/mL.[217]

SCUTELLARIA BAICALENSIS

SUGGESTED DOSE: Dried herb, 1–2 g three times per day; tea, 240 mL three times per day; or as a tincture, 2–4 mL three times per day

This is used as an adjunct to chemotherapy for lung cancer patients. Cell-based studies have demonstrated that *Scutellaria* inhibited nuclear factor kappa-beta formation, the primary mediating factor for inflammation, which could be beneficial to slow endometrial cancer.[218]

AGARICUS BLAZEI

SUGGESTED DOSE: 400 mg *Agaricus blazei* extract per day, containing 160 mg polysaccharides (approximately 25 percent beta-glucans)

Agaricus is a mushroom extract used in Chinese medicine for antitumor effects, potentially as a result of the beta-glucan content. A group of women with gynecological cancers were given *Agaricus* extract along with chemotherapy for at least 3 weeks for three cycles, and the women on the mushroom had higher natural killer cell activity.[219]

LYCOPENE

SUGGESTED DOSE: 30 mg per day

Lycopene has been used as an immune stimulant in a variety of cancers. Blood levels of lycopene were found to be inversely related to the risk of developing endometrial cancer in a group of females.[220] Additionally, cell studies show that lycopene can inhibit cancer progression in estrogen-affected cancer cells, such as the endometrial cells.[221]

BETA-CAROTENE

SUGGESTED DOSE: Experts recommend starting at 10,000 IU per day and going up to 83,000 IU per day for cancer prevention and treatment

Beta-carotene has been used as an immune stimulant for many diseases as well as cancer. Blood levels of beta-carotene were found to be inversely related to the risk of developing endometrial cancer in several studies upon review of intake and cancer development.[222, 223] Furthermore, endometrial cancer was inhibited in cells treated with beta-carotene and other carotenoids.[224] Many practitioners prefer beta-carotene–rich whole extracts of natural carotenoids from carotene-rich plant sources over isolated beta-carotene.

GREEN TEA EXTRACT

SUGGESTED DOSE: 1 g EGCG and mixed catechins per day

Catechins, antioxidants that are found in green tea, particularly EGCG (epigallocatechin-3-gallate), are known to have numerous antimetastatic and antiproliferative properties in cancers that are affected by estrogens. Cell studies demonstrated that EGCG inhibits cellular proliferation via inhibiting extracellular signal-regulated kinase activation and induces apoptosis (programmed cell death) in endometrial carcinoma cells.[225, 226]

OMEGA-3 FATTY ACIDS

SUGGESTED DOSE: 2–3 g combined EPA and DHA per day, with at least 1-2 g of a GLA source

Omega-3 fatty acids, DHA and EPA, have been shown to exert numerous anticancer effects on breast cancer cells. Human studies are limited on endometrial cancer, but one recently established that dietary polyunsaturated fatty acids and DHA inhibited endometrial cancer cell proliferation, colony formation, and migration, and promoted cell-programmed death (apoptosis) in animal and in-vitro models.[227] Additionally, GLA, another omega-3, helps to maintain balance in the fatty acids and enhances the anti-inflammatory effect.[228, 229]

Dietary Action Plan

EMPHASIZE

- Four or more daily servings of fruits and vegetables that are orange or yellow, to provide beta-carotene (peppers, squashes, and carrots, for example). Tomatoes and watermelon are rich sources of lycopene.
- Whole foods (foods that are as close to their natural form as possible)
- Low sugar/low glycemic diet; glycemic index and glycemic load are measures of the effect on blood glucose level after a food containing carbohydrates is consumed
- Omega-3 fatty acids, found in cold-water fish such as sardines, wild-caught salmon, cod, mackerel, and tuna
- High fiber, from whole grains, beans, vegetables, and fruits
- Healthy fats, from avocados, nuts, seeds, olive oil, coconut oil, and cold-water fish
- For animal protein, choose lean poultry and fish over red meat, and aim to view meat as a condiment rather than a staple. Try to choose grass-fed and organic meats and eggs whenever possible. Eat no fish larger than a salmon to minimize environmental contaminants, including mercury.[230]
- Having one to two servings of whole soy foods each day may prove beneficial (as long as the soy is GMO free). Try non-GMO soy milk as a beverage as well as edamame, tempeh, tofu, roasted soy nuts, and soy nut butter. Traditional fermented soy foods, such as miso, tempeh, and natto, are particularly beneficial.

AVOID

- Processed and grilled meats; try to limit intake of red meat to avoid excess estrogens
- Refined sugar, processed flours, artificial sweeteners, and sugary beverages—eliminate these to keep blood sugar under control (insulin plays a role in women's estrogen balance)
- Fast foods, fried foods, baked goods, and packaged, processed foods
- Alcohol—limit or avoid it; in most studies that have looked at alcohol consumption and risk of most cancer, regular consumption is linked with increased cancer risk
- Vegetable oils, shortening, margarine, and anything with hydrogenated or partially hydrogenated oils

Top 5 Lifestyle Interventions

1. Maintain a healthy weight, as obesity is related to an increased risk of estrogen-dependent cancers.

2. Drink green tea for the EGCG content, which may protect against endometrial cancer.[231]

3. Exercise often. It has been established that exercise reduces endometrial cancer risk.[232]

4. Practice mindfulness-based stress reduction, like breathing techniques, yoga, Pilates, and meditation.

5. Limit or avoid alcohol.

Important Nutrient/Drug Interactions

Given that many nutritional interventions have the potential to both increase the effectiveness of conventional treatments and possibly interfere with their effects, combined use should always be supervised. For example, beta-carotene has been shown to increase lung cancer in smokers, so do not use beta-carotene therapeutically if you are a smoker. Of course, anyone who has had any type of cancer will seriously damage his chances of long-term wellness if he continues to smoke tobacco or use smokeless tobacco products.

LEUKEMIA
Leukemia Basics

- Leukemia is a type of blood cancer that begins in the bone marrow and affects the white blood cells.

- Leukemia is relatively rare compared to most other cancers and is currently the 11th most common. According to the SEER 2008–2010 data, about 1.4 percent of men and women will be diagnosed with leukemia at some point during their lifetime.[233]

- Although rare compared to other cancers, acute leukemia is the most common cancer among children.

- Leukemia can be classified into two basic groups—acute and chronic. Acute types include acute myeloid leukemia (AML), acute lymphoblastic leukemia (ALL), and adult T-cell leukemia/lymphoma. Chronic types include chronic lymphocytic leukemia (CLL), chronic myelogenous leukemia (CML), and hairy cell leukemia.

Causes/Contributing Factors

Among the most well-established risk factors include:

- A history of leukemia in the family, particularly a first-degree relative
- Treatment for other cancers that used chemotherapy and radiation, especially as a child
- Additionally, exposure to radiation in the environment as found in certain industries and from x-rays[234, 235]
- Exposure to polycyclic aromatic hydrocarbons (PAHs). A human trial looked at PAH exposure and risk of childhood acute lymphoblastic leukemia (ALL) using concentrations in residential dust as an exposure indicator. It was found that ALL risk was increased with higher exposure to PAHs.[236]
- The toxin benzene is a known leukemogenic carcinogen.

Other risk factors include:

- Genetic disorders, such as Down syndrome
- Having a diagnosis of certain blood disorders, such as myelodysplastic syndrome
- Smoking cigarettes increases the risk of several types of leukemia, which may be influenced by specific gene variants.[237, 238]

Relevant Diagnostic Testing

SIGNS AND SYMPTOMS

- Fatigue
- Weight loss that is not intended and loss of appetite
- Bone and joint pain
- Swollen lymph nodes in the neck and groin
- Anemia or abnormalities of red or white blood cells (easy bruising)
- Pinpoint red spots on the skin (petechiae)

TESTING

- Labs will likely be ordered by your physician to assess red and white blood cell status and platelet count.
- If leukemia is suspected, then a bone marrow aspiration and biopsy may be performed, which is a test that looks for malignant cells in the bone marrow as well as certain changes in the cell chromosomes from a sample of blood or bone marrow (cytogenetic analysis).

- One test looks for genes that are "turned on" in several types of leukemia, such as acute myeloid leukemia (AML), called reverse transcription-polymerase chain reaction test, or RT-PCR.
- Another test compares the cancerous cells to normal blood cells to find the specific kind of leukemia, or immunophenotyping.

LEUKEMIA STAGING SYSTEMS

Most cancers are staged based on the size and spread of tumors. Unlike cancers of solid organs, there is no TNM system. Because leukemia already occurs in the developing blood cells within the bone marrow, leukemia staging is a little bit different. The stages of leukemia are often characterized by blood cell counts and the accumulation of leukemia cells in other organs, such as the liver or spleen.

Leukemia stages vary based on disease type. And some of the leukemias may be broken out into subtypes during the staging process.

The acute types of leukemia (AML and ALL) are sometimes staged based on the type of cell involved and how the cells look under a microscope. This is called the French-American-British (FAB) classification system.

Lymphocytic leukemias (CLL and ALL) occur in a type of white blood cell called lymphocytes. The white blood cell count at the time of diagnosis may be used to help stage the leukemia. Likewise, staging for myeloid leukemias (CML and AML) is based on the number of myeloblasts (immature white blood cells) found in the blood or bone marrow.

FACTORS AFFECTING LEUKEMIA STAGING AND PROGNOSIS

- White blood cell, red blood cell, and platelet count
- Age (advanced age may negatively affect prognosis)
- History of prior blood disorders
- Chromosome mutations or abnormalities in the cancer cell
- Bone damage
- Enlarged liver or spleen

Leukemia Supplement Program

Multiple nutritional supplements have been associated with reduced cancer occurrence and/or cancer progression. The list below contains those with the greatest evidence base and benefit, though it is not necessary that they all be included.

VITAMIN D

SUGGESTED DOSE: May require 5,000 IU per day or more, depending on blood levels

Human trials have shown that low levels of vitamin D are related to a higher risk of developing leukemia and also with a worsening prognosis following a diagnosis of AML.[239] Increased vitamin D level was associated with higher survival rate in elderly patients with AML.[240] Individuals with a history of lymphoma should also monitor 1,25-dihydroxyvitamin D levels, as rapid conversion to this active form has been observed in patients with lymphoma. The suggested dose is sufficient to raise 25-OH vitamin D levels to at least >40 ng/mL and preferably between 50 and 80 ng/mL.[241]

GRAPE SEED EXTRACT

SUGGESTED DOSE: 500 mg of a 90% oligomeric proanthocyanidin (OPC) extract

Grape seed extract used on leukemia cell lines decreased uncontrolled cell proliferation and survival and increased cell death in leukemia cells.[242, 243] Other studies indicate that the antioxidant in grape seeds called proanthocyanidins is likely to induce monocytic differentiation in leukemia cells (which prevents proliferation), mostly through decreasing reactive oxygen species, though many other mechanisms are possible.[244, 245]

CORDYCEPS

SUGGESTED DOSE: 3–6 g per day

Cordyceps is a fungus that has shown promising effects on immune stimulation, including aiding in cancer cell death. In cell studies, this plant induced apoptosis in human promyelocytic leukemia cells.[246] More recently, cell studies have shown that *Cordyceps* specifically suppresses proliferation in leukemia cells.[247]

ISOTHIOCYANATES AND DIM (3,3´-DIINDOLYLMETHANE)

SUGGESTED DOSE: DIM 250 mg, isothiocyanates 600 mcg per day

Isothiocyanates—especially indole-3-carbinol, or I3C, and DIM (3,3´-diindolylmethane)—are metabolites of substances known as glucosinolates, found in cruciferous vegetables such as broccoli, cauliflower, and cabbage. Both I3C and DIM have shown antitumor activity; treatment of four different T-ALL human cell lines with DIM in vitro significantly reduced cell proliferation and viability.[248] Other animal and in vitro tumor cell studies demonstrated that DIM induced cell death in myeloid cell leukemia.[249] I3C has shown antitumor activity in animals, and it has also been shown to be effective against human papillomavirus–mediated tumors in human patients.[250] Multiple activities of multiple members of the isothiocyanate family display anticarcinogenic activity and exhibit antitumor activity by affecting multiple pathways.[251]

CURCUMIN

SUGGESTED DOSE: 1–2 g per day of Meriva or Longvida curcumin

The active extract from the spice turmeric, curcumin has been shown to cause cell death in a variety of cancer cell lines. In trials with the human acute leukemia cell line THP-1, curcumin inhibited proliferation and induced apoptosis of these cancer cells.[252]

OLIVE LEAF EXTRACT

SUGGESTED DOSE: 250–500 mg of a standardized extract, one to three times per day

Olive leaf contains the antioxidants oleuropein and hydroxytyrosol, which are believed to have anticancer effects. Olive leaf extracts induced apoptosis as well as induction of differentiation (moving them toward a more normal phenotype) of human leukemia cells.[253, 254]

GREEN TEA EXTRACT

SUGGESTED DOSE: 1 g EGCG and mixed catechins per day

Catechins, antioxidants that are found in green tea, particularly EGCG (epigallocatechin-3-gallate), are known to have many antitumor effects. In human adult T-cell leukemia cells, EGCG reduced cancer cell proliferation.[255] In animal studies of leukemia cells a similar mechanism of tumor cell death was found.[256]

MILK THISTLE

SUGGESTED DOSE: At least 500 mg silymarin per day

Silymarin and silibinin from milk thistle have antiproliferative and antimetastatic properties, and may reduce the liver-damaging effects of chemotherapy, especially in children. In children with ALL and liver toxicity, milk thistle was associated with a trend toward significant reductions in liver toxicity.[257]

Dietary Action Plan

EMPHASIZE

- Brightly colored fresh vegetables, leafy greens, and fresh fruits (choose organic if possible)
- Cruciferous vegetables, such as broccoli, cauliflower, and cabbage, which have high levels of DIM
- Whole foods (foods that are as close to their natural form as possible)
- Low sugar/low glycemic diet; glycemic index and glycemic load are measures of the effect on blood glucose level after a food containing carbohydrates is consumed
- Omega-3 fatty acids, found in cold-water fish such as sardines, wild-caught salmon, cod, mackerel, and tuna
- High fiber, from whole grains, beans, vegetables, and fruits
- Healthy fats, from avocados, nuts, seeds, olive oil, coconut oil, and cold-water fish
- For animal protein, choose lean poultry and fish over red meat, and aim to

view meat as a condiment rather than a staple. Try to choose grass-fed and organic meats and eggs whenever possible. Eat no fish larger than a salmon to minimize environmental contaminants, including mercury.

AVOID

- Processed and grilled meats; try to limit intake of red meat
- Fast foods, fried foods, baked goods, and packaged, processed foods
- Sugar, sweeteners, and artificial sweeteners
- Vegetable oils, shortening, margarine, and anything with hydrogenated or partially hydrogenated oils

Top 5 Lifestyle Interventions

1. Stop smoking cigarettes—smoking has been associated with a greater risk and worse prognosis.
2. Move away from areas of high radiation, such as near nuclear power plants, and limit medical x-ray exposure.
3. Engage in stress reduction via meditation and yoga.
4. Maintain a healthy body weight, as obesity can worsen the prognosis of leukemia and increase drug resistance.[258]
5. Incorporate regular physical activity into your life—the risk for cardiovascular disease is increased in survivors of leukemia but may be mitigated by regular exercise.[259, 260]

Important Nutrient/Drug Interactions

Given that many nutritional interventions have the potential to both increase the effectiveness of conventional treatments and possibly interfere with their effects, combined use should always be supervised. For example, vitamin D has been shown to have synergistic effects when used with the iron chelating medication deferasirox for patients with acute myeloid leukemia, and to increase overall survival.[261] Leukemia patients should avoid supplements with iron in them, unless an actual iron deficiency has been medically documented.

LYMPHOMA
Lymphoma Basics

- Non-Hodgkin's lymphoma (NHL) is the most common type of lymphoma. Lymphomas are a heterogeneous group of lymphocyte cancers with close to

50 subtypes of varying aggressiveness, responsiveness to treatment, and survivals. They range from some of the slowest growing cancers (marginal zone lymphomas) to the most aggressive, rapidly dividing human malignancy (Burkitt's lymphoma). Hodgkin's lymphoma is less common and has a slightly higher cure rate. According to SEER data,[262] in 2011 there were 530,919 people living with NHL in the United States. There has been a 73 percent rise between 1973 and 1991 in NHL, with continued increases ever since.

- Approximately 2.1 percent of men and women will be diagnosed with NHL at some point during their lifetime, based on 2008–2010 SEER data, and the 5-year survival rate is approximately 70 percent.

- The survival rate for lymphoma has greatly increased in the past 40 years, especially in children. The 5-year relative survival rate for NHL patients has risen from 31 percent in Caucasians from 1960 to 1963 to approximately 70 percent for all races from 2003 to 2009. In youths under 20, the 5-year survival rate is 84.5 percent, which is a significant improvement since most youths did not survive 5 years in the 1970s. NHL and Hodgkin's lymphoma account for 11 percent of total cancer diagnoses in children.[263]

- Some of the many subtypes of NHL include: indolent (slow-growing) lymphomas, such as follicular lymphoma; aggressive lymphomas, such as diffuse large B-cell lymphoma; or highly aggressive types, such as Burkitt's lymphoma and lymphoblastic lymphoma. Other lymphomas may be named for their site of presentation, such as CNS lymphoma.

Causes/Contributing Factors

A number of risk factors are known to be associated with lymphoma. Among the most well-established ones include:

- Being Caucasian and male in the United States[264]

- Aging, although there are some lymphomas that occur more commonly in childhood

- Exposure to environmental radiation, or being treated with radiation and chemotherapy for other diseases

- Having HIV or other immune system problems, including other cancers and viral infections such as cytomegalovirus (CMV) and Epstein-Barr virus (EBV);[265] infection with hepatitis C nearly doubles the risk

Other risk factors include:

- Obesity and high BMI have been found to be a predictor of worse outcomes specifically for small lymphocytic lymphoma (versus diffuse large B-cell lymphoma and follicular lymphoma).[266]

- Pesticide and herbicide exposure. Human studies are demonstrating that exposure to pesticides increases the risk of NHL, especially in individuals who work and live on or near farms.[267, 268] Specifically, diffuse large B-cell lymphoma was positively associated with phenoxy herbicide exposure.[269] Glyphosate is a major concern with lymphoma risk.[270] Additionally, home pesticide use has been associated with a several-fold increase in risk for NHL in children.[271]
- A number of genetic variants have been associated with risk, particularly when combined with environmental toxin exposure.[272]
- Smoking, alcohol use, and sedentary lifestyle
- A number of autoimmune diseases have been associated with a higher risk of NHL, although the absolute risk is still small.[273]

Relevant Diagnostic Testing

- **SYMPTOMS:** Patients may often present with swollen lymph nodes (neck and groin typically) or abdominal masses as a primary symptoms. Different parts of the lymphatic system can present for different types of lymphomas. Burkitt's lymphoma may have a large abdominal mass. B-cell or lympho-blastic lymphoma may show up in the mediastinum or testicles. Some types of T-cell lymphomas can also present with skin lesions. Other physical signs and symptoms include:
    - Swollen abdomen (signs of a mass in the abdomen)
    - Feeling full even after just a small amount of food (from lymphoma pressing on the organs)
    - Confusion and headaches (from lymphoma in the brain)
    - Chest pain or pressure (from lymphoma pressing on the trachea)
    - Shortness of breath, chronic cough
    - Unexplained persistent fever (over 100.4°F), weight loss exceeding 10 percent of body weight, drenching night sweats, shaking chills, and fatigue. These are known as the B symptoms of lymphoma and are actually used in staging.
    - Symptoms from low blood cell counts, such as easy bruising and frequent infections
- **IMAGING, BIOPSY, AND LAB TESTING:** A biopsy of the swollen lymph node(s) is recommended and is often preceded by imaging of the body part affected, which can include x-ray, ultrasound, positron-emission tomography (PET), computed tomography (CT), or magnetic resonance imaging (MRI). Once the disease has been detected, other testing of the cancer cells includes cytogenetics and flow cytometry. Blood testing to assess white and

red blood cells and liver function is also routinely part of the diagnosis and monitoring of lymphomas. Initial staging and response to treatment are typically monitored by PET/CT scan.

ANN ARBOR STAGING SYSTEM FOR LYMPHOMA

Note: The staging system does not take into account the grade (growth rate) of the tumor tissue or prognostic factors, such as bulky disease, LDH (an enzyme measured in the blood called lactic acid dehydrogenase), or age. Bone marrow involvement and other so-called extranodal involvement are not unexpected for lymphoma and can often be reversed with treatment.

• **Stage I:** Disease is in a single lymph node or lymph node region.

• **Stage II:** Disease is in two or more lymph node regions on the same side of the diaphragm.

• **Stage III:** Disease is in lymph node regions on both sides of the diaphragm.

• **Stage IV:** Disease is widespread, including multiple involvement at one or more extranodal (beyond the lymph node) sites, such as the bone marrow (which is commonly involved), pleura (thin membrane that contains and protects the lungs), liver, or other organ.

Lymphoma Supplement Program

Multiple nutritional supplements have been associated with reduced cancer occurrence and/or cancer progression. The list below contains those with the greatest evidence base and benefit, though it is not necessary that they all be included.

VITAMIN D

SUGGESTED DOSE: May require 5,000 IU per day or more, depending on blood levels, but usually not until complete remission has been achieved; vitamin D must be used very cautiously at first in people who have lymphoma active in their body (see below).

Human trials have shown that low levels of vitamin D are related to a higher risk of developing T-cell lymphoma.[274] Epidemiological findings demonstrate that the time of year Hodgkin's lymphoma is diagnosed affects survival rates, with 20 percent lower fatality rates if diagnosed in autumn rather than winter. The survival rate was 60 percent better for those under 30 years old. This may reflect the positive influence that vitamin D levels have on the immune system and cancer fatality.[275] In addition to monitoring 25-OH levels, 1,25-dihydroxyvitamin D levels also must be measured, as individuals with lymphoma may have a rapid conversion to this active form and are at risk for vitamin D toxicity, even with modest doses of vitamin D.

The suggested dose is sufficient to raise 25-OH vitamin D levels to at least >40 ng/mL and optimally between 50 and 80 ng/mL, as long as serum 1,25-dihydroxyvitamin D remains within the normal range.[276]

INDOLE-3-CARBINOL (I3C)
SUGGESTED DOSE: 200–400 mg daily

I3C was found to increase cell death in adult T-cell leukemia/lymphoma (ATLL) cells in both human and cell studies.[277] Pregnant animals fed I3C resulted in lower incidences of lymphoma in their offspring.[278]

DIM (3,3'-DIINDOLYLMETHANE)
SUGGESTED DOSE: 250 mg per day

DIM significantly reduced human T-cell acute lymphoblastic leukemia (T-ALL) cells as well as reduced lymphoma tumors in mice by as much as 44 percent.[279]

CURCUMIN
SUGGESTED DOSE: 1–2 g per day of Meriva or Longvida curcumin

The active extract from the spice turmeric, curcumin has high anticancer effects on many cell lines, including lymphoma. In studies, curcumin inhibited the growth of HL cell lines and increased the sensitivity to the chemotherapy drug cisplatin.[280] Lymphoma tumor growth in mice was inhibited by curcumin.[281, 282]

QUERCETIN
SUGGESTED DOSE: 200–400 mg three times per day

Quercetin is a flavonoid that has been shown to induce cell death in lymphoma cell lines.[283] One cell study showed that quercetin combined with the drug rituximab enhanced the effectiveness of this drug in inhibiting diffuse large B-cell lymphoma cells.[284] TRAIL is an important cytokine needed for cell death that is often decreased in lymphoma cell lines. Quercetin restores TRAIL-induced cell death in resistant transformed follicular lymphoma B-cell lines.[285]

RESVERATROL
SUGGESTED DOSE: 100–200 mg per day

This antioxidant found in red wine and grapes inhibited Epstein-Barr virus in Burkitt's lymphoma cells.[286] Additionally it induced cell death in Hodgkin's lymphoma.[287]

COQ10
SUGGESTED DOSE: 100 mg per day

This antioxidant has been stated to improve survival rates in various forms of cancer as well as having cardioprotective influence on children with lymphoma.[288] Cell studies show that coenzyme Q10 reduced cell activity of malignant cells in Burkitt's lymphoma.[289]

FORSKOLIN

SUGGESTED DOSE: 10 mg, taken twice per day

Forskolin appears to have an immune regulatory effect on lymphoma cell lines and inhibits a key phase of cell division.[290, 291] Burkitt's lymphoma cancer cells treated with forskolin had higher rates of cell death.[292]

Dietary Action Plan

EMPHASIZE

- Cruciferous vegetables, such as broccoli, cauliflower, and cabbage, which contain compounds metabolized into DIM and I3C
- Whole foods (foods that are as close to their natural form as possible)
- Low sugar/low glycemic diet; glycemic index and glycemic load are measures of the effect on blood glucose level after a food containing carbohydrates is consumed
- Omega-3 fatty acids, found in cold-water fish such as sardines, wild-caught salmon, cod, mackerel, and tuna
- High fiber, from whole grains, beans, vegetables, and fruits
- Healthy fats, from avocados, nuts, seeds, olive oil, coconut oil, and cold-water fish
- For animal protein, choose lean poultry and fish over red meat, and aim to view meat as a condiment rather than a staple. Try to choose grass-fed and organic meats and eggs whenever possible. Eat no fish larger than a salmon to minimize environmental contaminants, including mercury.

AVOID

- Foods that have been treated with pesticides and herbicides, especially glyphosate
- Processed and grilled meats; try to limit intake of red meat
- Fast foods, fried foods, baked goods, and packaged, processed foods
- Sugar, sweeteners, and artificial sweeteners
- Vegetable oils, shortening, margarine, and anything with hydrogenated or partially hydrogenated oils

Top 5 Lifestyle Interventions

1. Maintain a healthy weight. Not only does obesity contribute to a higher incidence of lymphoma, it is also associated with a lower survival rate.

2. Do not smoke, especially if you have hepatitis C. In general, heavy smoking doubles the risk of having NHL. But heavy smokers who are hepatitis C–positive have a nearly fourfold higher risk of developing NHL than nonsmokers.[293]

3. If you are diabetic or prediabetic, eat a low glycemic diet and exercise regularly and vigorously.[294, 295]

4. Exercise is a well-established way to prevent cancer development, including lymphoma. One study found that women who sat for 6 hours a day had a 28 percent higher risk of NHL than those who sat for 3 hours per day.[296]

5. Meditation, stress relief, yoga, and other modalities to reduce overall emotional and physical stress have positive effects on lymphoma.[297]

Important Nutrient/Drug Interactions

Given that many nutritional interventions have the potential to both increase the effectiveness of conventional treatments and possibly interfere with their effects, combined use should always be supervised. For example, DIM has been shown to potentiate the effects of several types of chemotherapy in cell-based studies and may increase the effectiveness of therapy.[298, 299]

MELANOMA
Melanoma Basics

- Melanoma is a deadly form of skin cancer that accounts for only 2 to 4 percent of all skin cancer cases yet 79 percent of all skin cancer–related deaths.

- In 2011, there were an estimated 960,231 people living with melanoma of the skin in the United States.[300]

- Despite its deadly nature, when melanoma is diagnosed early, it is considered very survivable. According to the 2004–2010 SEER data, 91.3 percent of early diagnosed melanoma cases survive without recurrence at the 5-year mark.[301]

- The incidence for melanoma is currently increasing at a rate of 3 percent per year, the fastest of any cancer.[302]
- Although the incidence of melanoma is highest among older adults, it can occur in any age group. For example, it is the most common cancer among women ages 20 to 30.

Causes/Contributing Factors

A number of risk factors are known to be associated with melanoma, primarily based on genetics (such as skin tone, eye color, and hair color) and on level of sunburn and tanning.

Among the most well-established risk factors include:

- A history of melanoma in the family, particularly a first-degree relative. Ten percent of people with melanoma have a family history of the cancer.[303] A BRCA 2 gene (breast cancer mutation) also increases melanoma risk.
- Having a fair-skinned complexion—freckles, skin that burns easily, green or blue eyes, or red or blonde hair
- Having a history of sunburns (especially blistering sunburns in childhood) and long-term exposure to tanning

Other known risk factors include:

- Exposure to radiation, solvents, vinyl chloride, and PCBs
- Smoking
- Having a family history of unusual moles (atypical nevus syndrome)[304]

Relevant Diagnostic Testing

- **PHYSICAL EXAM:** Melanomas can occur in sun-exposed skin as well as areas not normally exposed to the sun, such as the abdomen, soles of the feet, and genital areas. Despite the fair complexion and white genetic profile for melanoma, there is one type found more frequently in African Americans and Asians: acral lentiginous melanoma, which occurs on the palms of the hands, soles of the feet, and nailbeds. With all melanomas, there is often a change in an existing mole or a new mole is discovered. Physicians perform the ABCDEs of mole identification to assess:
  - **ASYMMETRY:** One half doesn't match the appearance of the other half.
  - **BORDER IRREGULARITY:** The edges are ragged or blurred.
  - **COLOR:** The pigmentation is not uniform. Shades of tan, brown, and

black are present. Dashes of red, white, and blue make the appearance mottled.

- **DIAMETER**: The size of the mole is greater than 6 mm, or about the size of a pencil eraser. Any growth of a mole should be evaluated immediately.

- **EVOLUTION**: There is a change in the size, shape, symptoms (itching or tenderness, for example), surface (primarily bleeding), or color of a mole (especially darkening).

- **BIOPSY**: In this procedure, the abnormal tissue and a small amount of normal tissue around it are removed. A pathologist will examine the biopsied tissue microscopically. Patients may want to have the sample of tissue checked by a second pathologist. If the abnormal mole or lesion is malignant, the sample of tissue may also be tested for certain gene changes.

- **GENETIC EVALUATION**: Genetic evaluation may be recommended, as a number of genetic mutations have been associated with prognosis (outlook) and help to predict how beneficial different treatments may be.[305]

CANCER STAGING

Staging is the process of finding out how much cancer there is in a person's body and where it's located. Melanoma stages are assigned based on the size or thickness of the tumor, whether or not it has spread to the lymph nodes or other organs, and certain other characteristics, such as growth rate. Physical exams, imaging procedures, laboratory tests, pathology reports, and surgical reports provide information to determine the stage of a cancer. Very thin melanomas (less than 0.75 mm in thickness) are associated with very high cure rates from surgery alone, so early diagnosis is very valuable.

MELANOMA STAGING SYSTEM

- **Stage 0: TIS, N0, M0**: The melanoma is in situ, meaning that it is in the epidermis but has not spread to the dermis (lower layer).

- **Stage IA: T1A, N0, M0**: The melanoma is less than 1.0 mm in thickness. It is not ulcerated (under microscope) and has a mitotic rate of less than $1/mm^2$. It has not been found in lymph nodes or distant organs.

- **Stage IB: T1B or T2A, N0, M0**: The melanoma is less than 1.0 mm in thickness and is ulcerated or has a mitotic rate of at least $1/mm^2$; or it is between 1.01 and 2.0 mm and is not ulcerated. It has not been found in lymph nodes or distant organs.

- **Stage IIA: T2B or T3A, N0, M0**: The melanoma is between 1.01 mm and 2.0 mm in thickness and is ulcerated; or it is between 2.01 and 4.0 mm and is not ulcerated. It has not been found in lymph nodes or distant organs.

- **Stage IIB: T3B or T4A, N0, M0:** The melanoma is between 2.01 mm and 4.0 mm in thickness and is ulcerated; or it is thicker than 4.0 mm and is not ulcerated. It has not been found in lymph nodes or distant organs.
- **Stage IIC: T4B, N0, M0:** The melanoma is thicker than 4.0 mm and is ulcerated. It has not been found in lymph nodes or distant organs.
- **Stage IIIA: T1A to T4A, N1A or N2A, M0:** The melanoma can be of any thickness, but it is not ulcerated. It has spread to one to three lymph nodes near the affected skin area, but the nodes are not enlarged, and the melanoma is found only when they are viewed under the microscope. There is no distant spread.
- **Stage IIIB:** One of the following applies:
  » **T1B to T4B, N1A or N2A, M0:** The melanoma can be of any thickness and is ulcerated. It has spread to one to three lymph nodes near the affected skin area, but the nodes are not enlarged, and the melanoma is found only when they are viewed under the microscope. There is no distant spread.
  » **T1A to T4A, N1B or N2B, M0:** The melanoma can be of any thickness, but it is not ulcerated. It has spread to one to three lymph nodes near the affected skin area. The nodes are enlarged because of the melanoma. There is no distant spread.
  » **T1A to T4A, N2C, M0:** The melanoma can be of any thickness, but it is not ulcerated. It has spread to small areas of nearby skin or lymphatic channels around the original tumor, but the nodes do not contain melanoma. There is no distant spread.
- **Stage IIIC:** One of the following applies:
  » **T1B to T4B, N1B or N2B, M0:** The melanoma can be of any thickness and is ulcerated. It has spread to one to three lymph nodes near the affected skin area. The nodes are enlarged because of the melanoma. There is no distant spread.
  » **T1B to T4B, N2C, M0:** The melanoma can be of any thickness and is ulcerated. It has spread to small areas of nearby skin or lymphatic channels around the original tumor, but the nodes do not contain melanoma. There is no distant spread.
  » **Any T, N3, M0:** The melanoma can be of any thickness and may or may not be ulcerated. It has spread to four or more nearby lymph nodes, or to nearby lymph nodes that are clumped together—or it has spread to nearby skin or lymphatic channels around the original tumor and to nearby lymph nodes. The nodes are enlarged because of the melanoma. There is no distant spread.

- **Stage IV: Any T, any N, M1(A, B, or C):** The melanoma has spread beyond the original area of skin and nearby lymph nodes to other organs such as the lung, liver, or brain, or to distant areas of the skin, subcutaneous tissue, or distant lymph nodes. Although neither the spread nor the thickness is considered in this stage, typically the melanoma is thick and has also spread to distant lymph nodes or organs.

Melanoma Supplement Program

Multiple nutritional supplements have been associated with reduced cancer occurrence and/or cancer progression. The list below contains those with the greatest evidence base and benefit, though it is not necessary that they all be included.

ASTRAGALUS
SUGGESTED DOSE: Use of extract: 250–500 mg, three to four times a day standardized to 0.4% 4-hydroxy-3-methoxy isoflavones; powdered root: 250–500 mg, three to four times per day; tincture (1:5) in 30% ethanol: 20–60 drops, three times a day

In vivo and in vitro studies demonstrate that astragalus significantly inhibits the growth of melanoma.[306, 307]

GREEN TEA EXTRACT
SUGGESTED DOSE: 1 g EGCG and mixed catechins per day

Catechins, antioxidants that are found in green tea, particularly EGCG (epigallocatechin-3-gallate), are known to have numerous antimetastatic and antiproliferative properties. Studies on melanoma in animal cells have shown that EGCG causes cellular death and inhibition of cell cycles.[308, 309]

COPTIS
SUGGESTED DOSE: 2–10 g of whole herb in either tincture or capsule form

Coptis extract inhibited human metastatic melanoma cells in vitro.[310] The berberines from this traditional Chinese medicine herb are the active ingredients believed to have the anticancerous effects.

BERBERINE
SUGGESTED DOSE: 500 mg, three times per day

Berberine used in conjunction with the chemotherapy medication doxorubicin decreased melanoma tumor cell volume and replication of metastatic cells.[311, 312, 313]

RESVERATROL
SUGGESTED DOSE: 100 mg per day

Malignant melanoma cells exposed to resveratrol had disruption in cell signaling pathways in both human and animal cell studies.[314, 315]

MAITAKE MUSHROOM

SUGGESTED DOSE: Capsules range from 100 to 500 mg, with at least 12–25 mg of standardized extract, one to three times per day

Studies on melanoma in animal cells demonstrate powerful anticancer properties of the mushroom.[316]

RETINOL

SUGGESTED DOSE: 1,200 IU per day (the dose used in human trials for reducing the risk of melanoma)

Large human studies have shown that the use of vitamin A in the form of retinol significantly reduces the risk of melanoma, especially in sun-exposed areas of the body such as the head and neck.[317, 318]

CHAGA

SUGGESTED DOSE: In active treatment, 3 capsules, 500 mg each, of a hot water extract, two times per day, 30 minutes before meals; for prevention, 1 capsule, two times per day; for significant risk of relapse, 2 capsules, two times per day

In vitro studies of chaga have demonstrated potent anticancer effects on melanoma and liver cancer cells.[319, 320]

VITAMIN D

SUGGESTED DOSE: May require 5,000 IU per day or more, depending on blood levels

Meta-analysis on individuals with cutaneous melanoma demonstrated an inverse relationship between levels of vitamin D and the thickness of the tumors, as well as a poorer prognosis with deficient levels.[321, 322] Genetic analysis of melanoma patients also showed that certain common mutations in the vitamin D receptor gene are considered potential biomarkers for melanoma susceptibility, with low vitamin D levels in melanoma patients indicating the need for vitamin D supplementation.[323] The suggested dose is sufficient to raise 25-OH vitamin D levels to >40 ng/mL and optimally between 50 and 80 ng/mL.[324]

Dietary Action Plan

EMPHASIZE

- Foods high in beta-carotene, which can then convert to retinol, such as pumpkin, tomato, melon, kale, broccoli, mango, grapefruit, papaya, guava, carrots, spinach, peppers, and squash
- Cruciferous vegetables, such as broccoli, cauliflower, and cabbage
- Whole foods (foods that are as close to their natural form as possible)

- Low sugar/low glycemic diet; glycemic index and glycemic load are measures of the effect on blood glucose level after a food containing carbohydrates is consumed
- Omega-3 fatty acids, found in cold-water fish such as sardines, wild-caught salmon, cod, mackerel, and tuna
- High fiber, from whole grains, beans, vegetables, and fruits
- Healthy fats, from avocados, nuts, seeds, olive oil, coconut oil, and cold-water fish
- For animal protein, choose lean poultry and fish over red meat, and aim to view meat as a condiment rather than a staple. Try to choose grass-fed and organic meats and eggs whenever possible. Eat no fish larger than a salmon to minimize environmental contaminants, including mercury.

AVOID
- Processed and grilled meats; try to limit intake of red meat
- Fast foods, fried foods, baked goods, and packaged, processed foods
- Sugar, sweeteners, and artificial sweeteners
- Vegetable oils, shortening, margarine, and anything with hydrogenated or partially hydrogenated oils

Top 5 Lifestyle Interventions

1. Do not overtan or sunburn.[325] Even tanning without risk of sunburn contributes to the risk of developing melanoma.
2. Avoid obesity. High-fat diets and obesity combine to increase the risk for melanoma.[326, 327]
3. Consume a vegetable-rich, Mediterranean-style diet, emphasizing whole foods and cruciferous vegetables (such as broccoli, cauliflower, kale, and Brussels sprouts).
4. Practice mindfulness-based stress reduction, like breathing techniques, yoga, Pilates, and meditation.[328]
5. Maintain a regular physical activity schedule.[329]

Important Nutrient/Drug Interactions

Given that many nutritional interventions have the potential to both increase the effectiveness of conventional treatments and possibly interfere with their effects, combined use should always be supervised, especially if chemotherapy protocols are being utilized. For example, retinol (the active form of vitamin A) may enhance the effects of the chemotherapy agent doxorubicin, so those agents should be monitored when used in combination.[330]

RENAL CANCER
Renal Cancer Basics

- Renal cancer makes up 3.8 percent of all new cancer cases, with an estimated death rate in 2014 of 13,860.[331]

- Approximately 1.6 percent of men and women will be diagnosed with kidney and renal pelvis cancer at some point during their lifetime, based on 2008–2010 data.[332]

- Renal cell carcinoma is the most common type of kidney cancer (90 to 95 percent). It usually starts in one kidney and rarely occurs in both kidneys at the same time.[333]

- When the cancer has not spread (metastasized) beyond the kidney, the 5-year survival rate is 60 to 70 percent.[334]

Causes/Contributing Factors

Risk factors associated with renal cancer are primarily related to lifestyle factors such as obesity, hypertension, and diabetes. In fact, the combination of smoking, obesity, and hypertension has been estimated to cause at least 50 percent of renal cancers.[335]

Among the most well-established risk factors include:

- Cigarette smoking. This is the most common factor behind developing renal cancer. Additionally, individuals with renal cancer who are current smokers have lower rates of survival.[336]

- Obesity and high blood pressure.[337] Visceral obesity correlated with a higher rate of having recurrent renal cell carcinoma.[338] Obesity is a known contributing factor to development of chronic kidney disease as well as a factor in worsening the prognosis of those with renal cancer.[339] This risk appears higher in obese women than in men in some studies.[340]

- Having diabetes mellitus, types 1 and 2.[341]

Risk factors also include:

- Exposure to asbestos, cadmium, and trichloroethylene, found in occupational dusts.[342, 343]

- Women who have undergone a hysterectomy have at least double the risk of developing renal cancer in their lifetime compared to those who have not had the surgery.[344]

Relevant Diagnostic Testing

- **SYMPTOMS**: Renal cancer is often asymptomatic for years until it becomes advanced. However, the physical symptoms that most commonly occur initially include: blood in the urine (occurring in 40 percent of affected persons at the time they first seek medical attention for the symptom), flank pain (40 percent), a mass in the abdomen (25 percent), weight loss (33 percent), fever (20 percent), high blood pressure (20 percent), night sweats, and a feeling that something is "not right" or fatigue.[345]

  Renal cancer is also associated with a number of paraneoplastic syndromes (PNSs), which are conditions caused either by the hormones produced by the tumor or by the body's immune response to the tumor, and are present in about one-quarter of individuals with renal cell carcinoma.[346] These syndromes most commonly affect tissues that have not been invaded by the cancer. The most common PNSs seen in people with renal cell cancer are: anemia, high blood calcium, polycythaemia (the opposite of anemia, an overproduction of erythropoietin), and other blood abnormalities.

- **LAB STUDIES** used for diagnosis of renal cell carcinoma include the following:
  » Urinalysis
  » Complete blood cell count with differential
  » Electrolytes (sodium, potassium chloride, phosphorus)
  » Renal profile (creatinine, BUN)
  » Liver function tests (aspartate aminotransferase and alanine aminotransferase)
  » Serum calcium

- **IMAGING STUDIES** used to evaluate and stage renal masses include the following:
  » Excretory urography
  » CT scan
  » PET scan
  » Ultrasonography
  » Arteriography
  » Venography
  » MRI

CANCER STAGING

Staging is the process of finding out how much cancer there is in a person's body and where it's located. There are four stages of renal cancer and recurrent status:

• **Stage I:** The tumor is 7 cm or smaller and found only in the kidney.

• **Stage II:** The tumor is larger than 7 cm and is found only in the kidney.

• **Stage III:** The tumor is any size, and cancer is found in the kidney and also in one or more lymph nodes.

• **Stage IV:** The cancer has spread beyond the kidney to other organs such as the lungs, liver, bones, or brain and throughout the lymph nodes.

• **Recurrent:** Cancer has returned after it has been treated.

Renal Cancer Supplement Program

Multiple nutritional supplements have been associated with reduced cancer occurrence and/or cancer progression. The list below contains those with the greatest evidence base and benefit, though it is not necessary that they all be included.

ASTRAGALUS

SUGGESTED DOSE: Use of extract standardized to 0.4% 4-hydroxy-3-methoxy isoflavones: 250–500 mg, three to four times a day; powdered root: 250–500 mg, three to four times per day; tincture (1:5) in 30% ethanol: 20–60 drops, three times a day

A human cell study demonstrated that astragalus reduced oxidative damage to kidney cells.[347] Pretreatment of animal kidney cells with astragalus before the use of chemotherapy on these cells reduced the toxic effect of the chemotherapy without reducing its effectiveness.[348] Astragalus also slowed renal tumor progression in animal studies.[349]

LIGUSTRUM LUCIDUM

SUGGESTED DOSE: 5 mg, two to three times a day as a capsule or dried

When combined with astragalus, *Ligustrum*, a berry used in Chinese herbal medicine, also slowed renal tumor progression in animal studies.[350]

CAT'S CLAW (*UNCARIA TOMENTOSA*)

SUGGESTED DOSE: 250–350 mg per day of the ethanolic extract

Cat's claw has been used for decades to boost the immunity of the genito-urinary system. As a renal cancer therapy, it may prove useful, as it has anti-inflammatory effects in cancer cell line studies.[351]

MILK THISTLE EXTRACT (SILYMARIN)

SUGGESTED DOSE: 200 mg, two to three times per day

Human cells treated with milk thistle while undergoing chemotherapy demonstrated reduced toxicity from the chemotherapy.[352] Renal tumor size was significantly reduced in animals given milk thistle. Additionally, the use of milk thistle with common chemotherapy medications increased the effectiveness of the medications against the renal cancer.[353]

LICORICE ROOT

SUGGESTED DOSE: 100–600 mg per day, standardized at 25% glycyrrhizic acid[354]

An extract isolated from licorice root, called isoliquiritigenin, suppressed metastasis of renal cell cancer in an animal study. It also decreased the side effect of leukopenia from a common chemotherapy drug.[355] Animal studies also show that licorice root decreases the toxic side effects of the chemotherapy medication cisplatin on renal cells.[356]

LYCOPENE

SUGGESTED DOSE: 30 mg per day

Lycopene has been used as an immune stimulant in a variety of cancers. Blood levels of- lycopene were found to be inversely related to the risk of developing endometrial cancer in a group of females.[357]

BERBERINE

SUGGESTED DOSE: 500 mg, three times per day[358]

Human cell studies showed that mixing berberine with an immune peptide abbreviated as TRAIL (tumor necrosis factor–related apoptosis-inducing ligand) induced cell death in human renal cancer cells.[359] It has also demonstrated positive effects in animal studies with improvement to damaged kidney cells, and in human cell studies.[360, 361, 362]

VITAMIN D

SUGGESTED DOSE: May require 5,000 IU per day or more, depending on blood levels

A prospective study with a large human cohort found that higher plasma 25-OH vitamin D levels were associated with a significantly lower risk of renal cell cancer in men and women.[363] Additionally, research on the circulating vitamin D-binding protein (DBP) suggests a strong protective association observed between higher circulating DBP concentration and renal cancer risk.[364] The suggested dose is sufficient to raise 25-OH vitamin D levels to >40 ng/mL and optimally between 50 and 80 ng/mL.[365]

Dietary Action Plan

EMPHASIZE

- Antioxidant-rich, brightly colored fresh vegetables—especially broccoli, cauliflower, cabbage, onions, and garlic—leafy greens, and fresh fruits, especially berries (choose organic for all, if possible)

- Whole foods (foods that are as close to their natural form as possible)
- Research has shown that coconut oils protect kidney cells.[366]
- Low sugar/low glycemic diet due to the link between diabetes and renal cancer; glycemic index and glycemic load are measures of the effect on blood glucose level after a food containing carbohydrates is consumed.
- High fiber, from whole grains, beans, vegetables, and fruits
- For kidney cancer patients with significantly decreased renal function, it may be important to limit dietary intake of potassium, sodium, and phosphorus. In such situations, avoid meats, processed foods, and soda, which are high in phosphorus, and work with a nutritionist experienced in working with kidney disease patients. Or look up lists of low-potassium and high-potassium fruits and vegetables on the Internet, and choose the low-potassium ones. Also look up low-sodium and low-phosphorus diets—favor fresh and/or frozen produce over canned and processed food options.[367, 368]
- For animal protein, choose lean poultry and fish over red meat, and aim to view meat as a condiment rather than a staple. Try to choose grass-fed and organic meats and eggs whenever possible. Choose fish of salmon size or smaller to avoid excessive mercury and other environmental toxins that accumulate in large, long-lived fish.

AVOID
- Salty food that can contribute to hypertension
- Processed and grilled meats; try to limit intake of red meat. Managing excess proteins in the diet may also be critical for chronic kidney disease.[369]
- Fast foods, fried foods, baked goods, and packaged, processed foods
- Sugar, sweeteners, and artificial sweeteners, which can worsen diabetes
- Vegetable oils, shortening, margarine, and anything with hydrogenated or partially hydrogenated oils

Top 5 Lifestyle Interventions

1. Limit or eliminate alcohol. Alcohol is known to compromise liver function, and as a result this can exacerbate kidney disease.[370] Long-term alcohol consumption is also known to directly affect kidney cells.[371]

2. Do not smoke or expose yourself to secondhand smoke. Cigarette smoking is a known contributing factor to renal cancer.[372]

3. Avoid high glycemic foods (and sugar) and the risk of developing diabetes. However, even without diabetes the long-term ingestion of a high-sugar diet can lead to kidney damage.[373]

4. Maintain healthy cholesterol levels and ratios.[374, 375]

5. Stay in a healthy weight range.

Important Nutrient/Drug Interactions

Given that many nutritional interventions have the potential to both increase the effectiveness of conventional treatments and possibly interfere with their effects, combined use should always be supervised. For example, astragalus may increase urinary excretion due to its diuretic effect on the kidneys. Licorice root in large quantities can also lower potassium levels and may need monitoring. Additionally, licorice root may exacerbate hypertension in some individuals, so blood pressure should be monitored.[376]

THYROID CANCER
Thyroid Cancer Basics

- Approximately 1.1 percent of men and women will be diagnosed with differentiated thyroid cancer at some point during their lifetime, based on 2009–2011 SEER data.[377]

- In 2011, there were an estimated 566,708 people living with thyroid cancer in the United States, and thyroid cancer represented 3.8 percent of all new cancer cases.[378]

- Additionally, recent studies demonstrate that thyroid cancer rates seem to be rising, but some of this increase may be related to more aggressive diagnosis, and all of the increase represents papillary thyroid cancer, which is the least dangerous type.[379]

- The 5-year survival rate from differentiated thyroid cancer is estimated between 97 and 99 percent, although some less common forms of thyroid cancer have lower survival rates.[380] These are outlined ahead under the rather complex thyroid cancer staging system.

Causes/Contributing Factors

Among the most well-established risk factors include:

- Exposure to ionizing radiation in the head and neck, especially during childhood.[381] Telomere shortening, which can occur as a result of radiation and chemotherapy, appears to be a mechanism underlying the increased risk of thyroid cancer following these treatments.[382]

- Hereditary factors increase the risk of developing thyroid cancer. New research is focusing on the genetics and epigenetics of cancer development, and thyroid cancer may be linked to having the C677T polymorphism in the MTHFR gene, which means there is a mutation in the gene that codes for the enzyme that reduces folic acid to the form needed by the body.[383, 384] Thyroid cancer occurs more often in some families and is often seen at an earlier age when it runs in families, especially papillary thyroid cancer. Genes on chromosome 19 and chromosome 1 are suspected of causing these familial cancers.

Other risk factors include:

- Hormone influences of estrogen. The rate of thyroid cancer increases at puberty in females and only declines after menopause. Estrogen appears to be a growth factor for both benign and malignant thyroid cells.[385]

- Obesity is associated with risk of papillary thyroid cancer as well as more negative outcomes, such as severity of the cancer and metastases.[386, 387]

- Diabetes in females. Women with diabetes mellitus are at a greater risk for developing thyroid cancer.[388]

- Low dietary iodine intake. Follicular thyroid cancers are more common in areas of low iodine.

Relevant Diagnostic Testing

- **SYMPTOMS AND PHYSICAL EXAM:** Blood tests are not typically used to look for thyroid cancer, although a type of thyroid disease called Hashimoto's thyroiditis, which produces antibodies that can be measured via blood testing, is linked to a higher risk of thyroid cancer. It appears to be a less dangerous type of thyroid cancer.[389] Finding nodules or a mass in the neck near or on the thyroid gland is often the first sign of thyroid cancer that a physician will find. Physical symptoms can include a lump in the neck, swelling in the neck, pain in the neck (that can radiate up to the ears), hoarseness, trouble swallowing, or trouble breathing.

- **IMAGING AND SCANS:** A radioactive iodine uptake scan can detect the type of nodule that absorbs more radioactive iodine, known as hot nodules; these are more likely benign. A CT scan is a type of x-ray that can diagnose larger thyroid nodules or goiter. An MRI can locate tumors, assess tumor size, and look for tumor spread. A thyroid ultrasound can detect if a thyroid nodule is a fluid-filled cyst or a solid-filled mass.

- **NEEDLE BIOPSY:** Suspicious thyroid nodules will need to be biopsied to determine the type of tissue that's present. Typically thyroid nodules are biopsied using a needle, in a procedure known as fine needle aspiration biopsy, often guided by ultrasound imaging.

CANCER STAGING

Staging is the process of finding out how much cancer there is in a person's body and where it's located. Unlike most other cancers, thyroid cancers are grouped into stages in a way that also considers the subtype of thyroid cancer and the patient's age.

THYROID CANCER STAGING SYSTEM

Papillary or follicular (differentiated) thyroid cancer in patients younger than 45

• Younger people have a low likelihood of dying from differentiated (papillary or follicular) thyroid cancer. The TNM stage groupings for these cancers take this fact into account. So all people younger than 45 years with these cancers are stage I if they have no distant spread and stage II if they have distant spread.

• **Stage I (any T, any N, M0):** The tumor can be any size (any T) and may or may not have spread to nearby lymph nodes (any N). It has not spread to distant sites (M0).

• **Stage II (any T, any N, M1):** The tumor can be any size (any T) and may or may not have spread to nearby lymph nodes (any N). It has spread to distant sites (M1).

Papillary or follicular (differentiated) thyroid cancer in patients 45 years and older

• **Stage I (T1, N0, M0):** The tumor is 2 cm or less across and has not grown outside the thyroid (T1). It has not spread to nearby lymph nodes (N0) or distant sites (M0).

• **Stage II (T2, N0, M0):** The tumor is more than 2 cm but not larger than 4 cm across and has not grown outside the thyroid (T2). It has not spread to nearby lymph nodes (N0) or distant sites (M0).

• **Stage III:** One of the following applies:

   » **T3, N0, M0:** The tumor is larger than 4 cm across or has grown slightly outside the thyroid (T3), but it has not spread to nearby lymph nodes (N0) or distant sites (M0).

   » **T1 TO T3, N1A, M0:** The tumor is any size and may have grown slightly outside the thyroid (T1 to T3). It has spread to lymph nodes around the thyroid in the neck (N1a) but not to other lymph nodes or to distant sites (M0).

• **Stage IVA:** One of the following applies:

   » **T4A, any N, M0:** The tumor is any size and has grown beyond the thyroid gland and into nearby tissues of the neck (T4a). It might or might not have spread to nearby lymph nodes (any N). It has not spread to distant sites (M0).

> » **T1 TO T3, N1B, M0:** The tumor is any size and might have grown slightly outside the thyroid gland (T1 to T3). It has spread to certain lymph nodes in the neck (cervical nodes) or to lymph nodes in the upper chest (superior mediastinal nodes) or behind the throat (retropharyngeal nodes; N1b), but it has not spread to distant sites (M0).

• **Stage IVB (T4B, any N, M0):** The tumor is any size and has grown either back toward the spine or into nearby large blood vessels (T4b). It might or might not have spread to nearby lymph nodes (any N), but it has not spread to distant sites (M0).

• **Stage IVC (any T, any N, M1):** The tumor is any size and might or might not have grown outside the thyroid (any T). It might or might not have spread to nearby lymph nodes (any N). It has spread to distant sites (M1).

Medullary thyroid cancer (age is not a factor in the stage of medullary thyroid cancer)

• **Stage I (T1, N0, M0):** The tumor is 2 cm or less across and has not grown outside the thyroid (T1). It has not spread to nearby lymph nodes (N0) or distant sites (M0).

• **Stage II:** One of the following applies:

> » **T2, N0, M0:** The tumor is more than 2 cm but is not larger than 4 cm across and has not grown outside the thyroid (T2). It has not spread to nearby lymph nodes (N0) or distant sites (M0).

> » **T3, N0, M0:** The tumor is larger than 4 cm or has grown slightly outside the thyroid (T3), but it has not spread to nearby lymph nodes (N0) or distant sites (M0).

• **Stage III (T1 TO T3, N1A, M0):** The tumor is any size and might have grown slightly outside the thyroid (T1 to T3). It has spread to lymph nodes around the thyroid in the neck (N1a) but not to other lymph nodes or to distant sites (M0).

• **Stage IVA:** One of the following applies:

> » **T4A, any N, M0:** The tumor is any size and has grown beyond the thyroid gland and into nearby tissues of the neck (T4a). It might or might not have spread to nearby lymph nodes (any N). It has not spread to distant sites (M0).

> » **T1 TO T3, N1B, M0:** The tumor is any size and might have grown slightly outside the thyroid gland (T1 to T3). It has spread to certain lymph nodes in the neck (cervical nodes) or to lymph nodes in the upper chest (superior mediastinal nodes) or behind the throat (retropharyngeal nodes; N1b), but it has not spread to distant sites (M0).

- **Stage IVB (T4B, any N, M0):** The tumor is any size and has grown either back toward the spine or into nearby large blood vessels (T4b). It might or might not have spread to nearby lymph nodes (any N), but it has not spread to distant sites (M0).

- **Stage IVC (any T, any N, M1):** The tumor is any size and might or might not have grown outside the thyroid (any T). It might or might not have spread to nearby lymph nodes (any N). It has spread to distant sites (M1).

Anaplastic (undifferentiated) thyroid cancer—all anaplastic thyroid cancers are considered stage IV, reflecting the poor prognosis of this type of cancer

- **Stage IVA (T4A, any N, M0):** The tumor is still within the thyroid (T4a). It might or might not have spread to nearby lymph nodes (any N), but it has not spread to distant sites (M0).

- **Stage IVB (T4B, any N, M0):** The tumor has grown outside the thyroid (T4b). It might or might not have spread to nearby lymph nodes (any N), but it has not spread to distant sites (M0).

- **Stage IVC (any T, any N, M1):** The tumor might or might not have grown outside of the thyroid (any T). It might or might not have spread to nearby lymph nodes (any N). It has spread to distant sites (M1).

RECURRENT CANCER: This is not an actual stage in the TNM system. Cancer that comes back after treatment is called recurrent (or relapsed). If thyroid cancer returns, it is usually in the neck, but it may come back in another part of the body (for example, lymph nodes, lungs, or bones). Doctors may assign a new stage based on how far the cancer has spread, but this is not usually as formal a process as the original staging. The presence of recurrent disease does not change the original, formal staging.

Thyroid Cancer Supplement Program

Multiple nutritional supplements have been associated with reduced cancer occurrence and/or cancer progression. The list below contains those with the greatest evidence base and benefit, though it is not necessary that they all be included.

VITAMIN D
SUGGESTED DOSE: May require 5,000 IU per day or more, depending on blood levels

Vitamin D levels are associated with risk of several types of cancer, including thyroid cancer. Low 25-OH vitamin D blood levels were highly prevalent in people with solid tumors in a retrospective study of more than 30,000 individuals, despite levels infrequently being checked.[390] Individuals with a history of lymphoma should also monitor 1,25-dihydroxyvitamin D levels, as rapid conversion to this active form has been observed. The suggested dose is sufficient to raise 25-OH vitamin D levels to >40 ng/mL and optimally between 50 and 80 ng/mL.[391]

SELENIUM

SUGGESTED DOSE: 200 mcg, one to two times per day

Selenium is essential to keep an important antioxidant, called glutathione peroxidase, at proper levels. This enzyme serves to deactivate hydrogen peroxide (in concert with another enzyme called catalase) in thyroid cells. Hydrogen peroxide is a free radical–producing molecule created during the process of iodine and tyrosine combining to make the thyroid hormone thyroxine (T4). A human trial demonstrated that selenium levels were inversely correlated to more advanced thyroid disease.[392]

DIM (3,3′-DIINDOLYLMETHANE)

SUGGESTED DOSE: 300 mg per day

DIM, abundant in cruciferous vegetables, such as broccoli, cauliflower, and cabbage, has shown antitumor activity and inhibits cancer cell proliferation in estrogen receptor positive and negative cells. DIM displays antiestrogenic-like activity by inhibiting estradiol-enhanced thyroid cancer cell proliferation and in vitro metastasis–associated events, namely adhesion, migration, and invasion.[393, 394, 395]

GREEN TEA EXTRACT

SUGGESTED DOSE: 1 g EGCG and mixed catechins per day

Catechins, antioxidants that are found in green tea, particularly EGCG (epigallocatechin-3-gallate), are known to have numerous antimetastatic and anticancer effects in a variety of cancers that are hormone driven (such as breast and prostate cancer). A study on human thyroid cells supports the inhibitory role of EGCG on thyroid cancer cell proliferation and motility.[396]

CURCUMIN

SUGGESTED DOSE: 1–2 g per day of Meriva or Longvida curcumin

Cell studies researched the effects of curcumin on the cell viability, apoptosis, migration, and invasion of human thyroid cancer cell lines and found that curcumin produced antimetastatic activity. The findings project that curcumin might be an effective tumor growth reducing agent for the treatment of aggressive papillary thyroid carcinomas.[397, 398, 399]

MILK THISTLE

SUGGESTED DOSE: 500 mg silymarin per day

Silymarin and silibinin from milk thistle have antiproliferative and antimetastatic properties in various cancer cell lines. One study demonstrated that one of the active constituents of milk thistle, silibinin, decreased cell migration in thyroid cancer cells.[400]

Dietary Action Plan

EMPHASIZE

- Organic fruits and vegetables, as pesticides and bisphenol A may interact with thyroid health
- Whole foods (foods that are as close to their natural form as possible)
- Low sugar/low glycemic diet; glycemic index and glycemic load are measures of the effect on blood glucose level after a food containing carbohydrates is consumed
- High fiber, from whole grains, beans, vegetables, and fruits
- Healthy fats, from avocados, nuts, seeds, olive oil, coconut oil, and cold-water fish. Frequent adult consumption of saltwater fish decreases the risk of thyroid cancer.[401]
- For animal protein, choose lean poultry and fish over red meat, and aim to view meat as a condiment rather than a staple. Try to choose grass-fed and organic meats and eggs whenever possible. Eat no fish larger than a salmon to minimize environmental contaminants, including mercury.

AVOID

- Foods that contain substances called goitrogens, which have known effects on thyroid functioning. They are found in turnips, cabbages, rutabagas, mustard greens, soybeans, radishes, peanuts, pine nuts, and millet.
- Fast foods, fried foods, baked goods, and packaged, processed foods
- Sugar, sweeteners, and artificial sweeteners
- Vegetable oils, shortening, margarine, and anything with hydrogenated or partially hydrogenated oils

Top 5 Lifestyle Interventions

1. Maintain a healthy weight.
2. Engage in physical activity, which many studies suggest reduces risks of all hormone-driven cancers, including thyroid. (Differentiated thyroid cancers are driven by the pituitary hormone called TSH, not by the thyroid hormone itself.)
3. Avoid alcohol and smoking.

4. Focus on hormone-free, organic, whole foods to decrease exposure to pesticides and hormones.

5. Practice mindfulness-based stress reduction, like breathing techniques, yoga, Pilates, and meditation.

Important Nutrient/Drug Interactions

Given that many nutritional interventions have the potential to both increase the effectiveness of conventional treatments and possibly interfere with their effects, combined use should always be supervised. For example, DIM has been shown to potentiate the effects of several types of chemotherapy in cell-based studies and may increase the effectiveness of therapy.[402, 403]

PART THREE

EMOTIONAL
HEALTH

CHAPTER NINE

STRESS AND
MENTAL HEALTH

NTEGRATIVE MEDICINE, THE KIND WE ADVOCATE AND PRACTICE, VIEWS HUMANKIND THE
way Viktor Frankl, MD, the 20th-century Austrian neurologist and psychiatrist,
did: as spirit, mind, and body. Each of these areas has a profound effect. The terms
heartbroken and *sick at heart* are far more than romantic metaphors; they describe a
real physical condition, even though there may be no viral or bacterial cause. When
the heart is at ease, it is well. When it is *dis*-eased, the spirit, mind, and body—either
individually or in combination—need to be addressed. Broken heart syndrome—
often caused by an emotional trauma—is now a medically recognized cause of a
sudden decrease in heart pump function, also known as *takotsubo cardiomyopathy*.

In Western medicine, the body, spirit, and mind have traditionally been
segregated. Medicine's focus on the body, how its organs function and how its
blood flows, ignores the physical effects of the spirit and thus creates a purely
mechanistic view. To many doctors, our bodies are machines to be fixed, not
people to be healed.

In the 17th century, the French philosopher René Descartes concluded that
there were two separate substances in the world: matter, which behaved according to physical laws, and spirit, which was dimensionless and immaterial, with an
unbridgeable chasm between the two. Body and spirit; brain and mind—these
were two entities that were considered to be distinct and discrete parts of human
life that had to be looked at separately.

Descartes's concept dominated medical and religious thought for centuries. Usually, Western medicine does not treat the inner person, only the body; Western religion does not treat the body, only the spirit. Only now are doctors beginning to recognize the enormous role that the spirit, mind, and emotions play in wellness, disease, healing, and the maintenance of health.

While Western thought and practice remained blind to the correlation between spirit and body, societies in other parts of the world had long recognized a connection. More than 4,000 years ago in China, careful observers noticed that illness followed frustration. The Egyptians during the same period prescribed good cheer and an optimistic attitude as beneficial for health. The Greeks suggested rest and relaxation for illness, and the first-century Roman physician Galen observed that happy women had less incidence of breast cancer than those who were melancholy. And in the biblical book of Proverbs, you find the statement, "A merry heart maketh good medicine."

William James, the pioneering 19th-century American psychologist and philosopher, and Frankl both recognized humankind's search for a higher meaning and significance in life. "The pleasure principle might be termed the will to pleasure," Frankl writes in *Man's Search for Meaning*. "The status drive is equivalent to the will-to-power. But where do we hear of that which most deeply inspires man; where is the innate desire to give as much meaning as possible to one's life, to actualize as many values as possible—what I should like to call the will-to-meaning?"

The "will-to-meaning," he says, is the most distinctly human phenomenon of all, since no other animal is concerned about the meaning of its existence. Yet this life force—for that is exactly what it is—is ironically often overlooked by doctors whose purpose it is to maintain a patient's healthy life. Both James and Frankl understood that the body *and* the brain could be the source of sickness. They recognized a lack of spiritual fulfillment as predictive of illness; they understood the power of spirituality, the quest for life's purpose, the vital link between body and soul.

For humankind to be centered, whole, and fulfilled, the spiritual aspect of life must play a role. Whether in the context of organized religion, in support groups without particular religious affiliation, or by following an individual path of meditation and contemplation, some form of spiritual nourishment and solace is necessary. There is empirical scientific evidence that now supports this statement. According to new studies, not only does cancer cause stress, but stress promotes cancer once it's present. It's a vicious cycle that would be almost laughable if it weren't so deadly serious.

The cruel irony of stress and cancer is that while the nature of remission and follow-up monitoring is very anxiety provoking, we are now learning from basic research that stress can powerfully facilitate the process of metastasis in animal models.[1] In addition, it has been reported that stress-related psychosocial factors have led to higher cancer incidence in initially healthy people, poorer outcomes in patients diagnosed with cancer, and higher cancer mortality rates.

In a study in the *Journal of Psychosomatic Research* in 2007 from the University of Rochester, Dr. O. Palish reported that a history of stressful or traumatic life events may reduce resistance to tumor growth.[2] These findings were consistent with the possible long-lasting effect of previous life stress on stress response systems such as the hypothalamic-pituitary-adrenal (HPA) axis, the connection between the brain and the adrenals that coordinates stress response and release of hormones, proteins, and adrenaline, among other things.

In 2010, researchers at UCLA's Jonsson Comprehensive Cancer Center discovered that stress biologically reprograms the immune cells that are trying to fight the cancer, transforming them from soldiers protecting the body against disease into aiders and abettors of disease. They documented a thirtyfold increase in the spread of cancer throughout the bodies of stressed mice, compared to those that were not stressed. The researchers were able to halt these effects by treating the stressed animals with a drug that slows the metabolic process, called a beta-blocker. They also felt that healthy lifestyle behaviors such as exercise and stress-reduction techniques may influence biological pathways described in the study.[3]

The second part of this research, headed by Dr. Erica Sloan, showed that stress affected the metastatic cancer cells more than the primary tumor, thus emphasizing the role of stress in recurrence. When cancer recurs, the immune system sends out macrophages to try to repair the tissue damage caused by the uncontrolled growth of the cancer cells, while macrophages turn on inflammation genes that are part of the normal immune response to injury. However, the cancer cells feed on the growth factors involved in the normal immune response, causing increased bloodflow to the cancer, allowing it to grow and spread. Stress signals from the sympathetic nervous system enhance recruitment in this process and inadvertently facilitate escape of cancer cells into other parts of the body.

In the journal *Brain, Behavior, and Immunity*, Shamgar Ben-Eliyahu, PhD, a professor in the Department of Psychology of Tel Aviv University, reported that stress hormones can prevent healthy immune function, and stress and fear can affect cancer recurrence.[4] Psychological fear may be no less important than real physiologic tissue damage in suppressing immune competence during and after cancer therapy. Cancer surgery is a known immune suppressant, which takes place just when the immune system needs to be functioning at high levels to kill tumor tissue scattered throughout the body. In a study published in 1989, researchers at London's clinical oncology unit at Guy's Hospital found that women who had experienced life stressors were nine times more likely to have a relapse of breast cancer.

In a 2008 study by scientists at Ohio State University, breast cancer patients who had psychological intervention were documented to have a lower risk of cancer recurrence, and those who were taught relaxation methods had a 45 percent lower chance of cancer coming back than women who had only psychological assessment. In a follow-up study by the same group, an astounding 59 percent reduction in mortality was shown among women with recurrence who had an earlier psychological intervention to prevent stress.

Robert Cameron, MD, chief of thoracic surgery at UCLA Medical School, believes, "Many types of stress activate the body's endocrine system, which in turn can alter the way the immune system, the body's defense against infection and disease including cancer, functions. Uncontrolled emotional stress may lead to fatigue and lower the cancer patient's already compromised immune system." Additionally, when the body releases the stress hormone norepinephrine, it also stimulates production of compounds that contribute to aggressive tumor growth. Norepinephrine causes the tumor to produce two metalloproteinase compounds that break down part of the tumor structure to which the cancer cells adhere. Once such cells are no longer bound to the primary tumor, these cells spread through the body and metastasize elsewhere, causing rapid tumor growth. Norepinephrine also increases the production of growth factors that stimulate new blood vessels that feed cancer cells, a process called neo-angiogenesis. The resulting increased blood supply to cancer cells directly accelerates spread and growth of the tumor.

George Kulik, PhD, of Wake Forest University, reported in the *Journal of Biological Chemistry* that the levels of epinephrine that increase sharply in stressful situations can remain continuously elevated during persistent stress and depression. Studying prostate and breast cancer cells in the laboratory, Dr. Kulik and colleagues found that a protein, BCL-2-associated agonist of cell death, abbreviated as BAD, which causes cell death, becomes inactive when cancer cells are exposed to epinephrine.

Recent advances in medical technology have enabled us to visualize the brain's centers of emotion. This is achieved by the development of the functional MRI. Using this new technology, scientists are able to map out the areas of the brain that are functioning while a person is feeling, remembering, or thinking of a specific topic. Centers of negative emotions like fear, anxiety, and anger can be demarcated, as can centers of positive and pleasurable thoughts.

The areas identified in this process are in the midbrain and lower forebrain. Particularly involved is the hypothalamic–pituitary-adrenal (HPA) axis. It is immensely important, because this is the same axis through which messages to the rest of the body are sent from the brain by means of nerve impulse, neuro-peptide secretion, and circulation of hormones. Through this pathway, the 50 trillion cells of our body communicate and our nervous, endocrine, immune, and lymphatic systems interact.

The fight-or-flight reaction is evoked via this axis. Negative emotions can produce oxidative free radicals, cortisol, epinephrine, high blood sugar, high blood pressure, bone loss, and suppression of the immune system. In fact, recent studies have shown decreased recurrence risk of breast cancer in women who take a class of medication called beta-blockers for high blood pressure. These drugs essentially block the effect of adrenaline, the key molecule of the fight-or-flight response triggered by fear. (As mentioned earlier, beta-blockers were also found to be effective in laboratory mice at UCLA's Jonsson Compre-hensive Cancer Center.)

Unlike the gray-mattered cortex, which is our filter of the reality of space and time, this HPA axis responds to all information received as if it were real and happening now. Therefore, any negative events, thoughts, or feelings pro-cessed in these areas of the brain release a cascade of hormones, peptides, and sugars that create a chain reaction of activity in our body. Chronic triggering of this axis can lead to immune suppression, cell atrophy, RNA expression, and DNA mutation.

At the same time, studies done over the last 30 years that examined the relationship between stress and cancer have produced conflicting results. While some studies show a link between psychological factors and an increased risk of developing cancer, a direct cause-and-effect relationship has not been proven. However, evidence from both animal and human studies sug-gests that chronic stress weakens a person's immune system, which in turn may affect the incidence of cancer. Furthermore, it is difficult to separate stress from other physical or emotional factors when examining cancer risk. Behav-ioral factors such as using alcohol, smoking, and obesity are not only linked to cancer but often associated with the negative emotions that may accompany stressful situations.

The conundrum of how to manage stress to prevent recurrence of the very thing that is causing you stress is in itself, well, stressful.

So how is one to proceed in the face of inconclusive evidence? As physicians, we can quote the ancient Roman dictate *Primum nil nocere* (Above all, do no harm). Improving your attitude, outlook on life, and mental health can do noth-ing but improve your well-being. When recommending stress-management modalities, we can look at the risk-benefit ratio. Certainly incorporating stress-reducing techniques into your lifestyle can have great benefits with very little risk incurred. So, when one is trying to maximize and optimize health after cancer therapy, incorporating some stress-management modality into daily activities is really a no-brainer.

We're not alone in this thinking. The Commission on Cancer (COC), which accredits many cancer centers around the country, now mandates proper psychological distress management screening tools and treatments as part of its criteria for full accreditation beginning in 2015.

YOUR CANCER, YOUR STRESS

For patients who have completed cancer treatment and are in remission, one of the longest-lasting and ever-present factors of their new life is, in fact, stress. It may seem counterintuitive, but the stress following treatment can actually be worse than during treatment.

Being diagnosed with cancer and beginning treatment can be a whirlwind of emotion and activity. Everyone is focused on saving your life—your doctors, your family, your close friends, maybe even your colleagues and acquaintances. You have a team of supporters who are doing everything they can to help you win this battle against cancer.

Your days are filled with treatments and doctor visits. There are important decisions to make and big discussions to have with your doctors and family. Things like money, success at your job, and whether or not your child watches too much TV may seem trivial while you are in treatment. Every part of your being is focused on just being around to have these worries.

When treatment ends, however, you can be left feeling powerless and empty. Cancer survivors describe feeling everything from a sense of anticlimax to deep depression. Dr. Mehta estimates that 10 to 15 percent of his breast cancer patients opt to go on antidepressant medication at some point following their cancer treatment. Studies show that cancer survivors experience higher levels of anxiety and depression than the general population for years following their treatment, even when they remain in remission.

Once treatment is concluded, all the mundanities and typical life stressors— like paying your credit card bill or whether you get that promotion—become front and center again. Quite often they are exacerbated by the treatment and illness itself. Financial worries are a major stressor for people following cancer care. Many cancer patients go into debt during their treatment due to medical bills and time away from work. Another stressor is ongoing issues that may have seemed trivial when you were unsure of your prognosis. Now that you are healthy again, you and your spouse may fall back into a pattern of fighting and bickering, or your teenager, who was so uncharacteristically helpful while you were undergoing chemo, may slip right back into his precancer rebellious stage. In addition,

Ashley's Story

Ashley, who underwent a double mastectomy and 6 weeks of chemotherapy at age 33, likened the experience of her treatment ending to the feeling after a big wedding. Suddenly all the attention is no longer on you. Yet you are still feeling much of the stress, anxiety, and physical aftereffects of your illness. And for patients who have this reaction to the end of treatment, the feeling of depression can be exacerbated by feelings of guilt for having these feelings in the first place!

"You're in survival mode, and then everything settles down and you're left with all this baggage," said Ashley. "One, you're left with the fact that your body is defying you, and, two, my self-worth got wrapped up in that I had cancer—and then when I didn't have cancer, my self-worth was gone. And then that survival guilt is difficult: You got to live, and you're worrying about this?!"

Ashley's feelings following her treatment are common, which she discovered when speaking to other cancer survivors.

Cancer survivors may also feel anger and sadness about what they had to go through during their treatment, as well as anger over long-term effects of the cancer. And the hard parts aren't always what you think they will be. Ashley has had little long-term emotion about losing her breasts, but losing her hair affected her in very unexpected ways. "I think I handled the double mastectomy really well," she says, laughing. "I had my friends over and wore a Hooters tank top."

But almost 2 years after being declared cancer-free, she hates to look in the mirror and see her mid-length hair, which is only now long enough to pull into a stubby ponytail and is a reminder of everything she went through. "I always had long, blonde hair, and it grew back brunette. I wasn't a short hair person, and I'm not now. But I look in the mirror, and that's what I see. It's a reminder. It's like having a tattoo on your face."

for those who have finished treatment, scars or short hair can be ongoing reminders of what they've been through and what they could go through again.

The time following cancer may also feel like a strange letdown. For months or even years, everything has been about the cancer. Many cancer patients become invested in their view of themselves as someone fighting cancer. Suddenly, with no cancer, who are they?

One of the most stressful aspects of finishing cancer treatment is the knowledge that it can recur at any time. For most cancer survivors, the years following their treatment can feel like an endless waiting game. Unlike those treated for many diseases, cancer survivors are rarely told they are cured, but rather that they are in remission. Depending on the type, stage, and grade of cancer, each survivor is given a different prognosis or expectation that she will remain in remission. Many cancer survivors feel anxiety about recurrence, particularly when they visit their doctor for blood work and scans.

Feeling powerless over whether or not you are out of the woods can increase your anxiety. We are trapped by fears that can become self-fulfilling prophesies of future illness. As you continue to read this book and explore the relationship between emotion and health, you will learn ways to replace fear with confidence.

Many of the integrative oncology centers and treatment centers looking at postcancer protocols now take the emotional into consideration with the physical. To reduce the risk of recurrence, the Johns Hopkins Breast Center recommends taking care of yourself emotionally and physically by maintaining healthy weight, reducing stress, eating well, limiting alcohol consumption, quitting smoking, and staying involved in community activities, as well as checking your vitamin D level.

In *Radical Remission,* author Kelly A. Turner, PhD, analyzed more than 1,000 cases of radical remission (which she defines as "any cancer remission that is statistically unexpected") and found nine things that seemed to come up in almost every case: "radically changing your diet; taking control of your health; following your intuition; using herbs and supplements; releasing suppressed emotions; increasing positive emotions; embracing social support; deepening your spiritual connection; [and] having strong reasons for living." Surprising to her and many readers, only three of the nine factors were physical changes; the other six were emotional and mental. It appeared that the mental and emotional changes these patients made were as important, if not more important, than the physical changes.

We agree that the mind-body connection is vastly important for both the recovery of cancer patients and to help stave off both cancer recurrence and other disease. Additionally, the success of cancer survivors cannot be factored only in regard to whether they have no recurrence or how long they are healthy before recurrence, but also how they live the life they have left. All of us will die eventually; what truly matters is the quality of the life we lead while we are alive.

Our recommendations for improving your quality of life and spiritual and mental health loosely mirror Dr. Turner's six emotional factors for health for life after cancer. We recommend you: find a stress-management technique that works for you; find a spiritual connection; create a support system; find your balance; reduce the negatives and find the positives in your life; face death; and do for others. We'll expand upon each of these recommendations in the coming chapters.

DEPRESSION

One note before moving on to techniques for stress management and emotional wellness. A cancer diagnosis and treatment can exacerbate symptoms of previous emotional and mental illnesses such as depression, and can be especially debilitating for people who do not have a strong social support system. The treatments for cancer can also affect depression. Breast cancer, for example, involves hormonal treatment, and premenopausal women can be made postmenopausal in the space of a month.

Patients can also be pushed into a serious depression over concern about finances, inability to partake in activities they once cared about, changes in their looks, loss of control, and fear of death.

Depression can be extremely serious and even life threatening, and should not be treated lightly. Signs of serious depression include tearfulness and crying without provocation, withdrawal from activities you normally enjoy, difficulty sleeping at night or excessive sleeping during the day, and irritability. If you experience any of these symptoms, seek immediate medical advice from your primary doctor or your oncologist.

CHAPTER TEN

STRESS-
MANAGEMENT
TECHNIQUES

W E KNOW THAT CANCER AND ITS TREATMENT ARE EXTREMELY STRESSFUL FOR patients, and that this stress can factor into the chances for recurrence. Fortunately, we also know that there are many effective methods for managing stress.

There are complementary medicine techniques such as biofeedback, massage, acupuncture and acupressure, and use of specific botanicals known as adaptogens. There are even prescription beta-blockers, conventionally used to treat high blood pressure, which have been shown to improve cancer survival—very likely because they block the effects of stress hormones such as adrenaline and cortisol.

There are also stress relievers that are based in body movement and breathing, such as yoga, qigong, tai chi, Reiki, HeartMath, meditation, guided imagery, and progressive muscle relaxation. Any of these techniques can not only limit your anxiety and affect your happiness, but also keep you healthier.

There have been a number of studies addressing stress management and cancer. The best studied example of relaxation training comes from the research led by Barbara Andersen, PhD, of Ohio State University's James Cancer Center, in which 227 randomized patients who had been surgically treated for stage II (node positive) or III (locally advanced +/- node positive) breast cancer were followed for more than 11 years.[1] The relaxation training used was progressive muscle relaxation. Half of the patients were enrolled in the intervention program, while the other half were simply assessed on a regular basis. All received their regular medical treatments as well.

Those in the intervention group met weekly in groups of 8 to 12 with a clinical psychologist. During these weekly sessions, which continued for 4 months, participants learned progressive muscle relaxation for stress reduction; problem solving for common difficulties (such as fatigue); exercise and diet tips; and how to find support from family and friends, deal with treatment side effects, and keep up with medical treatment and follow-up.

After 4 months of weekly sessions, participants met monthly for 8 months. Researchers did a follow-up analysis in which they excluded people who were put in the intervention group but who attended fewer than 20 percent of the sessions (16 of the 114 participants fit this requirement).

When the infrequent attendees were excluded, the remainder had a 68 percent reduced risk of breast cancer death, compared to the 56 percent risk reduction for the whole participant group, which included those 16 who attended fewer than 20 percent of the sessions. Among patients who died of breast cancer, those who participated in the intervention program lived longer—an average of 6.1 years for program participants versus 4.8 years for those who were simply assessed. Any cancer drug that produced such a dramatic survival difference after breast cancer recurrence would be big news.

Intervention participants were also less likely to die from other causes such as heart disease or other cancers than breast cancer. For those who died of any cause, participants in the intervention lived an average of 6 years compared to 5 years for those who weren't. As Dr. Andersen commented, "Many of the strategies patients learned in the intervention program, such as stress reduction, may have protected them from heart disease and other causes of death."

Yoga

Although now extremely popular for both fitness and stress management throughout the West, yoga got its start some 5,000 years ago in India. While yoga has eight elements to it, when we talk about yoga today, we are generally referring to asanas, or postures. Yoga postures are undertaken to strengthen and purify the body. The asanas align the physical parts of your body—bones, muscles, soft tissues—while opening up channels of energy. Yoga is beneficial for physical strength and endurance, relieves muscle strain, provides flexibility, and increases your heart rate while lowering your blood pressure. It is also said to help regulate your adrenal glands and flush your lymph system, which are good things for those who have been treated for cancer.

The upside to yoga's popularity is that even if you live in a rural area, you should be able to find a local yoga studio—or barring that, you can buy a DVD or subscribe to an online yoga class. The downside is that not all yoga studios are created alike. Look for one where students are encouraged to listen to their bodies and where the values of breathing and meditation are encouraged more than how challenging your postures are. And although handstands may look intimidating, yoga can be done by anyone, including those with physical challenges. Find a yoga studio that embraces students of all levels.

Qigong

Not well known in the West, qigong is practiced in China, Japan, and Korea, and is related to Daoism, Buddhism, and Confucianism. The practice combines physical postures, breathing, and mental focus. Qigong is considered a health care practice and can manifest as the soft, slower practice of tai chi or the more intense practice of kung fu.

Tai Chi

Tai chi has been described as moving meditation. The practice combines gentle postures with breathing and mental concentration. It has been shown to have aerobic, balance, and muscle-strengthening benefits, as well as reduce anxiety and help with sleep. Tai chi is low impact, so it is accessible for practitioners of any age or physical ability. You can find a tai chi group to practice with in most urban areas, but it can also be done on your own at home. There are many tai chi resources available on the Internet.

Reiki

Reiki is a spiritual alternative medicine methodology developed in Japan. It utilizes the laying on of hands and purports to circulate life force from the practitioner to the client. Japanese and Western Reiki diverge in several ways, with Western Reiki using the concept of the seven chakras. While there is no evidence that Reiki treats any disease, it does provide relaxation benefits. You can find Reiki centers in most urban areas.

HeartMath

In HeartMath, you learn to moderate your body's responses to anxiety and stress by monitoring your heart rhythms. The Institute of HeartMath sells heart-monitoring equipment and books. Some people find it easier to connect to the quantitative aspect of HeartMath than to meditation or more traditional methods of relaxation.

Meditation

Meditating is defined as a state of thought-less awareness, in which the mind is emptied of worries and is calm but alert. You can meditate alone or with a group. Adherents recommend making a daily practice of meditation, even just 15 or 20 minutes a day. You might also start your day with a short meditation of just 5 or 10 minutes, and then meditate for a longer period later in the day. Some practitioners find listening to Indian ragas helps, while others find that acknowledging and forgiving worries or nagging thoughts can clear the mind.

Guided Imagery

Guided imagery is a therapy that uses the imagination to make a mind-body connection. You can use guided imagery for anything, such as athletic achievement (visualizing yourself winning a race or finishing an arduous run), but it is often used in alternative medicine for pain management and stress reduction. Consult with your doctor or alternative health care provider for a local referral, or you can find downloadable guided imagery transcripts and books through the Internet.

Progressive Muscle Relaxation

Progressive muscle relaxation is a simple technique where muscle groups are systematically tensed and then relaxed from one end of the body to the other. Progressive muscle relaxation may be used by physical therapists on its own or as part of biofeedback therapy, in which sensors are used to monitor the effect on blood pressure, heart rate, temperature, and muscle tenseness. This technique is popular for use in pain management but also for stress relief. Your doctor should be able to refer you to a local therapist who can guide you in this therapy.

OTHER STRESS-MANAGEMENT TECHNIQUES

Not every method for managing stress will work equally well for every patient. Stress management is highly individual. For a type-A personality, trying to meditate might be frustrating and just cause more stress. This person may find forms of biofeedback, such as HeartMath, to be more fulfilling. For other patients, a combination of techniques works best. Other therapeutic techniques to try include cognitive behavior therapy, music therapy, imagery therapy, laughter therapy, hypnosis, and time shifting.

And the best technique may not even be a regimented stress-management method. For some people, the best way to relax is a solitary form of exercise like swimming or running, watching a funny movie, taking walks in the outdoors, writing in a journal, or reading. Whatever works for you is the best technique.

"I try to control my stress," says Jay. "I practice meditation and yoga, and enjoy the meditative effects of swimming and walking. I try not to watch the news before I go to sleep. I try to laugh more. The power of laughter is huge. . . . I've started tapping into Jon Stewart, Colbert, Bill Maher. It's lighthearted and I want to laugh more."

Jay adds that he also manages stress through creative pursuits, art, and hobbies. "I read a lot and I write a lot. I write a lot of poems and I write letters to people," he says. "Music is a big part of my life and I listen to beautiful music—classical, jazz, or American or classic rock or opera. I'm a believer that music is a positive force."

Reading, writing, playing an instrument or listening to music, drawing or painting, and dancing can all be very powerful ways to relax and de-stress. The best relaxation methods may also be the best ways to keep active.

As with your diet and your exercise, it is important to choose stress-management techniques that you enjoy and can build upon. Following your intuition is key. It will help you find the technique that you enjoy, that works for you, and that you will stick with.

When exploring techniques, do your research but also find a reputable practitioner to learn from. There are many forms of yoga and meditation, for example, and you may be more suited to one than another. If the first class or teacher doesn't appeal to you, don't assume that no practitioner or form will be a good fit for you.

The best stress-management techniques will help you stay focused and in the present to avoid the places where all negative thoughts originate: the past and the future. Ironically, neither of these states exists. By keeping your mind in the present and avoiding the past and the future, these disciplines prevent the production of the harmful products of negative thoughts and emotions.

All of the various techniques of stress management affect the release of proteins and amino acids in the individual cells. The mystery, up until a decade or so ago, was how it works. With the exciting new scientific discoveries in epigenetics that have shown that simple life changes can open up avenues for change in our bodies, we now know that these techniques aren't just good for the mind, but good for the body as well.

As Dr. Moshe Frenkel stated in an article in *Cancer Strategies Journal*: "We are looking for magic but we already have the magic—we're simply not recognizing and applying it."[2]

CHAPTER ELEVEN

CREATING A SUPPORT SYSTEM

A STRONG SOCIAL SUPPORT SYSTEM IS VITAL FOR BOTH YOUR MENTAL AND physical health following cancer. Your social support system will provide guidance, advice, and assistance; offer shoulders to cry on; and help relieve stress. Whether your social support is a formal cancer support group, an informal group of friends or family, or a group that convenes around a shared interest, it will give you incentive to get out of the house and a way to form powerful connections. Even joining a bowling league has been found to provide physical as well as social and psychological benefits. Human beings are gregarious by nature, and being part of a group can have very positive effects.

There are a number of types of social support groups that you might consider seeking out when you are in remission. All have benefits, but not all will meet everyone's needs equally.

SPIRITUAL GROUPS

Whether you find your spiritual calling through a religious group or a secular spiritual group, studies have demonstrated that prayer can facilitate healing. Others have shown that people who regularly attend church have better immune systems than those who do not. A study of patients with a religious background showed a lower diastolic blood pressure, fewer admissions to the hospital, less coronary vascular disease, and fewer complications in cardiac catheterizations than in the general population. Another study of 10,000 male civil servants in Israel showed that, independent of lifestyle considerations, religious orthodoxy alone lowered the risk of coronary heart disease.

When 230 patients over 55 years old were studied in 1995, researchers found that those deriving no comfort, sustenance, or strength from religious beliefs had more than a threefold increased mortality following open-heart surgery. In 1990, another study demonstrated a significant relationship between a low incidence of cardiovascular disease and a high level of spiritual practice. In a 1991 analysis of 27 studies, 22 showed a positive relationship between health and religious commitment. Heart disease, hypertension, and overall mortality were improved by going to church. Finally, a 1994 survey of hospitalized patients reported that 98 percent believed in God and almost as many had a conviction that spiritual and physical well-being were equally important. Seventy-five percent prayed daily and felt their spiritual needs should be addressed by their physicians; 48 percent also wanted their physicians' prayers.

Some doctors bring faith healers into the operating room with them; others make sure that their patients are seen by a spiritual counselor before and after major surgery. Mehmet Oz, a Harvard-trained cardiac surgeon, started the Complementary Care Center at Columbia Presbyterian Hospital in New York, where he uses therapeutic touch, aromatherapy, and hypnosis on his heart transplant and other surgical patients.

Many of the doctors at Johns Hopkins Hospital pray with their patients and stop to pray at the huge statue of Christ in its main rotunda, where hundreds of religious messages are left in support of patients—not only by their families but by doctors and nurses as well.

We cite these examples to show that science can even be applied to so mystical a facet of our beings as spirituality. A deep belief in some higher power or cosmological force, whether it is the God of any denomination or the simple belief in human goodness and the capacity to love, can clearly be a factor in good health and rapid recovery. You must go outside yourself, see yourself in the context of the universe, and be able to love, care for, and give to yourself and others. This is one important path to physical health.

The holistic psychotherapist Daniel J. Benor, MD, defined spiritual healing as the intentional influence of one or more people on another living system without the use of any known physical means of intervention. Some individuals can, though perhaps with greater difficulty, do this by themselves. Spiritual intervention, Dr. Benor says, is nonlocal; it is not necessarily confined to the present moment or specific place. Doctors at Johns Hopkins Hospital, for instance, encourage a patient's family to set up prayer groups in their hometown while the operation is going on in Baltimore. At Duke University, concrete evidence has been shown of the effectiveness of such distant healing.

If the patient is able to participate, so much the better. However, even when the person being prayed for is unaware of it, prayer may make a difference. A double-blind randomized study on the effects of prayer on coronary care patients showed that the group being prayed for required fewer diuretics and antibiotics and less ventilator assistance than the control group.

"I worked with a spiritual teacher who used a kind of combination Hindu-based psychological gestalt therapy," says Cheryl. "There is a lot of symbolism with cancer, and she helped me separate what was my history and what was the disease. For me, it was feeling so helpless and out of control. I felt very childlike, very infantile. I just wanted this parental soothing, and it really wasn't appropriate or available. I wasn't 3. I had to kind of tease that apart to find my own equilibrium. It was coming to a sense of peace. There was a time there that I was just so fearful of dying. It was like I couldn't get a grip. The processes she devised allowed me to come to it on my own."

"Following treatment I saw a counselor for about a year," says Tara. "The counselor had a spiritual component, but it was not religious. She had the idea people had a purpose in life, and there is a time when they are meant to go. There are bigger forces than we have control of. I'm not a person who requires 100 percent certainty; I understand uncertainty. I've also read a lot of Taoism, which is more philosophical than religious, and I read a lot of Buddhism—how to work with your own mind, how to not let your erratic desires take control of you. I find that very helpful."

CANCER SUPPORT GROUP

Many cancer patients find a great deal of solace and help from cancer support groups. Groups come in many forms, from those available through the hospital where you received treatment to organizations like Gilda's Club to those that combine an interest or passion with cancer support. There are dragon boat groups throughout North America and Europe, where breast cancer survivors paddle the boats—which are similar to outrigger canoes and decorated as dragons—to build upper-body strength (helpful following a mastectomy and lymphadenectomy) and to provide social support. The movement has had such success that there are now dragon boat teams for survivors of many cancers. There are also knitting and quilting groups for cancer patients and survivors, as well as biking, swimming, skiing, and surfing groups that provide a hobby with cancer support.

OTHER SUPPORT GROUPS

Many people who find that cancer support groups are not right for them, or who find that cancer groups feel less comfortable for them after they are in remission, still have a desire to create social connections. Joining a biking or running club, a knitting or quilting group, a master's swim team, or any number of clubs and groups that revolve around a shared interest can be a tremendous way to create community and find support.

"My bike club was my support group," says Cheryl. "I never did get involved with a cancer support group. I always felt it was too much focus on the cancer. I just wanted to be with healthy people and feel healthy."

Some patients will need to try several groups before finding the right one for them, or they may find their needs change as they go from being a patient to being in remission. And then they may find their needs change yet again, 6 or 12 months out from treatment. It depends on the group, who's in it, and who's leading it, as well as where you are with your recovery. If you try one group and it doesn't speak to you, try another.

Many patients find that while cancer support groups are very helpful during and immediately following treatment, they become less effective the further into remission they get. For some people, cancer groups can feel like a double-edged sword. Although they provide a great deal of support and camaraderie, there can be a lot of fear when other members of the group relapse.

"My support group was very, very helpful," says Lise. "I went there for about three years. . . . Being in a group after cancer is really important. Sharing with people who have been through what you're going through . . . is very helpful. I only stopped because too many of the women were dying. . . . Developing a relationship with them and then going to see them when they're dying and then watching them die. It was too much."

In Lise's view, attending a cancer support group should be part of the protocol for cancer treatment. Despite the fact that she eventually moved away from the group, what she gained there was immeasurable.

"I think sharing your experience with other people is critical," says Lise. "I was in a women's support group, so sharing that with others, you become sisters. There's an immediate bond that you feel. I don't feel like it should be a suggestion. I think it's imperative that people after cancer are able to talk about it and hear other experiences and hear what other people are doing afterward. It's a community you wished you didn't belong to, but you do. It should be just part of what the doctor says: 'I'll see you in 6 months, but next week I've reserved a space for you. Here's the address. They know you're coming.'"

FRIENDS AND FAMILY

Some patients find that it's difficult to turn to family and close friends during and following treatment. There is too much shared anxiety and turmoil about the disease progression and prognosis. Other people find their family and friends are their biggest supporters, either in combination with or instead of other support groups.

"My support was my support group and my friends," says Lise. "The people who I consider friends are close enough that they are still very close friends. I think it strengthened relationships. When you are ill in that way, it's hard to ask for help. That created a vulnerability that allowed us to be closer."

Sherry agrees that both a cancer support group and supportive friends and family are ideal. "My immediate family and a group of close friends really have pitched in and helped. They are different than the people in the cancer support group. You need both. People in the cancer group really get you and know what's happening. Your friends don't understand what it's like, but they can take you away from it and let you have fun."

Jay did not attend any outside support groups, but looked instead to his wife and his brother, who'd also had cancer and was experienced in many of the complementary therapies that Jay also used. "I definitely looked to my family—my A team—as my closest support system," he said. "It's my wife and my brother. My wife was just unbelievable. She was right by me the whole time."

Having a close friend or family member who has also had cancer can be very beneficial in both gathering information and in sharing experiences. Tara turned to close friends who had had cancer instead of seeking support from a cancer support group. "I have a really close friend who's gone through breast cancer. She's the first person I called when I was diagnosed," she said. "Through all of the shock and fear, she was the living representation of 'look at me.' I had another friend who had gone through stage IV lung cancer, and that was incredibly empowering. . . . The best thing for me was to be with friends who had been there. I don't know if it would have helped me to be with a group of people in the same state of shock and fear as I was. Fear has a way of transmitting. It's hard not to get more frightened."

Ashley had friends who'd had cancer and knew what she was going through, but she also had other friends who could get her out of her head and help her stay positive. Both were helpful. Her seven best friends, who share her sense of humor, even formed a Facebook support group so that friends and family could stay updated on her health before and after treatment. They were there for her when she hit a rough patch emotionally about a year into remission, and they recently held a party to pick out new nipples for Ashley, who is undergoing breast reconstruction.

PETS

In addition to friends and family, many patients find solace, support, and connections through their pets. Pets have been shown to lower blood pressure and provide emotional support. They motivate their owners to get up in the morning and provide incentive for them to get out of the house. Pets need to be fed, walked, played with, and comforted, which in turn provides their owners comfort.

Dogs, in particular, can be great inspiration for getting in shape, but they can also provide an entrance for social connections. There are a number of dog-related activities that can introduce you to people with a shared love of animals—even if it's just fellow walkers in your neighborhood or at the dog park.

"My dogs were very important," says Lise. "The dogs motivated me to get out and still do. At least once a day we take a long hike, almost every day, at least five days a week. It's for their benefit, but I know it's also for my benefit. Plus the loving, the affection—pets are wonderful. When I was so sick, they knew it. They were very protective."

GOING HIGH TECH

The Internet has become one of the greatest sources of information and support for those diagnosed with cancer. Web site chat rooms can be a boon for patients who are seeking information and advice about both conventional and alternative treatments, as well as new trials for their particular type of cancer. Patients can connect and share insights with others who are facing the same cancer type and stage as they are. The Internet can also be very beneficial for patients who live in rural areas and don't have access to a local cancer support or survivors' group.

Many patients find that cancer Web sites can become less appropriate as they phase out of treatment because their value is in the information they provide versus support. Over time, people in remission may drift from online support groups in the same way that they move away from other cancer support groups.

"I joined an online metastatic breast cancer group called Crazy Sexy Cancer," says Sherry. "I got emotional support and a lot of information. It was great. Everybody was just very warm and friendly and close. But at one point, my healer said, 'You should step away. In order to be part of that group, you need to be sick, and you're healed.'"

CHAPTER TWELVE

FINDING YOUR BALANCE

W HEN WE SPEAK WITH CANCER SURVIVORS THROUGH OUR PRACTICES, WE OFTEN
hear the word *balance*.

Depending on the patient, this word may mean different things
in particular, but in a general sense it means that the person has achieved, or is
working to achieve, an equilibrium in life. In an applied sense, this may mean
she balances her work life with her family life and that she makes time for her
passions and her hobbies, while still engaging in the day-to-day activities that
keep her moving forward.

Physically, it may mean that patients eat healthfully and happily—that they
get the lion's share of their nutrition through locally grown, whole, mostly plant-
based foods, and still treat themselves on occasion to an ice cream cone or a glass
of their favorite red wine. Or it may mean that they exercise 3 days a week by
running on a treadmill to get their heart rate up, but that 2 days a week they
exercise by, say, surfing—an activity that provides them good exercise, a deep
spiritual satisfaction, and the thrill of catching a wave.

For patients to have balance, it also means that they have equilibrium
among the mind, body, and spirit. They are in good emotional, physical, and
spiritual health.

Whatever "balance" means to a particular person, we have seen time and
again that having gone through cancer treatments and coming out the other end

can help people to move toward a better sense of balance in their lives. And the better balanced they are, the better they are able to move forward and engage in happy and satisfying lives.

You have gone through something life threatening and life altering. After treatment is over, there is truly a new normal, and your perspective and motivations in life tend to change. Trying to figure out where that leaves you is difficult. Things in your life won't necessarily go back to the way they were before you had cancer. Sometimes relationships break up, and other times unexpected people become very close.

Following cancer, you have an opportunity to both accept and create the new you. This is a process, not a product. In his practice, Dr. McKee has seen the way cancer rapidly reorganizes his patients' priorities. Some of his patients leave a bad marriage or bad job; others pursue the things they always wanted to do, like painting or moving to the country.

He believes the word *balance* can mean many things to patients: a balance between taking care of themselves and taking care of other people, or a balance between work and recreation. Patients who are financially able may decide to quit working or cut down their work hours. Others may look into a different type of work. In some ways, cancer can be an invitation to change on many levels, and in Dr. McKee's experience, the more people change following a diagnosis, the better they seem to do.

A cancer diagnosis is a chance for a person to think deeply about what he's done in his life and what he wants to do in the future.

A NEW NORMAL

To find balance, it is important for cancer patients to realize that what they think is normal before treatment will not necessarily be their normal after treatment. Changes can include physical appearance, short- and long-term goals, and their view of the world.

For women going through breast cancer treatment, they may lose their breasts and their hair, both of which are symbols of femininity. This is not a small thing to overcome. And they may be surprised by what aspect of that loss affects them most—like Ashley, who breezed through the loss of her breasts but was devastated when she lost her hair.

Letting go of the idea of what you did and should look like and feel like can be an important step in moving on postcancer. You have climbed a mountain, and you are looking at the world from a different vantage point. In some ways, that's a good thing.

Even after the conclusion of your treatment, things continue to change. The *you* at the end of your treatment may not be the *you* 5 years out. Your scars will fade, and your hair will grow out. Some people become very depressed at the 5-year point post-treatment; some get survivor's guilt because they feel good while others don't. Being postcancer is not encapsulated in a week or a month or even a year.

"Once you have cancer, things truly are changed forever," says Lise. "You are looking at the world through different eyes. The balance for me, my life wasn't the way it was before, and I realized it never would be. Being balanced meant something different to me after than it did before."

For Lise, being balanced now means that she needs to be alone more than she ever has before. It also means that she has less interest in spending time with people with whom she is not close. "Now I'm very aware when I'm open with someone," said Lise. "I don't want to be around people I don't feel open with. I want to be around people who I want to connect with in some way."

Lise adds that she also notices her inner needs far more astutely. "I feel like I don't have the physical resources to expend. There's not really a lot of judgment about it—it's more that I don't have time," she says. "I don't want to be here, and I don't have to be here . . . I'm much more in tune to that. Being liked, being approved of, being accepted—that doesn't seem as important."

Ashley, now 35, has similarly recalibrated her life and comments that in many ways, she feels like she has more in common with people of retirement age than her peers.

"I try to live like I'm retired. I won't wait to do things," says Ashley, explaining that her job as a flight attendant gives her flexibility. "I'm housesitting in Hawaii and taking the time off work. Fortunately, I can do that. I spend a lot less time worrying about stuff. I rented my condo out so I don't have to pay my mortgage, and I hardly buy anything anymore. My priorities have changed. If I buy something, I'll have to work, and I don't want to work that much!

"After my treatment I thought, 'Why do people wait before they retire or get cancer to do this?' My plan for next year is to buy a Winnebago and travel. I'm more relaxed. I don't sweat the small stuff. There are bigger things in life."

Like Ashley, many cancer survivors find that they have a desire to refocus. This may mean cutting down their hours at work, changing jobs or retiring, spending more time with family or friends, or devoting more time to a hobby or passion.

"When I was very first diagnosed with CLL [chronic lymphocytic leukemia], I was working in a management role in health care," says Cheryl. "It was too stressful, and I was working too many hours. It was also stressful at home. My husband and I were going through a difficult time, so there was no relief. I told my boss I'm only going to work half-time, and to my surprise, they said okay.

Five years later, when I required treatment, I told my boss I needed to work from home, and again they said okay. They set me up with a computer at home, and I worked when I could. Even after I was done with treatment, I continued working at home, and I did that for 10 years until they asked me to come back into the office. I did that for 2 years and then left and started my own business. So now I'm in charge of my time, and I work 10 to 20 hours a week, but it's not stressful."

Although patients find equilibrium following cancer through a variety of means, we have some general recommendations. In our experience, patients who have resolved these matters in their lives seem to do better than patients who have not.

Reduce the Negatives

Many of us hold negative feelings and emotions from throughout our lives. These feelings may even stem from childhood or may arise from current relationships.

Patients who are mired in negative emotions have a more difficult time making positive changes in their physical and mental health. Optimizing your relationships is one of the best things you can do. This is something we tend to do as we age anyway. We tend to forgive more and carry resentments less. With a cancer diagnosis, it's an opportunity to put all of that into high gear. It's a chance to resolve all the unresolved relationships.

Dr. McKee encourages his patients to make a list of all the people they feel resentment toward and practice active forgiveness. If there are unresolved or chronic conflicts with your family or friends, take the lead in resolving them.

There are a number of programs that address finding forgiveness for life-shattering crimes, as well as for the petty grievances we collect throughout our lives. Some patients find working with a counselor to be helpful in this process.

Find the Positives

It has long been known that negative emotions are strong predictors of heart disease and other chronic degenerative diseases. What is not so well known, but is becoming increasingly evident, is that positive emotions—love, forgiveness, self-esteem, optimism, hope—can help prevent disease and even restore health after an illness. In a recent study of patients who had undergone successful angioplasty, patients who scored high in positive emotions and feelings were only one-third as likely as those with low scores to have another heart attack.

You can see negative versus positive emotions at work in yourself. The next time you feel anger, hatred, or pessimism, try to become aware of your body. Your muscles will be tight, particularly in your upper back and neck; your breathing will be shallow; your stomach will churn. Quite the opposite reaction happens if you can genuinely say, "I love you" or "I forgive you" or "I have hope." Your body feels lighter, your muscles relax, your breath is deep and regular.

It's more difficult to discern emotion if it has been hidden within your body. Resentments can fester, and swallowed anger can lodge in your stomach. Parental belittling when you were a child can affect your posture and self-esteem as an adult. A life scarred by unhappiness can determine the way you walk and talk and even the way you breathe. You may not be conscious of your feelings. They may be so embedded that they seem completely natural. If they're pointed out by a therapist or a friend, the response is often disbelief or denial. However, the feelings are there nevertheless, and—usually with the aid of a therapist but sometimes on your own—they can be changed.

Face Death

While it is important to view your future in a positive light, it is also important to face and accept death.

Accepting our mortality is, ironically, one of the best ways to avoid a premature death. The fear of cancer relapse is connected to the fear of death because most people are told if they relapse, there is little that can be done and they will die of their cancer. That just sits there, and the more afraid they are and the more stressed they are, the more likely they will die of their cancer.

The absence of guidance and empowerment only magnifies that stress. The most stressful thing is uncertainty. And every time you hear about a friend or a family member who gets cancer or relapses, the fear comes back.

Sometimes the fear of death is less about death itself and more about the other images in our heads that surround dying of cancer: fear of pain or fear of loss of independence.

We've worked with many people who ultimately died of their cancer but who were healed emotionally. This is one thing cancer provides us. If you drop dead of a heart attack, you don't have the chance to heal your life. With cancer you get a chance to resolve things.

"I try not to be fearful of persecution, death, injury, or pain," says Jay. "It becomes less powerful. Even if, God forbid, it recurs, I have all my personal things in order. I've written my directives and my will, and I've written poems and letters to the people in my life. It feels good. If I get hit by lightning or a UFO scoops me up, at least I know it'll be there written."

In Western culture and in our medical culture, we see death as a defeat, but if we think like that, then we will all be defeated. We all die. Use your cancer as an opportunity to face death, make amends, love fully, and live the fullest life you can.

Do for Others

True happiness is always accompanied by the characteristics of gratitude, usefulness, community, and something to look forward to.

If we don't have gratitude, we express resentment, which will never make us happy.

Usefulness is hardwired into our psyche, so we must always feel that what we're doing is important and helpful. Looking forward to a project or event on the horizon helps us start our day, week, or year, and even if we do not have family or close friends, we can create community through helping other people.

Many former cancer patients find that volunteering provides them with a deep spiritual satisfaction, a reason to get up and out of bed in the morning, and a way to turn their minds off themselves and their fears for the time they are volunteering.

Not all volunteering is formal. Many people who have gone through treatment become de facto cancer guides. Friends put them in touch with other people who have been recently diagnosed and who need some guidance and a positive model for treatment and recovery. This can be a way for people who have gone through cancer to impart the wisdom from their own experience. This can help patients feel like they've not gone through all of this in vain.

"I get a lot of e-mails from people who've just been diagnosed," says Ashley, who gives them advice on what to expect from their treatments and tells them her story. She also gives them advice about what to expect after they're in remission. "The advice I always tell them is that it's not over for the person when the treatment ends."

Lise lives in the Bay Area and was diagnosed with ovarian cancer when she was 60 years old. She is now 66 and cancer free. Before her diagnosis, she had been an active volunteer with a hospice program in a public hospital and at a hospice house. Although she went to a cancer support group for 3 years following her initial diagnosis, she ultimately pulled back from that group but continued to volunteer with the hospice program. "It was giving back, but it's also being able to connect deeply with people and experience compassion and love that sometimes we lose track of in our daily lives."

Lise adds, "When I go to the hospice, I'm so totally out of my own experience. It's like walking through a veil of one reality into another."

One of the worst things to do for a patient who has completed treatment is invest excessive amounts of time thinking about the what-ifs. One of the best ways to get out of your head is to do something for someone else.

Find Your Rhythm

Although no one would ask for a cancer diagnosis, surviving it can be an important wake-up call that allows you to make positive changes to both your physical and emotional life.

"A lot of people I know who have gone through cancer find their inner ground," says Tara. "They start to trust themselves more. This is incredibly helpful to relieve stress.

"One of the things you learn to do is support your health and not undermine it. I think people undermine their health by eating bad food. You need a regular lifestyle: You eat three meals a day at roughly the same time. You sleep 8 hours. You have regular sleeping hours and a regular eating schedule. You have a regular working schedule. Every single week, you have opportunities that you love. You have the opportunity to have heart-to-heart conversations with people you love. . . . People can only do so much. I think you learn that anyway, but with cancer you learn it in a hurry.

"I used to travel quite a bit, but now I'm cognizant that it's exhausting. It disrupts your rhythm. Now I travel every couple months rather than twice a month. I recognize I have a rhythm. I need to have time to produce and create and achieve. I need to have time to rest and to integrate and to do nothing and be quiet. I need that just as much as I need to do things. If I have both, I have my health."

Finding your balance means many things, but for a happy life—and one in which cancer recurrence is the least likely—balance means working less, playing more, smiling and laughing more often, spending more time with your friends and family, giving your body the food and exercise it needs, and providing your mind and spirit the nourishment they need through solitary walks, meditation, volunteering in a hospice, or other selfless activities that are meaningful to you.

We all only have one life. This is your chance to make the best of it.

CONCLUSION

YOU HAVE COME THROUGH A CANCER DIAGNOSIS AND ARE NOW IN REMISSION, and that means your life has been forever changed. However, this does not mean you are destined to have a recurrence or that the changes from having had cancer are necessarily negative.

We know now through the science of epigenetics that you are not stuck with your genetic history. Your choices in diet, exercise, and other aspects of your lifestyle can help determine whether your genes promote cancer—both for you and your descendants. You can "turn on" hundreds of genes that fight cancer and "turn off" the ones that encourage cancer by simply making the changes outlined in this book. Even small changes in your lifestyle can make a big difference in your risk for recurrence by reducing inflammation and boosting immune surveillance.

THE QUICK HITS:

Limit alcohol to one glass of red wine with food.

Quit smoking.

Walk or do some type of exercise 30 minutes a day, 6 days a week.

Do daily yoga stretching.

Lift weights or use exercise bands three times per week.

Find a stress-management practice that works for you.

Spend 10 minutes daily meditating or relaxing.

Support your immune system by getting enough sleep and practicing positive thinking.

Keep your weight under control and avoid obesity.

Avoid or eat only minimal amounts of organic meat.

Eat limited amounts of organic dairy products and organic poultry.

Eat whole grains and avoid white flour.

Avoid sugar and high-fructose corn syrup. Substitute stevia, xylitol, or small amounts of honey.

Eat five to nine servings of colorful fresh fruits and vegetables daily.

Eat broccoli, cabbage, Brussels sprouts, or other cruciferous vegetables three times per week.

Liberally add herbs and spices to your foods, especially garlic, onions, cilantro, and turmeric.

Read labels carefully and avoid chemical additives.

Choose safe, organic household and personal products.

Buy organic when possible, and thoroughly wash pesticide residue off conventionally grown fruits and vegetables.

Avoid trans fats completely.

Let the sun shine in. For optimum vitamin D, allow 20 minutes of sun on your bare skin, without sunscreen, at least three times per week (just be certain never to let it burn). Get your vitamin D blood levels checked and keep them optimum.

Take a multivitamin (without iron) daily; take 500 mg mixed omega-3 daily, and 250–300 mg magnesium daily.

Get in touch with your spirituality.

Make social connections; join a support group.

Volunteer.

Work less.

Spend more time with your friends and family.

Look on yourself and others through a lens of compassion and kindness.

AFTER CANCER CARE
Recipes

BREAKFASTS

LUNCHES

SUPPERS

SAUCES AND DRESSINGS

Sunrise Tofu Scramble

2 tablespoons extra-virgin olive oil or coconut oil

1 small sweet onion, chopped

1 clove garlic, minced

1 teaspoon ground turmeric

Ground black pepper

$\frac{1}{2}$ green or red bell pepper, chopped

2 pounds tofu, crumbled and drained

2 tablespoons chopped fresh parsley or cilantro

Salt

POWER FOODS:

1. **Onion**
2. **Garlic**
3. **Green or red bell pepper**
4. **Turmeric**
5. **Black pepper**

In a large skillet, heat the oil over medium-high heat. Add the onion, garlic, and turmeric and season to taste with black pepper. Cook until fragrant.

Add the bell pepper and cook until softened.

Add the tofu to the skillet and cook for 5 to 7 minutes, until heated through. Remove the skillet from the heat and add the parsley or cilantro and salt to taste.

Makes 4 servings

Japanese Breakfast

DASHI

1 ounce dried kombu seaweed

7 cups cold water

1 cup bonito flakes

1 cup sliced shiitake mushrooms

MISO SOUP

¹/₄ cup mellow white miso

¹/₄ package silken tofu, diced into ¹/₂" cubes

2 teaspoons wakame seaweed flakes

2 scallions, finely chopped

2 tablespoons olive oil or coconut oil

4 (4-ounce) wild salmon fillets

4 cups cooked brown rice (organic)

4 cups green tea

POWER FOODS:

1. Scallions
2. Shiitake mushrooms
3. Seaweed
4. Brown rice

To make the dashi: Place the seaweed in a saucepan with 6 cups of the water. Bring to a boil, then simmer for 5 to 10 minutes. Remove the seaweed and discard. Add the bonito flakes and the remaining 1 cup water to the saucepan. Bring to a boil, then simmer for 5 minutes. Remove from the heat and let the bonito flakes settle to the bottom. Strain the stock and discard the bonito flakes.

To make the miso soup: Bring the strained dashi to a simmering boil. Add the mushrooms and cook for 5 minutes. Pour ¹/₂ cup of the dashi into a small bowl. Add the white miso and mix thoroughly. Add the miso-dashi paste back into the dashi mushroom mixture along with the tofu and wakame. Reduce the heat to low, and do not boil. Stir until the mixture is combined and the ingredients are warmed through, about 3 to 5 minutes. Ladle the soup into bowls and sprinkle with scallions.

Heat the oil in a skillet or preheat a grill, and cook or grill the salmon. Serve with the brown rice and green tea.

NOTE: For vegetarians, make the miso soup with shiitake mushrooms both in place of dashi and serve with white beans instead of salmon.

In a traditional Japanese breakfast, an egg and various pickles are included.

Makes 2 servings

It's Easy Being Green Smoothie (From Dr. Oz)

4 cups leafy greens, any of your favorites such as kale, spinach, and collard greens

2 tablespoons hemp seeds or flaxseeds

1 cup frozen blueberries

$1/4$ cup frozen cherries

$1/4$ cup frozen raspberries

$1/4$ cup frozen pineapple pieces

$1/4$ cup frozen mango chunks

1 medium frozen peeled banana, broken into pieces

2 cups unsweetened almond milk

POWER FOODS:
1. **Greens**
2. **Flax**
3. **All fruit, especially berries**

In a high-powered blender, combine the greens, seeds, blueberries, cherries, raspberries, pineapple, mango, banana, and almond milk. Blend on high speed for 60 seconds, or until smooth. Enjoy icy cold.

Makes 2 servings

Total Body Restart Green Juice (From Dr. Oz)

2 cups spinach

2 cups peeled and chopped cucumber

2 ribs celery

$1/2$ teaspoon grated fresh ginger

1 bunch parsley

2 apples, finely chopped

Juice of 1 lime

Juice of $1/2$ lemon

POWER FOODS:
1. **Greens**
2. **Ginger**
3. **Parsley**

In a blender, combine the spinach, cucumber, celery, ginger, parsley, apples, lime juice, and lemon juice. Blend on high speed until smooth. Enjoy!

Makes 2 servings

LUNCHES

George and Martha's Split Pea Soup

1 cup dried yellow split peas

1/4 cup extra-virgin olive oil

1 teaspoon ground cumin

1 teaspoon ground turmeric

1/4 teaspoon ground red pepper

1/2 teaspoon ground black pepper

4 cloves garlic, minced

1 medium sweet onion, chopped

4 cups water or vegetable stock

1 teaspoon coarse salt

1 tablespoon fresh lime juice

1 cup finely chopped kale or spinach

1/2 teaspoon smoked paprika

Chopped scallions, avocado slices, crumbled veggie bacon (optional)

POWER FOODS:

1. **Onion**
2. **Garlic**
3. **Cumin**
4. **Turmeric**
5. **Red and black pepper**
6. **Kale or spinach**
7. **Scallions**
8. **Avocado**

Place the split peas in a medium saucepan. Cover with several inches of water and soak overnight. Drain.

In a large saucepan, heat 2 tablespoons of the oil over medium heat. Add the cumin, turmeric, red pepper, and black pepper and cook, stirring, for 2 minutes. Add the garlic and cook until softened. Add the onion and cook until it starts to soften. Add the split peas, water or stock, and salt and bring to a boil.

Reduce the heat, cover, and simmer for 1 hour, or until the split peas are softened but not mushy. Add the lime juice, then stir in the kale or spinach, and simmer for 3 to 5 minutes.

In a small bowl, combine the remaining 2 tablespoons oil with the smoked paprika and stir well. Spoon the soup into bowls, drizzle a teaspoon of the paprika mix over the soup, and top with the scallions, avocado slices, or veggie bacon, if desired.

Makes 4 servings

Carrot and Ginger Soup

1 tablespoon extra-virgin olive oil

1 large onion, chopped

1 tablespoon grated fresh ginger

3 cups carrots, chopped

1 teaspoon mild curry powder

1 medium potato, peeled and cut into small cubes

6 cups water or vegetable stock

1 cup orange juice

Salt and ground black pepper

Chopped fresh cilantro

POWER FOODS:

1. **Onion**
2. **Ginger**
3. **Carrots**
4. **Curry powder**

In a large skillet, heat the oil over medium-high heat. Add the onion and ginger and cook for 5 minutes, or until translucent. Add the carrots and curry powder and continue cooking for 5 minutes. Add the potato and water or stock. Bring to a boil, reduce the heat, cover, and simmer for 30 minutes, or until the carrots soften.

Stir in the orange juice. Pour the mixture into the bowl of a blender. Puree until smooth. If too thick, add more water or stock.

Season to taste with salt and pepper. Serve garnished with cilantro.

Makes 6 servings

Cream of Mushroom Soup

(From Conner Middelmann-Whitney)

SOUP

1 ounce dried porcini mushrooms

1 tablespoon olive oil

1 small yellow onion

4 whole shiitake mushrooms

15 ounces cremini or white button mushrooms

$\frac{1}{2}$ teaspoon dried thyme

1 quart chicken stock or vegetable broth

Salt and ground black pepper

Squeeze of lemon juice

Red-pepper flakes

Chopped fresh parsley

POWER FOODS:
1. **Mushrooms**
2. **Onion**
3. **Thyme**
4. **Black pepper**
5. **Red pepper**

CASHEW CREAM TOPPING

$\frac{1}{2}$ cup raw, unsalted cashews

$\frac{1}{2}$ cup water

Pinch of salt

To make the soup: Place the dried porcini mushrooms in a bowl and cover with hot water. Rehydrate for 15 minutes.

In a heavy pot over low heat, warm the oil and cook the onion for 4 to 5 minutes until translucent. Add the fresh mushrooms and thyme and cook for 4 to 5 minutes, or until the mushrooms are soft and release their juices.

With a slotted spoon, remove the rehydrated mushrooms from their soaking water, chop coarsely, and add to the mushroom mixture in the pot. Add the stock or broth. Strain the mushroom-soaking water through a cheesecloth to remove any grit and add to the mushroom mixture. Simmer for another 15 minutes.

Either serve the soup as is, or blend partially or completely. To blend, ladle the soup into a blender and process in two batches. Season to taste with salt, pepper, and lemon juice.

To make the cashew cream topping: Soak the cashews for at least 10 minutes in cold water. Drain the soaking water. Combine the nuts, the fresh water, and the salt in a small blender. Puree for 2 minutes, or until the mixture is smooth and velvety. Add a little more water for a thinner consistency.

Ladle the soup into serving bowls, drizzle with the cashew cream, and sprinkle with pepper flakes and parsley. Store any leftover cashew cream in a sealable container in the refrigerator. It keeps for up to 3 days.

Makes 4 servings

Blue Bell Inn Lentil Salad

2 cups French lentils

5 cups vegetable broth

2 small onions, 1 coarsely chopped,
1 finely chopped

1 rib celery, coarsely chopped

1/4 bunch flat-leaf parsley, coarsely chopped

1/4 cup tarragon vinegar

1 cup light olive oil

Salt and ground black pepper

A few hot cherry peppers, finely chopped

POWER FOODS:

1. **French lentils**
2. **Onion**
3. **Celery**
4. **Black pepper**

Wash the lentils and pick out any debris. Drain and place them in a large pot. Add the broth and bring to a boil. Cover, reduce the heat to medium-low, and cook for 1 hour.

Place the coarsely chopped onion, the celery, and parsley in a cheesecloth bag. Add to the pot and return the mixture to a boil. Reduce the heat to a simmer and cook for 10 minutes, or until the lentils are tender. Drain the lentils and let cool, then place in a large bowl.

In a small bowl, whisk together the vinegar, oil, and salt and pepper to taste. Add to the lentils and toss together.

Serve with the finely chopped onion and hot cherry peppers.

Makes 4 servings

Zorba's Chopped Salad

1 clove garlic

4 tablespoons extra-virgin olive oil

1 head romaine lettuce, chopped into bite-size pieces

2 cucumbers, peeled and chopped

2 tomatoes, chopped

1 red onion, chopped

1 green bell pepper, chopped

2 tablespoons chopped fresh mint

12 kalamata olives

4 ounces feta cheese, cut into cubes

1 tablespoon fresh lemon juice

1 tablespoon red wine vinegar

Salt and ground black pepper

A few pepperoncini (optional)

A few caper berries (optional)

POWER FOODS:

1. **Garlic**
2. **Romaine lettuce**
3. **Cucumbers**
4. **Tomatoes**
5. **Onion**
6. **Green bell pepper**
7. **Mint**
8. **Black pepper**
9. **Pepperoncini**
10. **Lemon**

In a large salad bowl, press or mince the garlic and add to the oil.

Add the lettuce, cucumbers, tomatoes, onion, bell pepper, and mint. Add the olives, cheese, lemon juice, and red wine vinegar. Season to taste with salt and black pepper.

Garnish with the pepperoncini and caper berries, if desired.

Makes 4 servings

Spinach, Avocado, and Pomegranate Salad

4 cups baby spinach

1 ripe avocado, sliced

1 grapefruit, divided into sections

Seeds of 1 pomegranate

1″ fresh ginger, peeled

Juice and zest of 1 lime

2 tablespoons apple cider vinegar

2 tablespoons extra-virgin olive oil

2 tablespoons chopped cilantro

POWER FOODS:

1. **Spinach**
2. **Avocado**
3. **Grapefruit**
4. **Pomegranate**
5. **Ginger**

Place the spinach, avocado, grapefruit, and pomegranate seeds in a large bowl.

In a medium bowl, combine the ginger, lime juice and zest, vinegar, oil, and cilantro. Mix well, then drizzle over the salad.

Makes 2 servings

Rainbow Asian Slaw
with Tangy Asian Dressing

1 small head red cabbage

1 small head green cabbage

2 large carrots, grated

$1/2$ cup chopped scallions

$1/4$ cup toasted sesame seeds

Tangy Asian Dressing (recipe below)

POWER FOODS:

1. **Cabbage**
2. **Carrots**
3. **Scallions**
4. **Sesame seeds**

Remove and discard the outer leaves of the cabbages. Shred or thinly slice the cabbages and place in a large bowl.

Add the carrots, scallions, sesame seeds, and Tangy Asian Dressing. Toss well and chill in the refrigerator.

Makes 4 servings

Tangy Asian Dressing

1 cup rice vinegar

2 tablespoons light soy sauce

3 tablespoons grated fresh ginger

$1/2$ tablespoon sesame oil

1 tablespoon orange juice

POWER FOOD:

Ginger

In a small bowl, combine the rice vinegar, soy sauce, ginger, oil, and orange juice. Whisk vigorously until well blended.

Makes 4 servings

Fig, Onion, and Goat Cheese Tart on a Flax-Almond Crust (From Conner Middelmann-Whitney)

TOPPING

3 tablespoons olive oil

3 red onions, finely sliced

1¼ teaspoons finely chopped fresh rosemary, divided

Salt and ground black pepper

2 tablespoons balsamic vinegar

8 fresh figs, stems removed, quartered

½ cup coarsely chopped walnuts

3.5 ounces fresh goat's cheese, coarsely crumbled

Handful of fresh arugula leaves

A few squirts of balsamic reduction (thick balsamic syrup in a bottle, available in most supermarkets), optional

POWER FOODS:
1. **Onions**
2. **Rosemary**
3. **Walnuts**
4. **Flaxseeds**
5. **Almonds**
6. **Garlic**

CRUST

3.5 ounces golden flaxseeds, finely ground

3.5 ounces finely ground almonds

1 teaspoon herbes de Provence

1 teaspoon baking powder

½ teaspoon salt

4 eggs

1 clove garlic, crushed

4 tablespoons olive oil

⅔ cup water

To make the topping: In a large skillet over medium heat, warm the oil. Add the onions and 1 teaspoon of the rosemary, sprinkle with salt, and cook for 20 to 25 minutes. To speed up the caramelizing, cover with a lid for the first 10 minutes, then remove the lid and continue cooking, stirring occasionally, to let the moisture evaporate. If the onions stick to the pot, add 1 to 2 tablespoons water to moisten.

Once the onions are very soft, add the balsamic vinegar and stir to combine. Season to taste with salt and pepper and remove from the heat.

Preheat the oven to 350°F. Cover a baking sheet or pie tin with parchment paper.

To make the crust: While the onions are cooking, make the crust. In a mixing bowl, combine the flaxseeds, almonds, herbs de Provence, baking powder, and salt. Make a well in the center and add the eggs, garlic, olive oil, and water. Whisk to obtain a smooth paste. Spread onto the baking sheet or pie tin, and bake for 20 to 25 minutes, or until golden on top.

Remove from the oven and increase the temperature to 400°F. Top the crust with the onions, figs, and walnuts. Return to the oven and bake for 10 minutes. Remove and scatter with goat cheese, arugula leaves, and the remaining ¼ teaspoon rosemary.

Serve immediately, drizzled with a little balsamic reduction, if desired.

Makes 4 servings

Grilled Shrimp with Salsa

6 large shrimp, peeled and deveined

$\frac{1}{4}$ cup extra-virgin olive oil

3 tablespoons lemon juice

Sea salt and ground black pepper

Juice of 1 lime

1 mango or papaya, sliced

3 red radishes, thinly sliced

1 onion, finely chopped

2 tablespoons chili powder

POWER FOODS:
1. **Lemon**
2. **Black pepper**
3. **Mango or papaya**
4. **Radishes**
5. **Onion**
6. **Chili powder**

In a large bowl, toss the shrimp with the oil and lemon juice and season with salt and pepper. Let marinate for about 30 minutes while you heat up the grill. Or use a grill pan on the stovetop. Grill or cook the shrimp.

In a large bowl, combine the lime juice, mango or papaya, radishes, onion, and chili powder. Mix well. Season with salt and pepper to taste.

Place the warm shrimp on a platter and top with the salsa.

Makes 2 servings

Tuscan Kale Salad (From Dr. Andrew Weil's *True Food*)

Juice of 1 lemon

3–4 tablespoons extra-virgin olive oil

2 cloves garlic, minced

Salt and ground black pepper

Red-pepper flakes

4–6 cups kale, loosely packed and sliced leaves
of Italian black Lacinato "dinosaur" cavolo nero
variety, with the midribs removed

$^2/_3$ cup grated Pecorino Toscano cheese, Asiago,
Parmesan, or veggie cheese shreds

$^1/_2$ cup fresh bread crumbs, made from lightly toasted bread

POWER FOODS:

1. **Kale**
2. **Lemon**
3. **Garlic**
4. **Red pepper**
5. **Black pepper**

In a small bowl, whisk together the lemon juice, oil, and garlic and season to taste with salt, black pepper, and a generous pinch (or more) of pepper flakes.

Place the kale in a serving bowl and pour the dressing over the top. Toss well. Add two-thirds of the cheese and toss again.

Let the kale sit for at least 5 minutes. Add the bread crumbs, toss again, and top with the remaining cheese.

Makes 6 to 8 servings

The Very, Very Best Veggie Burgers

$^1/_2$ cup brown rice (organic)

1 cup water

2 cans (16 ounces each) black beans, rinsed and drained

1 green bell pepper, halved and seeded

1 onion, quartered

$^1/_2$ cup sliced mushrooms

6 cloves garlic

$^3/_4$ cup shredded mozzarella or veggie cheese

2 eggs

1 tablespoon chili powder

1 tablespoon ground cumin

1 tablespoon garlic salt

1 teaspoon hot sauce

$^1/_2$ cup dry bread crumbs

POWER FOODS:

1. **Brown rice**
2. **Black beans**
3. **Green bell pepper**
4. **Onion**
5. **Mushrooms**
6. **Garlic**
7. **Chili powder**
8. **Cumin**

In a saucepan over high heat, bring the brown rice and water to a boil. Reduce the heat to medium-low, cover, and simmer for 45 to 50 minutes, or until the rice is tender and the liquid is absorbed.

Preheat an outdoor grill on high heat. Lightly oil a sheet of aluminum foil. Or coat a large skillet with olive or coconut oil.

In a large bowl, mash the beans with a fork until thick. Set aside.

In the bowl of a food processor, combine the bell pepper, onion, mushrooms, and garlic. Process until finely chopped. Stir the mixture into the mashed beans. Place the brown rice and cheese in the bowl of a food processor. Process until combined. Add to the black bean mixture and stir.

In a small bowl, whisk together the eggs, chili powder, cumin, garlic salt, and hot sauce. Stir it into the black bean mixture. Stir in the bread crumbs, adding more bread crumbs as needed until the mixture is sticky and holds together. Divide into 8 large patties.

Place the patties onto the prepared foil or skillet. Grill for 8 minutes per side, or until browned and heated through.

Makes 8 servings

Portuguese Baked Wild Halibut with Rice

2 tablespoons extra-virgin olive oil

2 tomatoes, chopped

2 cloves garlic, minced

1 small onion, finely chopped

½ cup chopped black olives

2 tablespoons chopped cilantro, plus a few sprigs for garnish

1 pound halibut

1 cup cooked brown rice (organic)

Salt and ground black pepper

2 cups dry white wine

POWER FOODS:

1. **Tomatoes**
2. **Garlic**
3. **Onion**
4. **Brown rice**
5. **Black pepper**

Preheat the oven to 350°F.

Pour the oil into a shallow baking dish. Scatter half the tomatoes, garlic, onion, olives, and cilantro in the dish. Put the fish and rice on top, season with salt and pepper, and cover with the rest of the tomatoes, garlic, onion, olives, and cilantro. Pour the wine on top.

Bake for 30 to 40 minutes, basting often. Place on a warm serving plate. Boil the drippings to desired thickness and pour over the fish to further moisten it. Garnish with the cilantro sprigs.

Makes 6 servings

Salmon and Vegetable Curry

(From Conner Middelmann-Whitney)

2 tablespoons coconut oil

1 onion, chopped

2 cloves garlic, finely chopped

1 tablespoon grated fresh ginger

1 teaspoon curry powder

1 tablespoon freshly grated turmeric
or 1 teaspoon ground

1 teaspoon ground coriander

Pinch of red-pepper flakes or chili powder

2 carrots, peeled and thinly sliced

2 cups fish, chicken, or vegetable stock

1 large leek, washed (make sure you rinse out any grit beneath
the top leaves) and sliced

1 head broccoli, separated into small florets

$1^3/_4$ cups coconut milk or reconstituted creamed coconut

Pinch of finely grated lime zest and a squeeze of lime juice
(from an organic lime)

A few squirts of Thai fish sauce

Salt

3–4 fresh salmon fillets (about 5–6 ounces per person), skinless, boneless
(remove any remaining bones with tweezers), cut into cubes of about 1″ x 1″

2 tablespoons chopped fresh cilantro

POWER FOODS:

1. **Coconut oil**
2. **Garlic**
3. **Ginger**
4. **Curry powder**
5. **Turmeric**
6. **Carrots**
7. **Broccoli**
8. **Cilantro**
9. **Salmon**

In a large, heavy-bottomed pot over medium heat, heat the oil and cook the onion for 4 to 5 minutes, or until translucent. Add the garlic and ginger and cook, stirring, for 1 minute. Add the curry, turmeric, coriander, and pepper flakes or chili powder and stir for 1 minute.

Add the carrots and stock, cover, and simmer for 5 minutes. Add the leek and broccoli and simmer for 5 minutes, or until the vegetables begin to soften. (The more finely you chop the vegetables, the faster they will soften and the more nutrients will be preserved.)

Stir in the coconut milk and remove from the heat. Your soup base is ready. (You can prepare this several hours in advance or, better still, make a double batch and freeze half of it for later.)

When you are ready to eat, bring the soup base to a gentle simmer, add the zest, and season to taste with fish sauce, salt, and a few drops of lime juice. Immerse the salmon cubes in the hot soup, cover, and simmer for 5 minutes (without stirring), or until the fish is cooked through.

Ladle the soup into bowls, sprinkle with the cilantro, and serve immediately. If desired, serve with steamed basmati rice or quinoa.

Makes 4 servings

Apple Sauerkraut with Honey-Mustard Salmon (From Conner Middelmann-Whitney)

2 tablespoons fine Dijon-style mustard

2 tablespoons coarse wholegrain mustard

1 teaspoon honey, plus extra for drizzling

1 teaspoon finely chopped fresh rosemary

3 tablespoons olive oil

1 white onion, finely chopped

1 apple (organic), skin-on, finely chopped

1 pound raw sauerkraut, drained in a strainer

4 wild-caught salmon fillets (remove any bones with tweezers)

Salt and ground black pepper

4 sprigs fresh rosemary

POWER FOODS:

1. **Rosemary**
2. **Onion**
3. **Apples**
4. **Sauerkraut**
5. **Salmon**

In a small bowl, mix the mustards, honey, and chopped rosemary.

In a medium pot over medium heat, warm 2 tablespoons of the oil and cook the onion for 5 minutes, or until translucent. Add the apple and cook, covered, for 10 minutes, or until the onion and apple are soft. Remove from the heat and add the sauerkraut. Toss to combine, cover, and keep warm.

Preheat the broiler. Warm the remaining 1 tablespoon oil in a small cast-iron skillet over medium-low heat. Sprinkle the salmon fillets with salt and pepper and place in the skillet, flesh side down. Cook for 2 minutes, then gently turn with a spatula and cook for another 2 minutes.

Smear the tops of the fish with the mustard sauce. Slide the skillet under the broiler for 1 minute, or until the mustard crust turns golden.

To serve, spoon the sauerkraut mixture evenly onto 4 plates, top each with a salmon fillet, drizzle a little honey over the top (if desired), and decorate each with a sprig of fresh rosemary.

Makes 4 servings

Salmon in Parchment

(From Dr. Andrew Weil's *The Healthy Kitchen*)

8 ounces thin spaghetti

1 tablespoon extra-virgin olive oil

$^3/_4$ teaspoon salt

2 tablespoons chopped fresh dill or parsley

4 salmon fillets (6 ounces each)

2 tablespoons Dijon mustard

1 cup julienned carrots

1 cup julienned zucchini

1 cup asparagus tips

1 cup julienned red bell peppers

POWER FOODS:

1. **Carrots**
2. **Zucchini**
3. **Asparagus**
4. **Red bell peppers**
5. **Mustard**

Preheat the oven to 400°F. Cut 4 large sheets of parchment paper. Fold each piece in half. Using scissors, cut the shape of half a heart from the folded side. (Remember the valentine you made in grade school?) Set aside.

In a large pot of rapidly boiling water, cook the spaghetti until al dente. Drain and toss with the oil, salt, and dill or parsley.

Rinse the salmon fillets and pat dry. Spread the mustard evenly over the top of each.

Open the 4 parchment paper heart shapes. Place one-quarter of the pasta in the center of the paper. Top with a salmon fillet and one-quarter each of the carrots, zucchini, asparagus, and bell peppers. Bring the sides of the heart over the filling and fold the edges together, starting at the top of the heart and overlapping the folded edges as you go. Fold the tip several times to secure it.

Place the pouches in the middle of the oven and bake for 10 minutes. Serve immediately in the sealed pouches, opening them just before eating.

Makes 4 servings

Moroccan Chicken Stew with Apricots
and Plums (From Conner Middelmann-Whitney)

2 tablespoons olive oil

4 chicken quarters (leg and thigh portions),
halved, or 1 pound boneless chicken thighs,
cut into bite-size cubes

2 red onions, halved and sliced lengthwise

1 tablespoon finely grated fresh ginger

1 tablespoon ground coriander

1 tablespoon paprika powder

2 teaspoons ground cumin

1 teaspoon ground cinnamon

1 teaspoon ground turmeric

Pinch of saffron strands or powder

1 tablespoon lemon juice, plus additional for seasoning

1 cup chicken stock

8 dried apricots, halved

8 dried plums, halved

1 preserved lemon, finely chopped (available from health food stores,
spice shops, or online), or finely grated zest of 1 organic lemon

10 green, pitted olives, sliced

Salt and ground black pepper

$\frac{1}{2}$ cup coarsely chopped walnuts

3 tablespoons chopped fresh cilantro or parsley

POWER FOODS:
1. **Onions**
2. **Ginger**
3. **Coriander**
4. **Cumin**
5. **Turmeric**
6. **Saffron**
7. **Walnuts**
8. **Cilantro**

In a large, wide pot over medium heat, warm the oil. Cook the chicken portions (or cubes) on both sides until golden. Transfer to a plate.

In the remaining oil, cook the onions over medium heat for 5 minutes, or until translucent. Add the ginger, coriander, paprika, cumin, cinnamon, turmeric, and saffron and cook for 1 minute, stirring so they don't burn. Add the 1 tablespoon lemon juice and stock, stir, and return the chicken to the pot. Cover with a lid and cook for 30 minutes, either on the stovetop at medium heat, stirring gently after 15 minutes, or in the oven at 350°F.

After 30 minutes, add the apricots, plums, chopped lemon or lemon zest, and olives, submerging these in the sauce and gently stirring to combine. Continue cooking (or return to the oven) for 20 minutes, or until the chicken is done. (If using free-range, pastured chicken, this may need an extra 30 minutes of cooking time.)

When the chicken is cooked through, remove from the heat (or oven) and season with salt, pepper, and lemon juice. Sprinkle with the walnuts and cilantro or parsley and serve. This is even better the next day when the flavors have had time to infuse.

Makes 4 servings

Fish Tajine (From Conner Middelmann-Whitney)
HERB AND SPICE PASTE (CHERMOULA)

$1/2$ cup chopped fresh cilantro

$1/2$ cup chopped fresh parsley

5–6 tablespoons olive oil

2 cloves garlic, minced

1 tablespoon paprika powder

1 tablespoon ground coriander

1 teaspoon ground cumin

1 teaspoon ground turmeric

1 teaspoon salt

1 teaspoon finely grated fresh ginger

Juice of $1/2$ lemon

Pinch of grated lemon zest

Pinch of chili powder (optional)

POWER FOODS:
1. **Cilantro**
2. **Parsley**
3. **Garlic**
4. **Coriander**
5. **Cumin**
6. **Turmeric**
7. **Ginger**
8. **Onion**
9. **Sweet potatoes**
10. **Tomato paste**
11. **Tomatoes**
12. **Lemon**
13. **Salmon**

VEGETABLES AND FISH

4 fish fillets, such as wild-caught sockeye salmon, mahi-mahi, cod, or halibut

Juice of 2 lemons

8 tablespoons olive oil, divided

1 large red onion, finely sliced

3 cloves garlic, minced

1 red bell pepper, sliced

1 green bell pepper, sliced

1 sweet potato, peeled and very thinly sliced

$1/2$ teaspoon paprika powder

1 tablespoon tomato paste

$1/2$ cup water

Salt and ground black pepper

4 tomatoes, sliced $1/8$" thick

1 preserved lemon, finely chopped (available from health food stores, spice shops, or online), or a drizzle of lemon juice (optional)

To make the herb and spice paste: In a small blender, combine the cilantro, parsley, oil, garlic, paprika, coriander, cumin, turmeric, salt, ginger, lemon juice, lemon zest, and chili powder (if desired). Blend until it makes a creamy paste.

To make the vegetables and fish: Combine the lemon juice and 4 tablespoons of the olive oil. Marinate the fish (ideally this is done at least an hour before cooking, but even 5 to 10 minutes is good). Pat the fish dry, place in a dish, and smear the herb and spice paste on all sides.

In a large pot over medium-high heat, warm 2 tablespoons of the oil. Add the onion and garlic and cook for 5 to 6 minutes, or until translucent. Add the bell peppers, sweet potato, paprika, tomato paste, and water. Season lightly with salt and pepper. Cover and cook for 10 minutes, stirring occasionally, until the sweet potatoes are al dente.

Preheat the oven to 350°F.

Transfer the vegetables to an ovenproof baking dish, lay the fish on top, and press lightly into the vegetables. Top the fish with the tomato slices, chopped lemon or lemon juice (if desired), and the remaining 2 tablespoons oil. Season to taste with salt and pepper.

Cover with foil or a lid and bake for 30 minutes, uncovering the dish after 15 minutes.

Makes 4 servings

Don't Worry Curry

2 tablespoons olive oil

1–2 tablespoons curry powder

Ground black pepper

1 cup brown or green lentils, picked and washed (organic)

1 cup brown rice, rinsed (organic)

4 cups water or vegetable broth

4 tablespoons vegetable broth

4 thin slices fresh ginger

3 ribs celery, finely chopped

3 cloves garlic, finely chopped

1 red bell pepper, chopped

Salt

2 tablespoons fresh cilantro

POWER FOODS:

1. **Lentils**
2. **Ginger**
3. **Celery**
4. **Garlic**
5. **Bell pepper**
6. **Curry powder**

In a large saucepan, heat the oil over medium heat. Add the curry powder and season to taste with black pepper. Add the lentils, rice, water or broth, broth, ginger, celery, garlic, and bell pepper. Season to taste with salt.

Bring to a boil, then simmer for 45 minutes, or until the lentils are softened and the rice is done. Dish into bowls and garnish with the cilantro.

Makes 4 servings

Sweet Zoe's Potatoes

10 ounces sweet potatoes, cut into 1″ cubes

2–3 tablespoons olive oil

1 teaspoon ground cinnamon

1 teaspoon salt

POWER FOODS:

1. **Sweet potatoes**
2. **Cinnamon**

Preheat the oven to 350°F. Line a baking sheet with parchment paper.

Place the potatoes in a large bowl. Add the oil, cinnamon, and salt and toss. Place the potatoes on the sheet. Bake for 30 to 45 minutes, or until fork tender.

Makes 4 servings

Broccoli Baobabs

¹/₃ cup olive oil

2 cloves garlic, chopped

Red-pepper flakes

1 large head broccoli, separated into florets

¹/₂ lemon

Salt and ground black pepper

POWER FOODS:

1. **Garlic**
2. **Red pepper**
3. **Broccoli**
4. **Black pepper**
5. **Lemon**

In a small skillet, heat the oil over medium heat. Add the garlic and cook until golden but not browned. Add the pepper flakes to taste (start with a pinch). Remove from the heat.

Place a steamer basket in a large pot with 2″ of water. Bring to a boil over high heat. Steam the broccoli in the basket for 5 minutes, or until bright green and tender. Drizzle the garlic mixture over the broccoli. Finish with a squeeze of lemon and season to taste with salt and pepper.

Makes 4 servings

SAUCES AND DRESSINGS

Snazzy Salsa

4 large tomatoes

1 sweet onion

1–2 cloves garlic

2 fresh jalapeño chile peppers, sliced, or if they are too hot for you, use canned chile peppers

$^1/_2$ cup chopped fresh cilantro leaves

2 tablespoons fresh lime juice

Salt and ground black pepper

POWER FOODS:
1. **Tomatoes**
2. **Onion**
3. **Garlic**
4. **Peppers**
5. **Black pepper**

If a chunky salsa is desired, chop the tomatoes, onion, garlic, and chile peppers and mix together in a large bowl. Add the cilantro and lime juice and mix well.

If a smoother salsa is desired, combine the tomatoes, onion, garlic, chile peppers, cilantro, and lime juice in a food processor. Process until blended.

Season to taste with salt and black pepper and adjust other seasonings as needed.

Serve with organic chips or as a condiment.

Makes 4 servings

Mariachi Guacamole

4 ripe avocados

1 red onion, finely chopped

1 large tomato, chopped

4 tablespoons finely chopped fresh cilantro

Hot chiles or 1 jalapeño chile pepper, if you like it hot, or hot pepper sauce to taste

$^{1}/_{3}$ cup fresh lime or lemon juice

Salt and ground black pepper

POWER FOODS:

1. **Avocados**
2. **Onion**
3. **Tomato**
4. **Peppers**
5. **Black pepper**

In a large bowl, mash the avocados with a fork. Add the onion, tomato, cilantro, chile peppers, and juice. Season to taste with salt and black pepper and adjust to desired hotness.

Cover lightly with plastic wrap, refrigerate, and let the flavors marry for at least 1 hour.

Makes 4 servings

Hector's Hummus

2 cups chickpeas (canned or cooked)

1 tablespoon tahini (sesame seed paste)

2–3 cloves garlic, minced

1 tablespoon extra-virgin olive oil

Juice of 1 large lemon

Salt and ground black pepper

Paprika

Chopped parsley

POWER FOODS:
1. **Chickpeas**
2. **Sesame seeds (tahini)**
3. **Garlic**
4. **Black pepper**
5. **Lemon**

In a blender or food processor, combine the chickpeas, tahini, garlic, oil, and lemon juice. Puree until smooth, then place in a bowl. Season to taste with salt and pepper. Sprinkle with paprika and chopped parsley.

Serve at room temperature or chilled as a dip for pitas.

Makes 4 servings

Fresh Tomato Sauce

4 large ripe tomatoes, chopped

³/₄ cup shredded fresh basil leaves

2 cloves garlic, minced

¹/₂ cup extra-virgin olive oil

Salt and ground black pepper

POWER FOODS:
1. **Tomatoes**
2. **Basil**
3. **Garlic**

Place the tomatoes in a large mixing bowl and stir in the basil, garlic, and oil. Season to taste with salt and pepper.

Serve over whole wheat or gluten-free pasta.

Makes 2 servings

Jean Bean's Roma Pasta Sauce

2 cups water

8–9 Roma tomatoes

$\frac{1}{2}$ cup extra-virgin olive oil

3–4 cloves garlic, minced

1 cup chopped mild onion

1 teaspoon red-pepper flakes

Salt and ground black pepper

$\frac{1}{4}$ cup chopped fresh Italian parsley

$\frac{1}{4}$ cup finely chopped fresh thyme

POWER FOODS:

1. **Tomatoes**
2. **Garlic**
3. **Onion**
4. **Red pepper**
5. **Thyme**

Preheat the oven to 225°F.

Place the water in a medium saucepan, bring it to a boil, and remove from the heat. Hot-bathe the tomatoes for 1 minute, then plunge them into cold water and peel off skin. Cut them in half.

In a roasting pan, heat the oil over medium-high heat on the stovetop. Add the garlic, onion, and pepper flakes and cook until the onions are translucent.

Lay the tomatoes, cut sides up, in the pan and cook over medium heat for 5 minutes. Season to taste with salt and black pepper, then carefully turn the tomatoes over. Place in the oven and roast for $2\frac{1}{2}$ hours.

Remove from the oven and sprinkle the parsley and thyme on top. Roast for 30 minutes. (If the tomatoes are too dry, add white wine for the last 30 minutes of cooking.) Toss with pasta.

Makes 6 servings

Cilantro-Walnut Pesto

(from Dr. Andrew Weil's *The Healthy Kitchen*)

1 cup walnut pieces

2 cups cilantro leaves, stems removed

1 jalapeño chile pepper, seeded and chopped

$\frac{1}{2}$ teaspoon cider vinegar

$\frac{1}{4}$ cup water

Salt

POWER FOODS:

1. **Walnuts**
2. **Pepper**

Put the walnuts in a food processor and process them until fine. Add the cilantro, chile pepper, vinegar, and 2 to 3 tablespoons of the water and season to taste with salt. Process, blending in a little more water if necessary to make a thick sauce. Taste and correct the seasoning, adding more salt if necessary.

Keep any leftover pesto in the refrigerator in a tightly covered container. Use as a dip or spread.

Makes 6 servings

Lemon Vinaigrette

1 cup extra-virgin olive oil

$\frac{1}{4}$–$\frac{1}{2}$ cup fresh lemon juice

1 clove garlic, minced

1 tablespoon finely chopped fresh chives

Salt and ground black pepper

POWER FOODS:

1. **Garlic**
2. **Chives**
3. **Black pepper**

Put the oil, lemon juice, garlic, and chives in a jar. Cover and shake until emulsified. Season to taste with salt and pepper. Keep in the refrigerator.

Makes 4 servings

Cilantro-Avocado Dressing

$\frac{1}{2}$ ripe avocado

$\frac{3}{4}$ cup packed fresh cilantro

$\frac{1}{2}$ cup fat-free plain yogurt

2 scallions, chopped

1 clove garlic, quartered

1 tablespoon lime juice

$\frac{1}{2}$ teaspoon sugar

$\frac{1}{2}$ teaspoon salt

POWER FOODS:
1. **Avocado**
2. **Scallions**
3. **Garlic**

In a blender, combine the avocado, cilantro, yogurt, scallions, garlic, lime juice, sugar, and salt. Blend until smooth.

Makes 4 servings

Christopher's Marinade

$\frac{1}{2}$ cup ponzu sauce or low-sodium organic soy sauce

$\frac{1}{2}$ cup rice vinegar

1 tablespoon light brown sugar or xylitol

1 teaspoon dark roasted sesame oil

1 teaspoon lemon or lime juice

2 cloves garlic, minced

1 tablespoon ginger juice

POWER FOODS:
1. **Garlic**
2. **Ginger**

In a medium bowl, combine the ponzu sauce or soy sauce, rice vinegar, sugar or xylitol, oil, lemon or lime juice, garlic, and ginger juice. Mix well. Use as a marinade.

Makes about 1 cup

ACKNOWLEDGMENTS

Dr. Lemole would like to thank:

Chris Conway as a facilitator and consultant; Sandra McLanahan for her medical and editorial skills; Emilyjane Lemole and Eileen McKiernan for recipe overview.

Dr. Mehta would like to thank:

My fellow authors, Drs. Gerald Lemole and Dwight McKee, for your collaboration, knowledge, and friendship.

Emily Jane Lemole for your guidance, your flurry of books and DVDs in the mail, and for encouraging me to put down the soda and introducing me to a new way of looking at health.

Our wordsmith, Kristin Mehus-Roe, for seamlessly bringing together three distinct voices, helping me to understand our audience, and speaking to what's most relevant and interesting.

Holy Redeemer Hospital administration for always supporting an integrative approach to patient care and recognizing leadership qualities in me before I had the confidence or experience to do so myself.

My parents, Kulin and Kishori Mehta, and my in-laws, Vinod and Sudha Parikh, for being vocal proponents of an integrative approach decades before it was en vogue.

Chris Conway for your boundless enthusiasm, support, and introductions.

Steve Parks for first putting the idea in my head of writing a book, not a pamphlet, as I had originally intended.

Dr. McKee would like to thank:

My dear friends Janie and Jerry Lemole, MD, for conceiving of this book, and to Pallav Mehta, MD, for his enthusiasm and energy in helping to manifest it.

The hematology-oncology division of the Scripps Clinic, La Jolla, California, for my hematology-oncology education.

Susan and Jeffrey Bland, PhD, David Jones, MD, and Mark Hyman, MD, for founding and developing the Institute for Functional Medicine, and all my friends and colleagues involved with IFM, who have created a robust holistic approach to healing, and its profound influence on my thinking.

The founders of Life Plus International, who have supported me throughout my career in pursuing my passions in medicine.

Donnie Yance and the ever-expanding Round Table Discussion Group for my extensive education in the field of botanical medicine and its application to cancer.

Joe Pizzorno, ND, and his research team for providing a solid evidence base for the use of nutritional-botanical supplementation in support of people with cancer challenges.

Kristin Mehus-Roe of Girl Friday Productions, and all of our editors at Rodale, who helped refine our ideas into engaging prose.

Chris Conway for connecting us to the wonderful people of Rodale.

ENDNOTES

CHAPTER 1

1   WHO, "10 Facts on Cancer," reviewed January 2013, www.who.int/features/factfiles/cancer/facts/en/index9.html.

2   J. Milford and F. Duran-Reynals, "Growth of a Chicken Sarcoma Virus in the Chick Embryo in the Absence of Neoplasia," *Cancer Research* 3 (1943): 578–84.

3   M. H. Sieweke, A. W. Stoker, and M. J. Bissell, "Evaluation of the Cocarcinogenic Effect of Wounding in Rous Sarcoma Virus Tumorigenesis," *Cancer Research* 49, no. 22 (November 15, 1989): 6419–24.

4   K. Pantel, C. Alix-Panabières, and S. Riethdorf, "Cancer Micrometastases," *Nature Reviews Clinical Oncology* 6, no. 6 (June 2009): 339–51.

5   D. Ornish et al., "Changes in Prostate Gene Expression in Men Undergoing an Intensive Nutrition and Lifestyle Intervention," *Proceedings of the National Academy of Sciences of the United States of America* 105, no. 24 (June 17, 2008): 8369–74.

CHAPTER 2

1   M. S. Linet et al., "Cancer Risks Associated with External Radiation from Diagnostic Imaging Procedures," *CA: A Cancer Journal for Clinicians* 62 (February 3, 2012): 75–100.

CHAPTER 3

1   C. M. Blanchard, K. S. Courneya, and K. Stein, "Cancer Survivors' Adherence to Lifestyle Behavior Recommendations and Associations with Health-Related Quality of Life: Results from the American Cancer Society's SCS-II," *Journal of Clinical Oncology* 26, no. 13 (May 2008): 2198–2204.

CHAPTER 4

1   G. W. Taylor et al., "Lymphatic Circulation Studied with Radioactive Plasma Proteins," *British Medical Journal* 1, no. 5011 (January 19, 1957): 133–37.

2   G. M. Lemole, *The Healing Diet* (New York: William Morrow, 2001): 78–92.

3   A. Cotonat and J. Cotonat, "Lymphagogue and Pulsatile Activities of Daflon 500 mg on Canine Thoracic Lymph Duct," *International Angiology* 8, no. S4 (October–December 1989): S15–18.

4   Lemole, *The Healing Diet,* 159–200.

5   H. Sinzinger, J. Kaliman, and A. Oguogho, "Eicosanoid Production and Lymphatic Responsiveness in Human Cigarette Smokers Compared with Non-smokers," *Lymphology* 33, no. 1 (March 2000): 24–31.

6   D. Porter et al., "Chimeric Antigen Receptor–Modified T Cells in Chronic Lymphoid Leukemia," *New England Journal of Medicine* 365 (August 25, 2011): 725–33.

7   W. Zou, "Immunosuppressive Networks in the Tumour Environment and Their Therapeutic Relevance," *Nature Reviews: Cancer* 5, no. 4 (2005): 263–74.

8   S. L. Topalian et al., "Nivolumab (anti-PD-1; BMS- 936558; ONO-4538) in Patients with Advanced Solid Tumors: Survival and Long-Term Safety in a Phase I Trial," presented at the 2013 American Society of Clinical Oncology Annual Meeting in Chicago, and in the *Journal of Clinical Oncology* 31, supplement: abstract 3002.

9   T. L. Whiteside, "Immune Suppression in Cancer: Effects on Immune Cells,

Mechanisms and Future Therapeutic Intervention," *Seminars in Cancer Biology* 16, no. 1 (February 2006): 3–15.

10   H. M. O'Hagan et al., "Oxidative Damage Targets Complexes Containing DNA Methyltransferases, SIRT1, and Polycomb Members to Promoter CpG Islands," *Cancer Cell* 20, no. 5 (November 15, 2011): 606–19.

CHAPTER 5

1   K. Y. Wolin et al., "Implementing the Exercise Guidelines for Cancer Survivor," *Journal of Supportive Oncology* 10, no. 5 (September–October 2012): 171–77.

2   D. W. Pekmezi and W. Demark-Wahnefried, "Updated Evidence in Support of Diet and Exercise Interventions in Cancer Survivors," *Acta Oncologica* 50, no. 2 (February 2011): 167–78.

3   J. A. Ligibel et. al., "American Society of Clinical Oncology Position Statement on Obesity and Cancer," *Journal of Clinical Oncology* 32, no. 31 (November 1, 2014): 3568–74.

4   C. L. Rock, "Nutrition and Physical Activity Guidelines for Cancer Survivors," *CA: A Cancer Journal for Clinicians* 62, no. 4 (July–August 2012): 243–74.

5   Moshe Frenkel, "Integrative Oncology Exceptional Patients: Thoughts and Reflections," *Cancer Strategies Journal* 1 no. 2 (Spring 2013): 2–7.

6   M. L. McCullough et al., "Following Cancer Prevention Guidelines Reduces Risk of Cancer, Cardiovascular Disease, and All-Cause Mortality," *Cancer Epidemiology, Biomarkers and Prevention* 20, no. 6 (June 2011): 1089–97.

7   M. Johansson et al., "Serum B Vitamin Levels and Risk of Lung Cancer," *Journal of the American Medical Association* 303, no. 23 (June 16, 2010): 2377–85.

8   A. Pan et al., "Red Meat Consumption and Mortality: Results from Two Prospective Cohort Studies," *Archives of Internal Medicine* 172, no. 7 (April 9, 2012): 555–63.

9   Ibid.

10   Ibid.

11   World Health Organization, "Breast Cancer: A Role for Trans Fatty Acids?" press release, April 11, 2008.

12   V. Chajès et al., "Association between Serum Trans-Monosaturated Fatty Acids and Breast Cancer Risk in the E3N-EPIC Study," *American Journal of Epidemiology* 167, no. 11 (June 2008): 1312–20.

13   S. E. Hankinson et. al., "Circulating Concentrations of Insulin-like Growth Factor-I and Risk of Breast Cancer," *Lancet* 351, no. 9113 (May 9, 1998): 1393–96.

14   J. M. Chan et al., "Plasma Insulin-like Growth Factor-1 and Prostate Cancer Risk: A Prospective Study," *Science* 179, no. 5350 (January 1998): 563–66.

15   M. L. Kwan et al., "Alcohol Consumption and Breast Cancer Recurrence and Survival among Women with Early-Stage Breast Cancer: The Life after Cancer Epidemiology Study," *Journal of Clinical Oncology* 28, no. 29 (October 10, 2010): 4410–16.

16   N. Hamajima, "Alcohol, Tobacco and Breast Cancer—Collaborative Reanalysis of Individual Data from 53 Epidemiological Studies, Including 58,515 Women with Breast Cancer and 95,067 Women without the Disease," *British Journal of Cancer* 87, no. 11 (November 18, 2002): 1234–45.

17   N. E. Allen et al., "Moderate Alcohol Intake and Cancer Incidence in Women," *Journal of the National Cancer Institute* 101, no. 5 (March 4, 2009): 296–305.

18   J. Zhou et al., "Soy Phytochemicals and Tea Bioactive Components

Synergistically Inhibit Androgen-Sensitive Human Prostate Tumors in Mice," *Journal of Nutrition* 133, no. 2 (February 2003): 516–21.

19   H. Yanagimoto et al., "Alleviating Function of Health Food (AHCC) for Side Effects in Chemotherapy Patients," 16th International Symposium of the AHCC Research Association, 2008.

20   S. Ohwada et al., "Adjuvant Immunochemotherapy with Oral Tegafur/Uracil plus PSK in Patients with Stage II or III Colorectal Cancer: A Randomised Controlled Study," *British Journal of Cancer* 90, no. 5 (March 8, 2004): 1003–10.

21   S. E. McCann et al., "Dietary Lignan Intakes in Relation to Survival among Women with Breast Cancer: The Western New York Exposures and Breast Cancer (WEB) Study," *Breast Cancer Research and Treatment* 122, no. 1 (July 2010): 229–35.

22   K. Buck et al., "Serum Enterolactone and Prognosis of Postmenopausal Breast Cancer," *Journal of Clinical Oncology* 29, no. 28 (October 1, 2011): 3730–38.

23   W. H. Tang et al., "Intestinal Microbial Metabolism of Phosphatidylcholine and Cardiovascular Risk," *New England Journal of Medicine* 368, no. 17 (April 25, 2013): 1575–84.

24   S. P. Fortmann, et al., "Vitamin and Mineral Supplements in the Primary Prevention of Cardiovascular Disease and Cancer: An Updated Systematic Evidence Review for the U.S. Preventive Services Task Force," *Annals of Internal Medicine* 159, no. 12 (December 17, 2013): 824–34.

25   T. C. Wallace, M. McBurney, V. L. Fulgoni, "Multivitamin/Mineral Supplement Contribution to Micronutrient Intakes in the United States, 2007–2010," *Journal of the American College of Nutrition* 33, no. 2 (2014): 94–102.

26   E. Guallar, et al., "Enough Is Enough: Stop Wasting Money on Vitamin and Mineral Supplements," *Annals of Internal Medicine* 159, no. 12 (December 17, 2013): 850–1.

27   T. C. Wallace, M. McBurney, V. L. Fulgoni, "Multivitamin/Mineral Supplement Contribution to Micronutrient Intakes in the United States, 2007–2010," *Journal of the American College of Nutrition* 33, no. 2 (2014): 94–102.

28   S. Hercberg, et al., "The SU.VI.MAX Study: A Randomized, Placebo-Controlled Trial of the Health Effects of Antioxidant Vitamins and Minerals," *Archives of Internal Medicine* 164, no. 21 (November 22, 2004): 2335–42.

29   J. M. Gaziano, et al., "Multivitamins in the Prevention of Cancer in Men: The Physicians' Health Study II Randomized Controlled Trial," *Journal of the American Medical Association* 308, no. 18 (November 14, 2012): 1971–80.

30   P. B. Bach and R. J. Lewis, "Multiplicities in the Assessment of Multiple Vitamins: Is It Too Soon to Tell Men That Vitamins Prevent Cancer?" *Journal of the American Medical Association* 308, no. 18 (November 14, 2012): 1916–7.

31   B. N. Ames, "A Role for Supplements in Optimizing Health: The Metabolic Tune-Up," *Archives of Biochemistry and Biophysics* 423, no. 1 (March 1, 2004): 227–34.

32   Cedric F. Garland, Christine B. French, Leo L. Baggerly, and Robert P. Heaney, "Vitamin D Supplement Doses and Serum 25-Hydroxyvitamin D in the Range Associated with Cancer Prevention," *Anticancer Research* 31, no. 2 (February 2011): 607–11.

CHAPTER 6

1   Moshe Frenkel, "Integrative Oncology Exceptional Patients: Thoughts and Reflections," *Cancer Strategies Journal* 1 no. 2 (Spring 2013): 2–7.

2   M. D. Holmes et al., "Physical Activity and Survival after Breast Cancer Diagnosis," *JAMA* 293, no. 20 (May 25, 2005): 2479–86.

3   C. M. Friedenreich et al., "Prospective Cohort Study of Lifetime Physical Activity and Breast Cancer Survival," *International Journal of Cancer* 124, no. 8 (April 15, 2009): 1954–62.

4   S. A. Kenfield, "Physical Activity and Survival after Prostate Cancer Diagnosis in the Health Professionals Follow-Up Study," *Journal of Clinical Oncology* 29, no. 6 (February 20, 2011): 726–32.

5   MacMillan Cancer Support, *The Importance of Physical Activity for People Living with and beyond Cancer: A Concise Evidence Review*, www.macmillan.org.uk/Documents/AboutUs/Commissioners/Physicalactivityevidencereview.pdf.

6   Collaborating for Health, "Exercise as Part of Cancer Care," August 8, 2011, www.c3health.org/alerts/alerts-physicalactivity/exercise-as-part-of-cancer-care/.

7   J. Ligibel et al., "Impact of a Mixed Strength and Endurance Exercise Intervention on Insulin Levels in Breast Cancer Survivors," *Journal of Clinical Oncology* 26, no. 6 (February 20, 2008): 907–12.

8   P. J. Goodwin et al., "Fasting Insulin and Outcome in Early-Stage Breast Cancer: Results of a Prospective Cohort Study," *Journal of Clinical Oncology* 20, no. 1 (January 1, 2002): 42–51.

9   M. D. Holmes et al., "Physical Activity and Survival after Breast Cancer Diagnosis," *JAMA* 293, no. 20 (May 25, 2005): 2479–86.

CHAPTER 7

1   L. Hardell and M. Carlberg, "Mobile Phone and Cordless Phone Use and the Risk for Glioma—Analysis of Pooled Case-Control Studies in Sweden, 1997–2003 and 2007–2009," *Pathophysiology* 22, no. 1 (March 2015): 1–13.

2   President's Cancer Panel, 2008–2009 Annual Report: *Reducing Environmental Cancer Risk: What We Can Do Now*, http://deainfo.nci.nih.gov/advisory/pcp/annualReports/pcp08-09rpt/PCP_Report_08-09_508.pdf.

CHAPTER 8

1   R. Siegel, D. Naishadham, A. Jemal, "Cancer Statistics, 2012," *CA: A Cancer Journal for Clinicians* 62, no. 1 (January–February 2012): 10–29.

2   D. R. Youlden et al., "The Descriptive Epidemiology of Female Breast Cancer: An International Comparison of Screening, Incidence, Survival and Mortality," *Cancer Epidemiology* 36, no. 3 (June 2012): 237–48.

3   H. D. Nelson et al., "Risk Factors for Breast Cancer for Women Aged 40 to 49 Years: A Systematic Review and Meta-Analysis," *Annals of Internal Medicine* 156, no. 9 (May 1, 2012): 635–48.

4   P. J. Goodwin et al., "Prognostic Effects of 25-Hydroxyvitamin D Levels in Early Breast Cancer," *Journal of Clinical Oncology* 27, no. 23 (August 10, 2009): 3757–63.

5   A. Vrieling et al., "Serum 25-Hydroxyvitamin D and Postmenopausal Breast Cancer Survival: A Prospective Patient Cohort Study," *Breast Cancer Research* 13, no. 4 (July 26, 2011): R74.

6   C. F. Garland et al., "Vitamin D Supplement Doses and Serum 25-Hydroxyvitamin D in the Range Associated with Cancer Prevention," *Anticancer Research* 31, no. 2 (February 2011): 607–11.

7   C. M. Alfano et al., "Fatigue, Inflammation, and Ð-3 and Ð-6 Fatty Acid Intake among Breast Cancer Survivors," *Journal of Clinical Oncology* 30, no. 12 (April 20, 2012): 1280–87.

8   Z. Ghoreishi et al., "Omega-3 Fatty Acids Are Protective against Paclitaxel-Induced Peripheral Neuropathy: A Randomized Double-Blind Placebo Controlled Trial," *BMC Cancer* 12 (August 15, 2012): 355.

9   Y. Xu and S. Y. Qian, "Anti-Cancer Activities of Ð-6 Polyunsaturated Fatty Acids," *Biomedical Journal* 37, no. 3 (May–June 2014): 112–19.

10   F. S. Kenny et al., "Gamma Linolenic Acid with Tamoxifen as Primary Therapy in Breast Cancer," *International Journal of Cancer* 85, no. 5 (March 1, 2000): 643–48.

11   P. Gupta and S. K. Srivastava, "Antitumor Activity of Phenethyl Isothiocyanate in HER2-Positive Breast Cancer Models," *BMC Medicine* 10 (July 24, 2012): 80.

12   Y. Jin, "3,3Ð-Diindolylmethane Inhibits Breast Cancer Cell Growth via miR-21-Mediated Cdc25A Degradation," *Molecular and Cellular Biochemistry* 358, no. 1–2 (December 2011): 345–54.

13   K. M. Dalessandri et al., "Pilot Study: Effect of 3,3Ð-Diindolylmethane Supplements on Urinary Hormone Metabolites in Postmenopausal Women with a History of Early-Stage Breast Cancer," *Nutrition and Cancer* 50, no. 2 (2004): 161–67.

14   A. T. Perez et al., "A Phase 1B Dose Escalation Trial of Scutellaria Barbata (BZL101) for Patients with Metastatic Breast Cancer," *Breast Cancer Research and Treatment* 120, no. 1 (February 2010): 111–18.

15   J. Klawitter et al., "Bezielle (BZL101)-Induced Oxidative Stress Damage Followed by Redistribution of Metabolic Fluxes in Breast Cancer Cells: A Combined Proteomic and Metabolomic Study," *International Journal of Cancer* 129, no. 12 (December 15, 2011): 2945–57.

16   M. Royt et al., "Curcumin Sensitizes Chemotherapeutic Drugs via Modulation of PKC, Telomerase, NF-kappaB and HDAC in Breast Cancer," *Therapeutic Delivery* 2, no. 10 (October 2011): 1275–93.

17   M. Bayet-Robert et al., "Phase I Dose Escalation Trial of Docetaxel plus Curcumin in Patients with Advanced and Metastatic Breast Cancer," *Cancer Biology and Therapy* 9, no. 1 (January 2010): 8–14.

18   T. H. Marczylo et al., "Comparison of Systemic Availability of Curcumin with That of Curcumin Formulated with Phosphatidylcholine," *Cancer Chemotherapy and Pharmacology* 60, no. 2 (July 2007): 171–77.

19   R. A. DiSilvestro et al., "Diverse Effects of a Low Dose Supplement of Lipidated Curcumin in Healthy Middle Aged People," *Nutrition Journal* 11 (September 26, 2012): 79.

20   G. Zhang et al. "Anti-Cancer Activities of Tea Epigallocatechin-3-Gallate in Breast Cancer Patients under Radiotherapy," *Current Molecular Medicine* 12, no. 2 (February 2012): 163–76.

21   S. F. Eddy, S. E. Kane, and G. E. Sonenshein, "Trastuzumab-Resistant HER2-Driven Breast Cancer Cells Are Sensitive to Epigallocatechin-3 Gallate," *Cancer Research* 67, no. 19 (October 1, 2007): 9018–23.

22   W. Zhu et al., "Trans-Resveratrol Alters Mammary Promoter Hypermethylation in Women at Increased Risk for Breast Cancer," *Nutrition and Cancer* 64, no. 3 (April 2012): 393–400.

23   R. Di Franco et al., "Skin Toxicity from External Beam Radiation Therapy in Breast Cancer Patients: Protective Effects of Resveratrol, Lycopene, Vitamin C and Anthocianin (Ixor®)," *Radiation Oncology* 7 (January 30, 2012): 12.

24   S. Kim et al., "Silibinin Prevents TPA-Induced MMP-9 Expression by Down-Regulation of COX-2 in Human Breast Cancer Cells," *Journal of Ethnopharmacology* 126, no. 2 (November 12, 2009): 252–57.

25   A. K. Tyagi et al., "Synergistic Anti-Cancer Effects of Silibinin with Conventional Cytotoxic Agents Doxorubicin, Cisplatin and Carboplatin against

Human Breast Carcinoma MCF-7 and MDA-MB468 Cells," *Oncology Reports* 11, no. 2 (February 2004): 493–99.

26   J. Duo J et al., "Quercetin Inhibits Human Breast Cancer Cell Proliferation and Induces Apoptosis via Bcl-2 and Bax Regulation," *Molecular Medicine Reports* 5, no. 6 (June 2012): 1453–56.

27   S. M. Mense, J. Chhabra, and H. K. Bhat, "Preferential Induction of Cytochrome P450 1A1 over Cytochrome P450 1B1 in Human Breast Epithelial Cells following Exposure to Quercetin," *Journal of Steroid Biochemistry and Molecular Biology* 110, no. 1–2 (May 2008): 157–62.

28   H. S. Seo et al., "Phytoestrogens Induce Apoptosis via Extrinsic Pathway, Inhibiting Nuclear Factor-KappaB Signaling in HER2-Overexpressing Breast Cancer Cells," *Anticancer Research* 31, no. 10 (October 2011): 3301–13.

29   X. Song et al., "Grape Seed Proanthocyanidin Suppression of Breast Cell Carcinogenesis Induced by Chronic Exposure to Combined 4-(Methylnitrosamino)-1-(3-Pyridyl)-1-Butanone and Benzo[a]pyrene," *Molecular Carcinogenesis* 49, no. 5 (May 2010): 450–63.

30   I. Kijima et al., "Grape Seed Extract Is an Aromatase Inhibitor and a Suppressor of Aromatase Expression," *Cancer Research* 66, no. 11 (June 1, 2006): 5960–67.

31   A. Cutando et al., "Role of Melatonin in Cancer Treatment," *Anticancer Research* 32, no. 7 (July 2012): 2747–53.

32   J. Ju et al., "Cancer-Preventive Activities of Tocopherols and Tocotrienols," *Carcinogenesis* 31, no. 4 (April 2010): 533–42.

33   C. S. Yang, N. Suh, and A. N. Kong, "Does Vitamin E Prevent or Promote Cancer?" *Cancer Prevention Research* (Philadelphia, Pa.) 5, no. 5 (May 2012): 701–5.

34   K. Nimptsch et al., "Dietary Vitamin K Intake in Relation to Cancer Incidence and Mortality: Results from the Heidelberg Cohort of the European Prospective Investigation into Cancer and Nutrition (EPIC-Heidelberg)," *American Journal of Clinical Nutrition* 91, no. 5 (May 2010): 1348–58.

35   K. Nimptsch, Rohrmann S, Linseisen J. "Dietary Intake of Vitamin K and Risk of Prostate Cancer in the Heidelberg Cohort of the European Prospective Investigation into Cancer and Nutrition (EPIC-Heidelberg)," *American Journal of Clinical Nutrition* 87, no. 4 (April 2008): 985–92.

36   H. Zhang et al., "Vitamin K2 Augments 5-Fluorouracil-Induced Growth Inhibition of Human Hepatocellular Carcinoma Cells by Inhibiting NF-ÐB Activation," *Oncology Reports* 25, no. 1 (January 2011): 159–66.

37   N. Parekh, U. Chandran, and E. V. Bandera, "Obesity in Cancer Survival," *Annual Review of Nutrition* 32 (August 21, 2012): 311–42.

38   P. D. Loprinzi et al., "Physical Activity and the Risk of Breast Cancer Recurrence: A Literature Review," *Oncology Nursing Forum* 39, no. 3 (May 1, 2012): 269–74.

39   O. Voevodina et al., "Association of Mediterranean Diet, Dietary Supplements and Alcohol Consumption with Breast Density among Women in South Germany: A Cross-Sectional Study," *BMC Public Health* 13 (March 7, 2013): 203.

40   L. E. Carlson et al., "Mindfulness-Based Stress Reduction in Relation to Quality of Life, Mood, Symptoms of Stress and Levels of Cortisol, Dehydroepiandrosterone Sulfate (DHEAS) and Melatonin in Breast and Prostate Cancer Outpatients," *Psychoneuroendocrinology* 29, no. 4 (May 2004): 448–74.

41   K. E. Calhoun et al., "Dehydroepiandrosterone Sulfate Causes Proliferation

of Estrogen Receptor-Positive Breast Cancer Cells Despite Treatment with Fulvestrant," *Archives of Surgery* 138, no. 8 (August 2003): 879–83.

42   L. J. Schurgers et al., "Vitamin K-Containing Dietary Supplements: Comparison of Synthetic Vitamin K1 and Natto-Derived Menaquinone-7," *Blood* 109, no. 8 (April 15, 2007): 3279–83.

43   A. F. Peery et al., "Burden of Gastrointestinal Disease in the United States: 2012 Update," *Gastroenterology* 143, no. 5 (November 2012): 1179–87.

44   D. A. Joseph et al., "Prevalence of Colorectal Cancer Screening among Adults—Behavioral Risk Factor Surveillance System, United States, 2010," supplement, *Morbidity and Mortality Weekly Report* 61 (June 15, 2012): S51–56.

45   E. A. Platz et al., "Proportion of Colon Cancer Risk That Might Be Preventable in a Cohort of Middle-Aged US Men," *Cancer Causes and Control* 11, no. 7 (August 2000): 579–88.

46   S. L. Stewart et al., "A Population-Based Study of Colorectal Cancer Histology in the United States, 1998-2001," supplement, *Cancer* 107, no. S5 (September 1, 2006): S1128–41.

47   Z. Fu et al., "Lifestyle Factors and Their Combined Impact on the Risk of Colorectal Polyps," *American Journal of Epidemiology* 176, no. 9 (November 1, 2012): 766–76.

48   C. A. Doubeni et al., "Socioeconomic Status and the Risk of Colorectal Cancer: An Analysis of More Than a Half Million Adults in the National Institutes of Health-AARP Diet and Health Study," *Cancer* 118, no. 14 (July 15, 2012): 3636–44.

49   J. Gong et al., "A Pooled Analysis of Smoking and Colorectal Cancer: Timing of Exposure and Interactions with Environmental Factors," *Cancer Epidemiology, Biomarkers and Prevention* 21, no. 11 (November 2012): 1974–85.

50   E. L. Jamin et al., "Combined Genotoxic Effects of a Polycyclic Aromatic Hydrocarbon (B(a)P) and an Heterocyclic Amine (PhIP) in Relation to Colorectal Carcinogenesis," *PLoS One* 8, no. 3 (2013): e58591.

51   P. Ferrari et al., "Lifetime and Baseline Alcohol Intake and Risk of Colon and Rectal Cancers in the European Prospective Investigation into Cancer and Nutrition (EPIC)," *International Journal of Cancer* 121, no. 9 (November 1, 2007): 2065–72.

52   N. F. Sanchez et al., "Physical Activity Reduces Risk for Colon Polyps in a Multiethnic Colorectal Cancer Screening Population," *BMC Research Notes* 5 (June 20, 2012): 312.

53   A. Chao et al., "Amount, Type, and Timing of Recreational Physical Activity in Relation to Colon and Rectal Cancer in Older Adults: The Cancer Prevention Study II Nutrition Cohort," *Cancer, Epidemiology, Biomarkers and Prevention* 13, no. 12 (2004): 2187–95.

54   K. Ng et al., "Circulating 25-Hydroxyvitamin D Levels and Survival in Patients with Colorectal Cancer," *Journal of Clinical Oncology* 26, no. 18 (June 20, 2008): 2984–91.

55   R. E. Stubbins, A. Hakeem, and N. P. Núñez, "Using Components of the Vitamin D Pathway to Prevent and Treat Colon Cancer," *Nutrition Reviews* 70, no. 12 (December 2012): 721–29.

56   Garland et al., "Vitamin D Supplement Doses and Serum 25-Hydroxyvitamin D in the Range Associated with Cancer Prevention."

57   M. Shakibaei et al., "Curcumin Enhances the Effect of Chemotherapy against Colorectal Cancer Cells by Inhibition of NF-ÐB and Src Protein Kinase Signaling Pathways," *PLoS One* 8, no. 2 (2013): e57218.

58   R. E. Carroll et al., "Phase IIa Clinical Trial of Curcumin for the Prevention of Colorectal Neoplasia," *Cancer Prevention Research* (Philadelphia, Pa.) 4, no. 3 (March 2011): 354–64.

59   Marczylo et al., "Comparison of Systemic Availability of Curcumin with That of Curcumin Formulated with Phosphatidylcholine."

60   DiSilvestro et al., "Diverse Effects of a Low Dose Supplement of Lipidated Curcumin in Healthy Middle Aged People."

61   G. Yang et al., "Prospective Cohort Study of Green Tea Consumption and Colorectal Cancer Risk in Women," *Cancer Epidemiology, Biomarkers and Prevention* 16, no. 6 (June 2007): 1219–23.

62   M. Shimizu et al., "Green Tea Extracts for the Prevention of Metachronous Colorectal Adenomas: A Pilot Study," *Cancer Epidemiology, Biomarkers and Prevention* 17, no. 11 (November 2008): 3020–25.

63   M. E. Juan, I. Alfaras, and J. M. Planas, "Colorectal Cancer Chemoprevention by Trans-Resveratrol," *Pharmacological Research* 65, no. 6 (June 2012): 584–91.

64   K. R. Patel et al., "Clinical Pharmacology of Resveratrol and Its Metabolites in Colorectal Cancer Patients," *Cancer Research* 70, no. 19 (October 2010): 7392–99.

65   S. Radhakrishnan et al., "Resveratrol Potentiates Grape Seed Extract Induced Human Colon Cancer Cell Apoptosis," *Frontiers in Bioscience* (elite edition) 3 (June 1, 2011): 1509–23.

66   M. Kaur et al., "Grape Seed Extract Upregulates p21 (Cip1) through Redox-Mediated Activation of $ERK_{1/2}$ and Posttranscriptional Regulation Leading to Cell Cycle Arrest in Colon Carcinoma HT29 Cells," *Molecular Carcinogenesis* 50, no. 7 (July 2011): 553–62.

67   M. A. Azcárate-Peril, M. Sikes, and J. M. Bruno-Bárcena, "The Intestinal Microbiota, Gastrointestinal Environment and Colorectal Cancer: A Putative Role for Probiotics in Prevention of Colorectal Cancer?" *American Journal of Physiology Gastrointestinal Liver Physiology* 301, no. 3 (September 2011): G401–24.

68   A. J. Cockbain, G. J. Toogood, and M. A. Hull, "Omega-3 Polyunsaturated Fatty Acids for the Treatment and Prevention of Colorectal Cancer," *Gut* 61, no. 1 (January 2012): 135–49.

69   J. A. Read et al., "Nutrition Intervention Using an Eicosapentaenoic Acid (EPA)-Containing Supplement in Patients with Advanced Colorectal Cancer. Effects on Nutritional and Inflammatory Status: A Phase II Trial," *Supportive Care in Cancer* 15, no. 3 (March 2007): 301–7.

70   Xu and Qian, "Anti-Cancer Activities of Ð-6 Polyunsaturated Fatty Acids."

71   F. S. Kenny et al., "Gamma Linolenic Acid with Tamoxifen as Primary Therapy in Breast Cancer," *International Journal of Cancer* 85, no. 5 (March 1, 2000): 643–48.

72   N. Bhatnagar et al., "3,3Ð-Diindolylmethane Enhances the Efficacy of Butyrate in Colon Cancer Prevention through Down-Regulation of Survivin," *Cancer Prevention Research* (Philadelphia, Pa.) 2 no. 6 (June 2009): 581–89.

73   A. Lerner et al., "The Indolic Diet-Derivative, 3,3Ð-Diindolylmethane, Induced Apoptosis in Human Colon Cancer Cells through Upregulation of NDRG1," *Journal of Biomedicine and Biotechnology* 2012 (2012): 256178.

74   H. Zhang et al., "Antitumor Activities of Quercetin and Quercetin-5Ð,8-Disulfonate in Human Colon and Breast Cancer Cell Lines," *Food and Chemical Toxicology* 50, no. 5 (May 2012): 1589–99.

75   C. P. Xavier et al., "Quercetin Enhances 5-Fluorouracil-Induced Apoptosis in MSI Colorectal Cancer Cells through p53 Modulation," *Cancer Chemotherapy and Pharmacology* 68, no. 6 (December 2011): 1449–57.

76   Cutando et al., "Role of Melatonin in Cancer Treatment."

77   Ju et al., "Cancer-Preventive Activities of Tocopherols and Tocotrienols."

78   Yang, Suh, and Kong, "Does Vitamin E Prevent or Promote Cancer?"

79   Nimptsch et al., "Dietary Vitamin K Intake in Relation to Cancer Incidence and Mortality."

80   Nimptsch, Rohrmann, and Linseisen, "Dietary Intake of Vitamin K and Risk of Prostate Cancer in the Heidelberg Cohort of the European Prospective Investigation into Cancer and Nutrition."

81   Zhang et al., "Vitamin K2 Augments 5-Fluorouracil-Induced Growth Inhibition of Human Hepatocellular Carcinoma Cells by Inhibiting NF-ÐB Activation."

82   J. A. Meyerhardt et al., "Dietary Glycemic Load and Cancer Recurrence and Survival in Patients with Stage III Colon Cancer: Findings from CALGB 89803," *Journal of the National Cancer Institute* 104, no. 22 (November 21, 2012): 1702–11.

83   J. A. Meyerhardt et al., "Association of Dietary Patterns with Cancer Recurrence and Survival in Patients with Stage III Colon Cancer," *JAMA* 298, no. 7 (August 15, 2007): 754–64.

84   C. Blair et al., "Cross-Sectional & Longitudinal Associations between Light-Intensity Physical Activity & Physical Function Among Cancer Survivors," *Cancer Epidemiology Biomarkers and Prevention* 22, no. 3 (March 2013): 475–76.

85   E. S. Rinella, E. D. Bankaitis, D. W. Threadgill, "Dietary Calcium Supplementation Enhances Efficacy but also Toxicity of EGFR Inhibitor Therapy for Colon Cancer," *Cancer Biology and Therapy* 13, no. 3 (February 1, 2012): 130–37.

86   Schurgers et al., "Vitamin K-Containing Dietary Supplements."

87   Siegel, Naishadham, and Jemal, "Cancer Statistics, 2012."

88   C. S. Dela Cruz, L. T. Tanoue, and R. A. Matthay, "Lung Cancer: Epidemiology, Etiology, and Prevention," *Clinics in Chest Medicine* 32, no. 4 (December 2011): 605–44.

89   R. W. Field and B. L. Withers, "Occupational and Environmental Causes of Lung Cancer," *Clinics in Chest Medicine* 33, no. 4 (December 2012): 681–703.

90   J. J. Erasmus and B. S. Sabloff, "CT, Positron Emission Tomography, and MRI in Staging Lung Cancer," *Clinics in Chest Medicine* 29, no. 1 (March 2008): 39–57, v.

91   S. Tretli et al., "Serum Levels of 25-Hydroxyvitamin D and Survival in Norwegian Patients with Cancer of Breast, Colon, Lung, and Lymphoma: A Population-Based Study," *Cancer Causes and Control* 23, no. 2 (February 2012): 363–70.

92   K. H. Allin and B. G. Nordestgaard, "Elevated C-Reactive Protein in the Diagnosis, Prognosis, and Cause of Cancer," *Critical Reviews in Clinical Laboratory Sciences* 48, no. 4 (July–August 2011): 155–70.

93   Garland et al., "Vitamin D Supplement Doses and Serum 25-Hydroxyvitamin D in the Range Associated with Cancer Prevention."

94   C. Finocchiaro et al., "Effect of n-3 Fatty Acids on Patients with Advanced

Lung Cancer: A Double-Blind, Placebo-Controlled Study," *British Journal of Nutrition* 108, no. 2 (July 2012): 327–33.

95   B. S. van der Meij et al., "Oral Nutritional Supplements Containing n-3 Polyunsaturated Fatty Acids Affect Quality of Life and Functional Status in Lung Cancer Patients during Multimodality Treatment: An RCT," *European Journal of Clinical Nutrition* 66, no. 3 (March 2012): 399–404.

96   R. A. Murphy et al., "Supplementation with Fish Oil Increases First-Line Chemotherapy Efficacy in Patients with Advanced Nonsmall Cell Lung Cancer," *Cancer* 117, no. 16 (August 15, 2011): 3774–80.

97   Xu and Qian, "Anti-Cancer Activities of Ð-6 Polyunsaturated Fatty Acids."

98   Kenny et al., "Gamma Linolenic Acid with Tamoxifen as Primary Therapy in Breast Cancer."

99   S. Y. Choi, J. H. Yu, and H. Kim, "Mechanism of Alpha-Lipoic Acid-Induced Apoptosis of Lung Cancer Cells," *Annals of the New York Academy of Sciences* 1171 (August 2009): 149–55.

100   G. Mantovani et al., "Restoration of Functional Defects in Peripheral Blood Mononuclear Cells Isolated from Cancer Patients by Thiol Antioxidants Alpha-Lipoic Acid and N-Acetyl Cysteine," *International Journal of Cancer* 86, no. 6 (June 15, 2000): 842–47.

101   X. Wu et al., "Isothiocyanates Induce Oxidative Stress and Suppress the Metastasis Potential of Human Non-Small Cell Lung Cancer Cells," *BMC Cancer* 10 (June 9, 2010): 269.

102   W. J. Wu et al., "Ð-Phenylethyl Isothiocyanate Reverses Platinum Resistance by a GSH-Dependent Mechanism in Cancer Cells with Epithelial-Mesenchymal Transition Phenotype," *Biochemical Pharmacology* 85, no. 4 (February 15, 2013): 486–96.

103   M. Suganuma, A. Saha, and H. Fujiki, "New Cancer Treatment Strategy Using Combination of Green Tea Catechins and Anticancer Drugs," *Cancer Science* 102, no. 2 (February 2011): 317–23.

104   H. Yin et al., "Synergistic Antitumor Efficiency of Docetaxel and Curcumin against Lung Cancer," *Acta Biochimica et Biophysica Sinica* (Shanghai) 44, no. 2 (February 2012): 147–53.

105   Marczylo et al., "Comparison of Systemic Availability of Curcumin with That of Curcumin Formulated with Phosphatidylcholine."

106   DiSilvestro et al., "Diverse Effects of a Low Dose Supplement of Lipidated Curcumin in Healthy Middle Aged People."

107   Y. S. Kim, J. W. Sull, and H. J. Sung, "Suppressing Effect of Resveratrol on the Migration and Invasion of Human Metastatic Lung and Cervical Cancer Cells," *Molecular Biology Reports* 39, no. 9 (September 2012): 8709–16.

108   T. K. Lam et al., "Dietary Quercetin, Quercetin-Gene Interaction, Metabolic Gene Expression in Lung Tissue and Lung Cancer Risk," *Carcinogenesis* 31, no. 4 (April 2010): 634–42.

109   S. Y. Zheng et al., "Anticancer Effect and Apoptosis Induction by Quercetin in the Human Lung Cancer Cell Line A-549," *Molecular Medicine Reports* 5, no. 3 (March 2012): 822–26.

110   Cutando et al., "Role of Melatonin in Cancer Treatment."

111   P. Lissoni et al., "Five Years Survival in Metastatic Non-Small Cell Lung Cancer Patients Treated with Chemotherapy Alone or Chemotherapy and Melatonin: A Randomized Trial," *Journal of Pineal Research* 35, no. 1 (August 2003): 12–15.

112   Ju et al., "Cancer-Preventive Activities of Tocopherols and Tocotrienols."

113   Yang, Suh, and Kong, "Does Vitamin E Prevent or Promote Cancer?"

114   Nimptsch et al., "Dietary Vitamin K Intake in Relation to Cancer Incidence and Mortality."

115   Nimptsch, Rohrmann, and Linseisen, "Dietary Intake of Vitamin K and Risk of Prostate Cancer in the Heidelberg Cohort of the European Prospective Investigation into Cancer and Nutrition (EPIC-Heidelberg)."

116   Zhang et al., "Vitamin K2 Augments 5-Fluorouracil-Induced Growth Inhibition of Human Hepatocellular Carcinoma Cells by Inhibiting NF-ÐB Activation."

117   M. E. Wright et al, "Intakes of Fruit, Vegetables, and Specific Botanical Groups in Relation to Lung Cancer Risk in the NIH-AARP Diet and Health Study," *American Journal of Epidemiology* 168, no. 9 (November 1, 2008): 1024–34.

118   K. Y. Christensen et al., "The Risk of Lung Cancer Related to Dietary Intake of Flavonoids," *Nutrition and Cancer* 64, no. 7 (2012): 964–74.

119   L. Solberg Nes, et al., "Physical Activity Level and Quality of Life in Long Term Lung Cancer Survivors," *Lung Cancer* 77, no. 3 (September 2012): 611–16.

120   Y. J. Jeon et al., "Effects of Beta-Carotene Supplements on Cancer Prevention: Meta-Analysis of Randomized Controlled Trials," *Nutrition and Cancer* 63, no. 8 (November 2011): 1196–1207.

121   Schurgers et al., "Vitamin K-Containing Dietary Supplements."

122   O. W. Brawley, "Trends in Prostate Cancer in the United States," *Journal of the National Cancer Institute. Monographs* 2012, no. 45 (December 2012): 152–56.

123   K. M. Wilson, E. L. Giovannucci, and L. A. Mucci, "Lifestyle and Dietary Factors in the Prevention of Lethal Prostate Cancer," *Asian Journal of Andrology* 14, no. 3 (May 2012): 365–74.

124   G. S. Sandhu and G. L. Andriole, "Overdiagnosis of Prostate Cancer," *Journal of the National Cancer Institute. Monographs* 2012, no. 45 (December 2012): 146–51.

125   J. Ma et al., "Prediagnostic Body-Mass Index, Plasma C-Peptide Concentration, and Prostate Cancer-Specific Mortality in Men with Prostate Cancer: A Long-Term Survival Analysis," *Lancet. Oncology* 9, no. 11 (November 2008): 1039–47.

126   R. Hurst et al., "Selenium and Prostate Cancer: Systematic Review and Meta-Analysis," *American Journal of Clinical Nutrition* 96, no. 1 (July 2012): 111–22.

127   B. Julin et al., "Dietary Cadmium Exposure and Prostate Cancer Incidence: A Population-Based Prospective Cohort Study," *British Journal of Cancer* 107, no. 5 (August 21, 2012): 895–900.

128   Y. S. Lin et al., "Increased Risk of Cancer Mortality Associated with Cadmium Exposures in Older Americans with Low Zinc Intake," *Journal of Toxicology and Environmental Health, Part A* 76, no. 1 (2013): 1–15.

129   T. P. Kilpeläinen et al., "Prostate Cancer Mortality in the Finnish Randomized Screening Trial," *Journal of the National Cancer Institute* 105, no. 10 (May 15, 2013): 719–25.

130   D. Ilic et al., "Screening for Prostate Cancer," *Cochrane Database Systematic Reviews* 1 (January 31, 2013): CD004720.

131   S. J. Freedland, "Screening, Risk Assessment, and the Approach to Therapy in Patients with Prostate Cancer," *Cancer* 117, no. 6 (March 15, 2011): 1123–35.

132   I. M. Shui et al., "Vitamin D-Related Genetic Variation, Plasma Vitamin D, and Risk of Lethal Prostate Cancer: A Prospective Nested Case-Control Study," *Journal of the National Cancer Institute* 104, no. 9 (May 2, 2012): 690–99.

133   F. Fang et al., "Prediagnostic Plasma Vitamin D Metabolites and Mortality among Patients with Prostate Cancer," *PLoS One* 6, no. 4 (April 6, 2011): e18625.

134   D. T. Marshall et al., "Vitamin D3 Supplementation at 4000 International Units per Day for One Year Results in a Decrease of Positive Cores at Repeat Biopsy in Subjects with Low-Risk Prostate Cancer under Active Surveillance," *Journal of Clinical Endocrinology Metabolism* 97, no. 7 (July 2012): 2315–24.

135   Garland et al., "Vitamin D Supplement Doses and Serum 25-Hydroxyvitamin D in the Range Associated with Cancer Prevention."

136   C. M. Yang et al., "Lycopene and the LXRÐ Agonist T0901317 Synergistically Inhibit the Proliferation of Androgen-Independent Prostate Cancer Cells via the PPARÐ-LXRÐ-ABCA1 Pathway," *Journal of Nutritional Biochemisty* 23, no. 9 (September 2012): 1155–62.

137   A. J. Teodoro et al., "Effect of Lycopene on Cell Viability and Cell Cycle Progression in Human Cancer Cell Lines," *Cancer Cell International* 12, no. 1 (August 6, 2012): 36.

138   E. Giovannucci, "Commentary: Serum Lycopene and Prostate Cancer Progression: A Re-consideration of Findings from the Prostate Cancer Prevention Trial," *Cancer Causes and Control* 22, no. 7 (July 2011): 1055–59.

139   H. S. Kim et al., "Effects of Tomato Sauce Consumption on Apoptotic Cell Death in Prostate Benign Hyperplasia and Carcinoma," *Nutrition and Cancer* 47, no. 1 (2003): 40–47.

140   K. Gupta et al., "Green Tea Polyphenols Induce p53-Dependent and p53-Independent Apoptosis in Prostate Cancer Cells through Two Distinct Mechanisms," *PLoS One* 7, no. 12 (2012): e52572.

141   J. McLarty et al., "Tea Polyphenols Decrease Serum Levels of Prostate-Specific Antigen, Hepatocyte Growth Factor, and Vascular Endothelial Growth Factor in Prostate Cancer Patients and Inhibit Production of Hepatocyte Growth Factor and Vascular Endothelial Growth Factor in Vitro," *Cancer Prevention Research* (Philadelphia, Pa.) 2, no. 7 (July 2009): 673–82.

142   S. Bettuzzi et al., "Chemoprevention of Human Prostate Cancer by Oral Administration of Green Tea Catechins in Volunteers with High-Grade Prostate Intraepithelial Neoplasia: A Preliminary Report from a One-Year Proof-of-Principle Study," *Cancer Research* 66, no. 2 (January 15, 2006): 1234–40.

143   P. H. Killian et al., "Curcumin Inhibits Prostate Cancer Metastasis in Vivo by Targeting the Inflammatory Cytokines CXCL1 and -2," *Carcinogenesis* 33, no. 12 (December 2012): 2507–19.

144   Marczylo et al., "Comparison of Systemic Availability of Curcumin with That of Curcumin Formulated with Phosphatidylcholine."

145   DiSilvestro et al., "Diverse Effects of a Low Dose Supplement of Lipidated Curcumin in Healthy Middle Aged People."

146   S. Sheth et al., "Resveratrol Reduces Prostate Cancer Growth and Metastasis by Inhibiting the Akt/MicroRNA-21 Pathway," *PLoS One* 7 no. 12 (2012): e51655.

147   Y. Fang, V. G. DeMarco, and M. B. Nicholl, "Resveratrol Enhances Radiation Sensitivity in Prostate Cancer by Inhibiting Cell Proliferation and Promoting Cell Senescence and Apoptosis," *Cancer Science* 103, no. 6 (June 2012): 1090–98.

148   M. M. Epstein et al., "Dietary Fatty Acid Intake and Prostate Cancer Survival in Örebro County, Sweden," *American Journal of Epidemiology* 176, no. 3 (August 2012): 240–52.

149   W. J. Aronson et al., "Phase II Prospective Randomized Trial of a Low-Fat

Diet with Fish Oil Supplementation in Men Undergoing Radical Prostatectomy," *Cancer Prevention Research* (Philadelphia, Pa.) 4, no. 12 (December 2011): 2062–71.

150 Xu and Qian, "Anti-Cancer Activities of Ð-6 Polyunsaturated Fatty Acids."

151 Kenny et al., "Gamma Linolenic Acid with Tamoxifen as Primary Therapy in Breast Cancer."

152 A. Vidlar et al., "The Safety and Efficacy of a Silymarin and Selenium Combination in Men after Radical Prostatectomy—A Six Month Placebo-Controlled Double-Blind Clinical Trial," *Biomedical Papers of the Medical Faculty of the University Palacky, Olomouc Czechoslovakia* 154, no. 3 (September 2010): 239–44.

153 T. W. Flaig et al., "A Study of High-Dose Oral Silybin-Phytosome Followed by Prostatectomy in Patients with Localized Prostate Cancer," *Prostate* 70, no. 8 (June 2010): 848–55.

154 L. M. Beaver et al., "3,3Ð-Diindolylmethane, but not Indole-3-Carbinol, Inhibits Histone Deacetylase Activity in Prostate Cancer Cells," *Toxicology and Applied Pharmacology* 263, no. 3 (September 15, 2012): 345–51.

155 T. T. Wang et al., "Broccoli-Derived Phytochemicals Indole-3-Carbinol and 3,3Ð-Diindolylmethane Exerts Concentration-Dependent Pleiotropic Effects on Prostate Cancer Cells: Comparison with Other Cancer Preventive Phytochemicals," *Molecular Carcinogenesis* 51, no. 3 (March 2012): 244–56.

156 K. Senthilkumar et al., "Quercetin Inhibits Invasion, Migration and Signalling Molecules Involved in Cell Survival and Proliferation of Prostate Cancer Cell Line (PC-3)," *Cell Biochemistry and Function* 29, no. 2 (March 2011): 87–95.

157 T. M. Brasky et al., "Specialty Supplements and Prostate Cancer Risk in the VITamins and Lifestyle (VITAL) Cohort," *Nutrition and Cancer* 63, no. 4 (2011): 573–82.

158 S. Y. Park et al., "Grape Seed Extract Regulates Androgen Receptor-Mediated Transcription in Prostate Cancer Cells through Potent Anti-Histone Acetyltransferase Activity," *Journal of Medicinal Food* 14, no. 1–2 (January–February 2011): 9–16.

159 Cutando et al., "Role of Melatonin in Cancer Treatment."

160 Ju et al., "Cancer-Preventive Activities of Tocopherols and Tocotrienols."

161 Yang, Suh, and Kong, "Does Vitamin E Prevent or Promote Cancer?"

162 Nimptsch et al., "Dietary Vitamin K Intake in Relation to Cancer Incidence and Mortality."

163 Nimptsch, Rohrmann, and Linseisen, "Dietary Intake of Vitamin K and Risk of Prostate Cancer in the Heidelberg Cohort of the European Prospective Investigation into Cancer and Nutrition."

164 Zhang et al., "Vitamin K2 Augments 5-Fluorouracil-Induced Growth Inhibition of Human Hepatocellular Carcinoma Cells by Inhibiting NF-ÐB Activation."

165 I. Drake et al., "Dietary Intakes of Carbohydrates in Relation to Prostate Cancer Risk: A Prospective Study in the Malmö Diet and Cancer Cohort," *American Journal of Clinical Nutrition* 96, no. 6 (December 2012): 1409–18.

166 S. J. Freedland and W. J. Aronson, "Dietary Intervention Strategies to Modulate Prostate Cancer Risk and Prognosis," *Current Opinion in Urology* 19, no. 3 (May 2009): 263–67.

167 Y. Song et al., "Whole Milk Intake Is Associated with Prostate Cancer-Specific Mortality among U.S. Male Physicians," *Journal of Nutrition* 143, no. 2 (February 2013): 189–96.

168 Blair et al., "Cross-Sectional & Longitudinal Associations between Light-Intensity Physical Activity & Physical Function Among Cancer Survivors."

169 A. D. Joshi et al., "Red Meat and Poultry, Cooking Practices, Genetic Susceptibility and Risk of Prostate Cancer: Results from a Multiethnic Case-Control Study," *Carcinogenesis* 33, no. 11 (November 2012): 2108-18.

170 C. Catsburg et al., "Polymorphisms in Carcinogen Metabolism Enzymes, Fish Intake, and Risk of Prostate Cancer," *Carcinogenesis* 33, no. 7 (July 2012): 1352–59.

171 C. Bosire et al., "Index-Based Dietary Patterns and the Risk of Prostate Cancer in the NIH-AARP Diet and Health Study," *American Journal of Epidemiology* 177, no. 6 (March 15, 2013): 504–13.

172 S. C. Gupta et al., "Chemosensitization of Tumors by Resveratrol," *Annals of the New York Academy of Sciences* 1215 (January 2011): 150–60.

173 L. Collins and S. Basaria. "Adverse Effects of Androgen Deprivation Therapy in Men with Prostate Cancer: A Focus on Metabolic and Cardiovascular Complications," *Asian Journal of Andrology* 14, no. 2 (March 2012): 222–25.

174 Schurgers et al., "Vitamin K-Containing Dietary Supplements: Comparison of Synthetic Vitamin K1 and Natto-Derived Menaquinone-7."

175 American Cancer Society, *Cancer Facts and Figures 2011* (Atlanta: American Cancer Society, 2011).

176 S. Sharma, P. Ksheersagar, and P. Sharma, "Diagnosis and Treatment of Bladder Cancer," *American Family Physician* 80, no. 7 (October 2009): 717–23.

177 D. M. Parkin et al., "Global Cancer Statistics, 2002," *CA: A Cancer Journal for Clinicians* 55, no. 2 (March–April 2005): 74–108.

178 S. F. Altekruse et al. (eds.), *SEER Cancer Statistics Review, 1975–2007* (Bethesda, MD: National Cancer Institute, 2010).

179 S.A. Strope and J. E. Montie, "The Causal Role of Cigarette Smoking in Bladder Cancer Initiation and Progression, and the Role of Urologists in Smoking Cessation," *Journal of Urology* 180, no. 1 (July 2008): 31–37.

180 N. D. Freedman et al., "Association between Smoking and Risk of Bladder Cancer among Men and Women," *JAMA* 306, no. 7 (August 17, 2011): 737–45.

181 J. W. Wu et al., "Dietary Intake of Meat, Fruits, Vegetables, and Selective Micronutrients and Risk of Bladder Cancer in the New England Region of the United States," *British Journal of Cancer* 106, no. 11 (May 22, 2012): 1891–98.

182 M. T. Brinkman et al., "Intake of Ð-Linolenic Acid and Other Fatty Acids in Relation to the Risk of Bladder Cancer: Results from the New Hampshire Case-Control Study," *British Journal of Nutrition* 106, no. 7 (October 2011): 1070–77.

183 A. M. Mondul et al., "Influence of Vitamin D Binding Protein on the Association between Circulating Vitamin D and Risk of Bladder Cancer," *British Journal of Cancer* 107, no. 9 (October 23, 2012): 1589–94.

184 A. N. Peiris, B. A. Bailey, and T. Manning, "Relationship of Vitamin D Monitoring and Status to Bladder Cancer Survival in Veterans," *Southern Medical Journal* 106, no. 2 (February 2013): 126–30.

185 Garland et al., "Vitamin D Supplement Doses and Serum 25-Hydroxyvitamin D in the Range Associated with Cancer Prevention."

186 F. Geng et al., "Allyl Isothiocyanate Arrests Cancer Cells in Mitosis, and Mitotic Arrest in Turn Leads to Apoptosis via Bcl-2 Protein Phosphorylation," *Journal of Biological Chemistry* 286, no. 37 (September 16, 2011): 32259-67.

187 J. Qin et al., "Epigallocatechin-3-Gallate Inhibits Bladder Cancer Cell

Invasion via Suppression of NF-ÐB-Mediated Matrix Metalloproteinase-9 Expression," *Molecular Medicine Reports* 6, no. 5 (November 2012): 1040–44.

188   K. M. Rieger-Christ et al., "The Green Tea Compound, (-)-Epigallocatechin-3-Gallate Downregulates N-Cadherin and Suppresses migration of Bladder Carcinoma Cells," *Journal of Cellular Biochemistry* 102, no. 2 (October 1, 2007): 377–88.

189   H. Mazdak and H. Zia, "Vitamin E Reduces Superficial Bladder Cancer Recurrence: A Randomized Controlled Trial," *International Journal of Preventive Medicine* 3, no. 2 (February 2012): 110–15.

190   E. J. Jacobs et al., "Vitamin C and Vitamin E Supplement Use and Bladder Cancer Mortality in a Large Cohort of US Men and Women," *American Journal of Epidemiology* 156, no. 11 (December 2002): 1002–10.

191   K. Kanai et al., "Vitamin E Succinate Induced Apoptosis and Enhanced Chemosensitivity to Paclitaxel in Human Bladder Cancer Cells in Vitro and in Vivo," *Cancer Science* 101, no. 1 (January 2010): 216–23.

192   A. Supabphol et al., "N-Acetylcysteine Inhibits Proliferation, Adhesion, Migration and Invasion of Human Bladder Cancer Cells," *Journal of the Medical Association of Thailand* 92, no. 9 (September 2009): 1171–77.

193   B. Tian et al., "Effects of Curcumin on Bladder Cancer Cells and Development of Urothelial Tumors in a Rat Bladder Carcinogenesis Model," *Cancer Letters* 264, no. 2 (June 18, 2008): 299–308.

194   A. M. Kamat et al., "Curcumin Potentiates the Antitumor Effects of Bacillus Calmette-Guerin against Bladder Cancer through the Downregulation of NF-kappaB and Upregulation of TRAIL Receptors," *Cancer Research* 69, no. 23 (December 1, 2009): 8958–66.

195   Marczylo et al., "Comparison of Systemic Availability of Curcumin with That of Curcumin Formulated with Phosphatidylcholine."

196   DiSilvestro et al., "Diverse Effects of a Low Dose Supplement of Lipidated Curcumin in Healthy Middle Aged People."

197   P. Q. Vinh et al., "Chemopreventive Effects of a Flavonoid Antioxidant Silymarin on N-Butyl-N-(4-Hydroxybutyl)Nitrosamine-Induced Urinary Bladder Carcinogenesis in Male ICR Mice," *Japanese Journal of Cancer Research* 93, no. 1 (January 2002): 42–49.

198   A. K. Tyagi et al., "Silibinin Down-Regulates Survivin Protein and mRNA Expression and Causes Caspases Activation and Apoptosis in Human Bladder Transitional-Cell Papilloma RT4 Cells," *Biochemical and Biophysical Research Communications* 312, no. 4 (December 26, 2003): 1178–84.

199   Y. Sun et al., "Inhibition of STAT Signalling in Bladder Cancer by Diindolylmethane: Relevance to Cell Adhesion, Migration and Proliferation," *Current Cancer Drug Targets* 13, no. 1 (January 2013): 57–68.

200   V. SekeroÐlu, B. Aydin, and Z. A. SekeroÐlu, "Viscum album L. Extract and Auercetin Reduce Cyclophosphamide-Induced Cardiotoxicity, Urotoxicity and Genotoxicity in Mice," *Asian Pacific Journal of Cancer Prevention* 12, no. 11 (2011): 2925–31.

201   Y. Kim, W. J. Kim, and E. J. Cha, "Quercetin-Induced Growth Inhibition in Human Bladder Cancer Cells Is Associated with an Increase in Ca-activated K Channels," *Korean Journal of Physiology and Pharmacology* 15, no. 5 (October 2011): 279–83.

202   Cutando et al., "Role of Melatonin in Cancer Treatment."

203   Nimptsch et al., "Dietary Vitamin K Intake in Relation to Cancer Incidence and Mortality."

204   Nimptsch, Rohrmann, and Linseisen, "Dietary Intake of Vitamin K and Risk of Prostate Cancer in the Heidelberg cohort of the European Prospective Investigation into Cancer and Nutrition."

205   Zhang et al., "Vitamin K2 Augments 5-Fluorouracil-Induced Growth Inhibition of Human Hepatocellular Carcinoma Cells by Inhibiting NF-ÐB Activation."

206   M. M. Ros et al., "Fruit and Vegetable Consumption and Risk of Aggressive and Non-Aggressive Urothelial Cell Carcinomas in the European Prospective Investigation into Cancer and Nutrition," *European Journal of Cancer* 48, no. 17 (November 2012): 3267–77.

207   Blair et al., "Cross-Sectional & Longitudinal Associations between Light-Intensity Physical Activity & Physical Function Among Cancer Survivors."

208   Jeon et al., "Effects of Beta-Carotene Supplements on Cancer Prevention: Meta-Analysis of Randomized Controlled Trials."

209   Schurgers et al., "Vitamin K-Containing Dietary Supplements: Comparison of Synthetic Vitamin K1 and Natto-Derived Menaquinone-7."

210   National Cancer Institute, "SEER Stat Fact Sheets: Endometrial Cancer," accessed August 2014, http://seer.cancer.gov/statfacts/html/corp.html.

211   K. Matsuo et al., "Significance of Adenomyosis on Tumor Progression and Survival Outcome of Endometrial Cancer," *Annals of Surgical Oncology* 21, no. 13 (December 2014): 4246–55.

212   A. T. Ali, "Reproductive Factors and the Risk of Endometrial Cancer," *International Journal of Gynecological Cancer* 24, no. 3 (March 2014): 384–93.

213   S. Furness et al., "Hormone Therapy in Postmenopausal Women and Risk of Endometrial Hyperplasia," *Cochrane Database of Systematic Reviews* 2012, no. 8: CD000402.

214   L. L. Moore et al., "Metabolic Health Reduces Risk of Obesity-Related Cancer in Framingham Study Adults," *Cancer Epidemiology, Biomarkers, and Prevention* 23, no. 10 (October 2014): 2057–65.

215   L. Bergadà et al., "Role of Local Bioactivation of Vitamin D by CYP27A1 and CYP2R1 in the Control of Cell Growth in Normal Endometrium and Endometrial Carcinoma," *Lab Investigation* 94, no. 6 (June 2014): 608–22.

216   H. Nguyen et al., "Progesterone and 1,25-Dihydroxyvitamin DÐ Inhibit Endometrial Cancer Cell Growth by Upregulating Semaphorin 3B and Semaphorin 3F," *Molecular Cancer Research* 9, no. 11 (November 2011): 1479–92.

217   Garland et al., "Vitamin D Supplement Doses and Serum 25-Hydroxyvitamin D in the Range Associated with Cancer Prevention."

218   L. Kavandi et al., "The Chinese Herbs Scutellaria baicalensis and Fritillaria cirrhosa Target NFÐB to Inhibit Proliferation of Ovarian and Endometrial Cancer Cells," *Molecular Carcinogenesis* (November 19, 2013), doi: 10.1002/mc.22107.

219   W. S. Ahn et al., "Natural Killer Cell Activity and Quality of Life Were Improved by Consumption of a Mushroom Extract, Agaricus blazei Murill Kyowa, in Gynecological Cancer Patients Undergoing Chemotherapy," *International Journal of Gynecological Cancer* 14, no. 4 (July–August 2004): 589–94.

220   N. H. Jeong et al., "Preoperative Levels of Plasma Micronutrients Are Related to Endometrial Cancer Risk," *Acta Obstetrica Gynecologica Scandinavica* 88, no. 4 (2009): 434–39.

221   K. Hirsch et al., "Lycopene and Other Carotenoids Inhibit Estrogenic Activity of 17Beta-Estradiol and Genistein in Cancer Cells," *Breast Cancer Research and Treatment* 104, no. 2 (August 2007): 221–30.

222   Jeong et al., "Preoperative Levels of Plasma Micronutrients Are Related to Endometrial Cancer Risk."

223   C. Pelucchi et al., "Dietary Intake of Carotenoids and Retinol and Endometrial Cancer Risk in an Italian Case-Control Study," *Cancer Causes and Control* 19, no. 10 (December 2008): 1209–15.

224   Hirsch et al., "Lycopene and Other Carotenoids Inhibit Estrogenic Activity of 17Beta-Estradiol and Genistein in Cancer Cells."

225   M. Manohar et al., "(-)-Epigallocatechin-3-Gallate Induces Apoptosis in Human Endometrial Adenocarcinoma Cells via ROS Generation and p38 MAP Kinase Activation," *Journal of Nutritional Biochemistry* 24, no. 6 (June 2013): 940–47.

226   S. B. Park et al., "Antiproliferative and Apoptotic Effect of Epigallocatechin-3-Gallate on Ishikawa Cells Is Accompanied by Sex Steroid Receptor Downregulation," *International Journal of Molecular Medicine* 30, no. 5 (November 2012): 1211–18.

227   H. Zheng et al., "Inhibition of Endometrial Cancer by n-3 Polyunsaturated Fatty Acids in Preclinical Models," *Cancer Prevention Research* 7, no. 8 (August 2014): 824–34.

228   Xu and Qian, "Anti-Cancer Activities of Ð-6 Polyunsaturated Fatty Acids."

229   Kenny et al., "Gamma Linolenic Acid with Tamoxifen as Primary Therapy in Breast Cancer."

230   H. Arem et al., "Omega-3 and Omega-6 Fatty Acid Intakes and Endometrial Cancer Risk in a Population-Based Case-Control Study," *European Journal of Nutrition* 52, no. 3 (April 2013): 1251–60.

231   L. M. Butler and A. H. Wu, "Green and Black Tea in Relation to Gynecologic Cancers," *Molecular Nutrition and Food Research* 55, no. 6 (June 2011): 931–40.

232   N. Keum et al., "Leisure-Time Physical Activity and Endometrial Cancer Risk: Dose-Response Meta-Analysis of Epidemiological Studies," *International Journal of Cancer* 135, no. 3 (August 1, 2014): 682–94.

233   National Cancer Institute, "SEER Stat Fact Sheets" Leukemia," accessed August 2014, http://seer.cancer.gov/statfacts/html/leuks.html.

234   T. Y. Shih et al., "Association between Leukaemia and X-ray in Children: A Nationwide Study," *Journal of Paediatrics and Child Health* 50, no. 8 (August 2014): 615–18.

235   M. Gillies and R. Haylock, "The Cancer Mortality and Incidence Experience of Workers at British Nuclear Fuels plc, 1946–2005," *Journal of Radiological Protection* 34, no. 3 (July 2014): 595–623.

236   N. C. Deziel et al., "Polycyclic Aromatic Hydrocarbons in Residential Dust and Risk of Childhood Acute Lymphoblastic Leukemia," *Environmental Research* 133 (August 2014): 388–95.

237   E. Milne et al., "Parental Prenatal Smoking and Risk of Childhood Acute Lymphoblastic Leukemia," *American Journal of Epidemiology* 175, no. 1 (January 1, 2012): 43–53.

238   K. M. Lee et al., "Paternal Smoking, Genetic Polymorphisms in CYP1A1 and Childhood Leukemia Risk," *Leukemia Research* 33, no. 2 (February 2009): 250–58.

239   H. J. Lee et al., "Low 25(OH) Vitamin D3 Levels Are Associated with Adverse Outcome in Newly Diagnosed, Intensively Treated Adult Acute Myeloid Leukemia," *Cancer* 120, no. 4 (February 15, 2014): 521–29.

240   E. Paubelle et al., "Deferasirox and Vitamin D Improves Overall Survival in Elderly Patients with Acute Myeloid Leukemia after Demethylating Agents Failure," *PLoS One* 8, no. 6 (June 20, 2013): e65998.

241   Garland et al., "Vitamin D Supplement Doses and Serum 25-Hydroxyvitamin D in the Range Associated with Cancer Prevention."

242   J. Espino et al., "Tempranillo-Derived Grape Seed Extract Induces Apoptotic Cell Death and Cell Growth Arrest in Human Promyelocytic Leukemia HL-60 Cells," *Food and Function* 4, no. 12 (December 2013): 1759–66.

243   N. Gao et al., "Induction of Apoptosis in Human Leukemia Cells by Grape Seed Extract Occurs via Activation of c-Jun NH2-Terminal Kinase," *Clinical Cancer Research* 15, no. 1 (January 2009): 140–49.

244   M. Wang et al., "Monocytic Differentiation of K562 Cells Induced by Proanthocyanidins from Grape Seeds," *Archives of Pharmacal Research* 35, no. 1 (January 2012): 129–35.

245   H. Hu and Y. M. Qin, "Grape Seed Proanthocyanidin Extract Induced Mitochondria-Associated Apoptosis in Human Acute Myeloid Leukaemia 14.3D10 Cells," *Chinese Medical Journal* 119, no. 5 (March 5, 2006): 417–21.

246   Q. X. Zhang and J. Y. Wu, "Cordyceps sinensis Mycelium Extract Induces Human Premyelocytic Leukemia Cell Apoptosis through Mitochondrion Pathway," *Experimental Biology and Medicine* (Maywood, N.J.) 232, no. 1 (January 2007): 52–57.

247   B. S. Ko et al., "Cordycepin Regulates GSK-3Ð/Ð-Catenin Signaling in Human Leukemia Cells," *PLoS One* 8, no. 9 (September 26, 2013): e76320.

248   L. E. Shorey et al., "3,3'-Diindolylmethane Induces G1 Arrest and Apoptosis in Human Acute T-Cell Lymphoblastic Leukemia Cells," *PLoS One* 7, no. 4 (2012): e34975.

249   N. Gao et al., "3,3'-Diindolylmethane Exhibits Antileukemic Activity In Vitro and In Vivo through a Akt-Dependent Process," *PLoS One* 7, no. 2 (2012): e31783.

250   H. L. Bradlow et al., "Multifunctional Aspects of the Action of Indole-3-Carbinol as an Antitumor Agent," *Annals of the New York Academy of Sciences* 889 (1999): 204–13.

251   X. Wu, Q. H. Zhou, and K. Xu, "Are Isothiocyanates Potential Anti-Cancer Drugs"? *Acta Pharmacologica Sinica* 30, no. 5 (May 2009): 501–12.

252   Y. Guo et al., "Curcumin Induces Apoptosis via Simultaneously Targeting AKT/mTOR and RAF/MEK/ERK Survival Signaling Pathways in Human Leukemia THP-1 Cells," *Die Pharmazie* 69, no. 3 (March 2014): 229–33.

253   I. Samet et al., "Olive (Olea europaea) Leaf Extract Induces Apoptosis and Monocyte/Macrophage Differentiation in Human Chronic Myelogenous Leukemia K562 Cells: Insight into the Underlying Mechanism," *Oxidative Medicine and Cellular Longevity* 2014 (2014): 927619.

254   L. Abaza et al., "Induction of Growth Inhibition and Differentiation of Human Leukemia HL-60 Cells by a Tunisian Gerboui Olive Leaf Extract," *Bioscience, Biotechnology, and Biochemistry* 71, no. 5 (May 2007): 1306–12.

255   S. Harakeh et al., "Epigallocatechin-3-Gallate Inhibits Tax-Dependent Activation of Nuclear Factor Kappa B and of Matrix Metalloproteinase 9 in Human T-Cell Lymphotropic Virus-1 Positive Leukemia Cells," *Asian Pacific Journal of Cancer Prevention* 15, no. 3 (2014): 1219–25.

256   A. C. Huang et al., "Epigallocatechin Gallate (EGCG), Influences a Murine WEHI-3 Leukemia Model In Vivo through Enhancing Phagocytosis of

Macrophages and Populations of T- and B-Cells," *In Vivo* 27, no. 5 (September–October 2013): 627–34.

257   E. J. Ladas et al., "A Randomized, Controlled, Double-Blind, Pilot Study of Milk Thistle for the Treatment of Hepatotoxicity in Childhood Acute Lymphoblastic Leukemia (ALL)," *Cancer* 116, no. 2 (January 2010): 506–13.

258   X. Sheng and S. D. Mittelman, "The Role of Adipose Tissue and Obesity in Causing Treatment Resistance of Acute Lymphoblastic Leukemia," *Frontiers in Pediatrics* 2 (June 5, 2014): 53.

259   L. S. Järvelä et al., "Endothelial Function in Long-Term Survivors of Childhood Acute Lymphoblastic Leukemia: Effects of a Home-Based Exercise Program," *Pediatric Blood and Cancer* 60, no. 9 (September 2013): 1546–51.

260   J. Chiang et al., "Comparison of Anti-Leukemic Immunity Against U937 Cells in Endurance Athletes versus Sedentary Controls," *International Journal of Sports Medicine* 21, no. 8 (November 2000): 602–7.

261   E. Paubelle et al., "Deferasirox and Vitamin D Improves Overall Survival in Elderly Patients with Acute Myeloid Leukemia after Demethylating Agents Failure," *PLoS One* 8, no. 6 (June 20, 2013): e65998.

262   National Cancer Institute, "SEER Stat Fact Sheets: Non-Hodgkin Lymphoma," accessed August 2014, http://seer.cancer.gov/statfacts/html/nhl.html.

263   S. M. Jaglowski et al., "Lymphoma in Adolescents and Young Adults," *Seminars in Oncology* 36, no. 5 (October 2009): 381–418.

264   X. C. Wu et al., "Incidence of Extranodal non-Hodgkin Lymphomas among Whites, Blacks, and Asians/Pacific Islanders in the United States: Anatomic Site and Histology Differences," *Cancer Epidemiology* 33, no. 5 (November 2009): 337–46.

265   H. A. Robbins et al., "Epidemiologic Contributions to Recent Cancer Trends among HIV-Infected People in the United States," *AIDS* 28, no. 6 (March 27, 2014): 881–90.

266   Q. J. Leo et al., "Obesity and Non-Hodgkin Lymphoma Survival in an Ethnically Diverse Population: The Multiethnic Cohort Study," *Cancer Causes and Control* 25, no. 11 (November 2014): 1449–59.

267   E. A. Salem, M. M. Hegazy, and E. A. El Khouley, "Pesticide Exposure as a Risk Factor for Lymphoproliferative Disorders in Adults," *Eastern Mediterranean Health Journal* 20, no. 6 (June 18, 2014): 363–71.

268   M. Pahwa et al., "0409 The North American Pooled Project (NAPP): Pooled Analyses of Case-Control Studies of Pesticides and Agricultural Exposures, Lymphohematopoietic Cancers and Sarcoma," *Occupational and Environmental Medicine*, supplement 1, 71 (June 2014): A116.

269   L. Schinasi and M. E. Leon, "Non-Hodgkin Lymphoma and Occupational Exposure to Agricultural Pesticide Chemical Groups and Active Ingredients: A Systematic Review and Meta-Analysis," *International Journal of Environmental Research and Public Health* 11, no. 4 (April 23, 2014): 4449–4527.

270   M. Eriksson et al., "Pesticide Exposure as Risk Factor for Non-Hodgkin Lymphoma Including Histopathological Subgroup Analysis," *International Journal of Cancer* 123, no. 7 (October 1, 2008): 1657–63.

271   J. D. Buckley et al., "Pesticide Exposures in Children with Non-Hodgkin Lymphoma," *Cancer* 89, no. 11 (December 1, 2000): 2315–21.

272   M. Kokouva et al., "Relationship between the Paraoxonase 1 (PON1) M55L and Q192R Polymorphisms and Lymphohaematopoietic Cancers in a Greek Agricultural Population," *Toxicology* 307 (May 10, 2013): 12–16.

273   M. Fallah et al., "Autoimmune Diseases Associated with Non-Hodgkin Lymphoma: A Nationwide Cohort Study," *Annals of Oncology* 25, no. 10 (October 2014): 2025–30.

274   M. T. Drake et al., "Vitamin D Insufficiency and Prognosis in Non-Hodgkin's Lymphoma," *Journal of Clinical Oncology* 28, no. 27 (September 20, 2010): 4191–98.

275   A. C. Porojnicu et al., "Season of Diagnosis Is a Prognostic Factor in Hodgkin's Lymphoma: A Possible Role of Sun-Induced Vitamin D," *British Journal of Cancer* 93, no. 5 (September 5, 2005): 571–74.

276   Garland et al., "Vitamin D Supplement Doses and Serum 25-Hydroxyvitamin D in the Range Associated with Cancer Prevention."

277   Y. Machijima et al., "Anti-Adult T-Cell Leukemia/Lymphoma Effects of Indole-3-Carbinol," *Retrovirology* 6 (January 16, 2009): 7.

278   Z. Yu et al., "Indole-3-Carbinol in the Maternal Diet Provides Chemoprotection for the Fetus Against Transplacental Carcinogenesis by the Polycyclic Aromatic Hydrocarbon Dibenzo[a,l]pyrene," *Carcinogenesis* 27, no. 10 (October 2006): 2116–23.

279   Shorey et al., "3,3'-Diindolylmethane Induces G1 Arrest and Apoptosis in Human Acute T-Cell Lymphoblastic Leukemia Cell."

280   S. Kewitz, I. Volkmer, and M. S. Staege, "Curcuma Contra Cancer? Curcumin and Hodgkin's Lymphoma," *Cancer Growth and Metastasis* 6 (August 8, 2013): 35–52.

281   L. Das and M. Vinayak, "Curcumin Attenuates Carcinogenesis by Down Regulating Proinflammatory Cytokine Interleukin-1 (IL-1Ð and IL-1Ð) via Modulation of AP-1 and NF-IL6 in Lymphoma Bearing Mice," *International Immunopharmacology* 20, no. 1 (May 2014): 141–47.

282   G. Zhu et al., "[Effect of Curcumin on Expressions of Mitogen-Activated Protein Kinases and Matrix Metalloproteinases in Jurkat Cells]." *Nan Fang Yi Ke Da Xue Xue Bao* 33, no. 12 (December 2013): 1792–95.

283   X. Peng et al., "A New Acylated Flavonoid Glycoside from the Flowers of Camellia Nitidissima and Its Effect on the Induction of Apoptosis in Human Lymphoma U937 Cells," *Journal of Asian Natural Products Research* 14, no. 8 (2012): 799–804.

284   X. Li et al., "Quercetin Potentiates the Antitumor Activity of Rituximab in Diffuse Large B-Cell Lymphoma by Inhibiting STAT3 Pathway," *Cell Biochemistry and Biophysics* 70, no. 2 (November 2014): 1357–62.

285   G. Jacquemin et al., "Quercetin-Mediated Mcl-1 and Survivin Downregulation Restores TRAIL-Induced Apoptosis in Non-Hodgkin's Lymphoma B Cells," *Haematologica* 97, no. 1 (January 2012): 38–46.

286   A. De Leo et al., "Resveratrol Inhibits Epstein Barr Virus Lytic Cycle in Burkitt's Lymphoma Cells by Affecting Multiple Molecular Targets," *Antiviral Research* 96, no. 2 (November 2012): 196–202.

287   R. Frazzi et al., "Resveratrol-Mediated Apoptosis of Hodgkin Lymphoma Cells Involves SIRT1 Inhibition and FOXO3a Hyperacetylation," *International Journal of Cancer* 132, no. 5 (March 1, 2013): 1013–21.

288   J. Bryant et al., "Cardioprotection against the Toxic Effects of Anthracyclines Given to Children with Cancer: A Systematic Review," *Health Technology Assessment* 11, no. 27 (July 2007): iii, ix-x, 1–84.

289   F. Bruge et al., "NAD(P)H:quinone Oxidoreductase (NQO1) Loss of

Function in Burkitt's Lymphoma Cell Lines," *BioFactors* 23, nos. 1–4 (2008): 71–81.

290   F. J. Darfler et al., "Stimulation of Forskolin of Intact S49 Lymphoma Cells Involves the Nucleotide Regulatory Protein of Adenylate Cyclase," *Journal of Biological Chemistry* 257, no. 20 (October 25, 1982): 11901–7.

291   K. B. Gützkow, S. Naderi, and H. K. Blomhoff, "Forskolin-Mediated G1 Arrest in Acute Lymphoblastic Leukaemia Cells: Phosphorylated pRB Sequesters E2Fs," *Journal of Cell Science* 115, pt. 5 (March 1, 2002): 1073–82.

292   S. Taga et al., "Intracellular Signaling Events in CD77-Mediated Apoptosis of Burkitt's Lymphoma Cells," *Blood* 90, no. 7 (October 1, 1997): 2757–67.

293   R. Talamini et al., "Smoking and Non-Hodgkin Lymphoma: Case-Control Study in Italy," *International Journal of Cancer* 115, no. 4 (July 1, 2005): 606–10.

294   J. Zhang et al., "Diabetes Mellitus Potentiates Diffuse Large B-Cell Lymphoma via High Levels of CCL5," *Molecular Medicine Reports* 10, no. 3 (September 2014): 1231–36.

295   J. Mitri, J. Castillo, and A. G. Pittas, "Diabetes and Risk of Non-Hodgkin's Lymphoma: A Meta-Analysis of Observational Studies," *Diabetes Care* 31, no. 12 (December 2008): 2391–97.

296   L. R. Teras et al., "Recreational Physical Activity, Leisure Sitting Time and Risk of Non-Hodgkin Lymphoid Neoplasms in the American Cancer Society Cancer Prevention Study II Cohort," *International Journal of Cancer* 131, no. 8 (October 15, 2012): 1912–20.

297   L. Cohen et al., "Psychological Adjustment and Sleep Quality in a Randomized Trial of the Effects of a Tibetan Yoga Intervention in Patients with Lymphoma," *Cancer* 100, no. 10 (May 15, 2004): 2253–60.

298   P. K. Kandala and S. K. Srivastava, "Diindolylmethane Suppresses Ovarian Cancer Growth and Potentiates the Effect of Cisplatin in Tumor Mouse Model by Targeting Signal Transducer and Activator of Transcription 3 (STAT3)," *BMC Medicine* 10 (January 26, 2012): 9.

299   A. Ahmad et al., "3, 3'-Diindolylmethane Enhances the Effectiveness of Herceptin against HER-2/neu-Expressing Breast Cancer Cells," *PLoS One* 8 no. 1 (2013): e54657.

300   National Cancer Institute, "SEER Stat Fact Sheets: Melanoma of the Skin," accessed August 2014, http://seer.cancer.gov/statfacts/html/melan.html.

301   F. Boriani et al., "Acral Lentiginous Melanoma—Misdiagnosis, Referral Delay and 5 Years Specific Survival according to Site," *European Review for Medical and Pharmacological Sciences* 18, no. 14 (2014): 1990–96.

302   N. Howlader et al., "SEER Cancer Statistics Review, 1975–2009 (Vintage 2009 Populations)," National Cancer Institute, updated August 20, 2012, http://seer.cancer.gov/archive/csr/1975_2009_pops09/.

303   C. M. Olsen, H. J. Carroll, and D. C. Whiteman, "Familial Melanoma: A Meta-Analysis and Estimates of Attributable Fraction," *Cancer Epidemiology, Biomarkers and Prevention* 19, no. 1 (January 2010): 65–73.

304   J. A. Usher-Smith et al., "Risk Prediction Models for Melanoma: A Systematic Review," *Cancer Epidemiology, Biomarkers and Prevention* 23, no. 8 (August 2014): 1450–63.

305   A. Kosiniak-Kamysz et al., "Increased Risk of Developing Cutaneous Malignant Melanoma Is Associated with Variation in Pigmentation Genes and VDR, and May Involve Epistatic Effects," *Melanoma Research* 24, no. 4 (August 2014): 388–96.

306   X. Y. Huang, S. Z. Zhang, and W. X. Wang, "Enhanced Antitumor Efficacy

with Combined Administration of Astragalus and Pterostilbene for Melanoma," *Asian Pacific Journal of Cancer Prevention* 15, no. 3 (2014): 1163–69.

307   D. T. Chu, J. R. Lin, and W. Wong, "[The In Vitro Potentiation of LAK Cell Cytotoxicity in Cancer and Aids Patients Induced by F3—A Fractionated Extract of Astragalus Membranaceus]," *Zhonghua Zhong Liu Za Zhi* 16, no. 3 (May 1994): 167–71.

308   I. A. Siddiqui et al., "Excellent Anti-Proliferative and Pro-Apoptotic Effects of (-)-Epigallocatechin-3-Gallate Encapsulated in Chitosan Nanoparticles on Human Melanoma Cell Growth Both In Vitro and In Vivo," *Nanomedicine* 10, no. 8 (November 2014): 1619–26.

309   C. C. Chen et al., "Improving Anticancer Efficacy of (-)-Epigallocatechin-3-Gallate Gold Nanoparticles in Murine B16F10 Melanoma Cells," *Drug Design, Development and Therapy* 8 (May 8, 2014): 459–74.

310   R. Liu et al., "Jatrorrhizine Hydrochloride Inhibits the Proliferation and Neovascularization of C8161 Metastatic Melanoma Cells," *Anti-Cancer Drugs* 24, no. 7 (August 2013): 667–76.

311   A. Mittal, S. Tabasum, and R. P. Singh, "Berberine in Combination with Doxorubicin Suppresses Growth of Murine Melanoma B16F10 Cells in Culture and Xenograft," *Phytomedicine* 21, no. 3 (February 15, 2014): 340–47.

312   H. S. Kim et al., "Berberine-Induced AMPK Activation Inhibits the Metastatic Potential of Melanoma Cells via Reduction of ERK Activity and COX-2 Protein Expression," *Biochemical Pharmacology* 83, no. 3 (February 1, 2012): 385–94.

313   T. P. Hamsa and G. Kuttan, "Berberine Inhibits Pulmonary Metastasis through Down-Regulation of MMP in Metastatic B16F-10 Melanoma Cells," *Phytotherapy Research* 26, no. 4 (April 2012): 568–78.

314   Y. H. Lee, N. C. Kumar, and R. D. Glickman, "Modulation of Photochemical Damage in Normal and Malignant Cells by Naturally Occurring Compounds," *Photochemistry and Photobiology* 88, no. 6 (November–December 2012): 1385–95.

315   Y. S. Habibie et al., "Survivin Suppression through STAT$_{3}$/β-Catenin Is Essential for Resveratrol-Induced Melanoma Apoptosis," *International Journal of Oncology* 45, no. 2 (August 2014): 895–901.

316   Y. Masuda et al., "Inhibitory Effect of MD-Fraction on Tumor Metastasis: Involvement of NK Cell Activation and Suppression of Intercellular Adhesion Molecule (ICAM)-1 Expression in Lung Vascular Endothelial Cells," *Biological and Pharmaceutical Bulletin* 31, no. 6 (June 2008): 1104–8.

317   Y. P. Zhang, R. X. Chu, and H. Liu, "Vitamin A Intake and Risk of Melanoma: A Meta-Analysis," *PLoS One* 9, no. 7 (July 21, 2014): e102527.

318   M. M. Asgari, T. M. Brasky, and E. White, "Association of Vitamin A and Carotenoid Intake with Melanoma Risk in a Large Prospective Cohort," *Journal of Investigative Dermatology* 132, no. 6 (June 2012): 1573–82.

319   M. J. Youn et al., "Potential Anticancer Properties of the Water Extract of Inonotus [corrected] Obliquus by Induction of Apoptosis in Melanoma B16-F10 Cells," *Journal of Ethnopharmacology* 121, no. 2 (January 21, 2009): 221–28.

320   M. J. Youn et al., "Chaga Mushroom (Inonotus obliquus) Induces G0/G1 Arrest and Apoptosis in Human Hepatoma HepG2 Cells," *World Journal of Gastroenterology* 14, no. 4 (January 28, 2008): 511–17.

321   S. Caini et al., "Vitamin D and Melanoma and Non-Melanoma Skin Cancer Risk and Prognosis: A Comprehensive Review and Meta-Analysis," *European Journal of Cancer* 50, no. 15 (October 2014): 2649–58.

322   S. Field et al., "Vitamin D and Melanoma," *Dermato-endocrinology* 5 no. 1 (January 1, 2013): 121–29.

323   K. Zeljic et al., "Melanoma Risk Is Associated with Vitamin D Receptor Gene Polymorphisms," *Melanoma Research* 24, no. 3 (June 2014): 273–79.

324   Garland et al., "Vitamin D Supplement Doses and Serum 25-Hydroxyvitamin D in the Range Associated with Cancer Prevention."

325   R. I. Vogel et al., "Exposure to Indoor Tanning without Burning and Melanoma Risk by Sunburn History," *Journal of the National Cancer Institute* 106, no. 7 (July 16, 2014).

326   J. I. Jung et al., "High-Fat Diet-Induced Obesity Increases Lymphangiogenesis and Lymph Node Metastasis in the B16F10 Melanoma Allograft Model: Roles of Adipocytes and M2-Macrophages," *International Journal of Cancer* 136, no. 2 (January 15, 2015): 258–70.

327   F. Skowron et al., "Role of Obesity on the Thickness of Primary Cutaneous Melanoma," *Journal of the European Academy of Dermatology and Venereology* 29, no. 2 (February 2015): 262–69.

328   A. R. Ragan et al., "Chronic Mild Stress Facilitates Melanoma Tumor Growth in Mouse Lines Selected for High and Low Stress-Induced Analgesia," *Stress* 16, no. 5 (September 2013): 571–80.

329   S. Radom-Aizik et al., "Impact of Brief Exercise on Peripheral Blood NK Cell Gene and MicroRNA Expression in Young Adults," *Journal of Applied Physiology* 114, no. 5 (March 1, 2013): 628–36.

330   E. Czeczuga-Semeniuk et al., "The Effect of Doxorubicin and Retinoids on Proliferation, Necrosis and Apoptosis in MCF-7 Breast Cancer Cells," *Folia Histochemica et Cytobiologica* 42, no. 4 (2004): 221–27.

331   National Cancer Institute, "SEER Stat Fact Sheets: Kidney and Renal Pelvis Cancer," accessed August 2014, http://seer.cancer.gov/statfacts/html/kidrp.html.

332   K. M. Sanfilippo et al., "Hypertension and Obesity and the Risk of Kidney Cancer in 2 Large Cohorts of US Men and Women," *Hypertension* 63, no. 5 (May 2014): 934–41.

333   K. Sachdeva et al., "Renal Cell Carcinoma," *Medscape*, updated July 30, 2014, http://emedicine.medscape.com/article/281340-overview.

334   T. R. Smith et al., "Survival after Surgery and Stereotactic Radiosurgery for Patients with Multiple Intracranial Metastases: Results of a Single-Center Retrospective Study," *Journal of Neurosurgery* 121, no. 4 (October 2014): 839–45.

335   C. Häggström et al., "Metabolic Factors Associated with Risk of Renal Cell Carcinoma," *PLoS One* 8, no. 2 (2013): e57475.

336   Y. Xu et al., "The Impact of Smoking on Survival in Renal Cell Carcinoma: A Systematic Review and Meta-Analysis," *Tumour Biology* 35, no. 7 (July 2014): 6633–40.

337   S. C. King et al., "Continued Increase in Incidence of Renal Cell Carcinoma, Especially in Young Patients and High Grade Disease: United States 2001 to 2010," *Journal of Urology* 191, no. 6 (June 2014): 1665–70.

338   Y. H. Park, "Visceral Obesity in Predicting Oncologic Outcomes of Localized Renal Cell Carcinoma," *Journal of Urology* 192, no. 4 (October 2014): 1043–49.

339   B. Stengel et al., "Lifestyle Factors, Obesity and the Risk of Chronic Kidney Disease," *Epidemiology* 14, no. 4 (July 2003): 479–87.

340   K. Odagiri et al., "Waist to Height Ratio Is an Independent Predictor for the

Incidence of Chronic Kidney Disease," *PLoS One* 9, no. 2 (February 12, 2014): e88873.

341 S. P. Psutka et al., "Diabetes Mellitus Is Independently Associated with an Increased Risk of Mortality Among Clear Cell Renal Cell Carcinoma Patients," *Journal of Urology* 192, no. 6 (December 2014): 1620–27.

342 G. Lewis and A. P. Maxwell, "Early Diagnosis Improves Survival in Kidney Cancer," *The Practitioner* 256, no. 1748 (February 2012): 13–16, 2.

343 S. Karami et al., "Occupational Exposure to Dusts and Risk of Renal Cell Carcinoma," *British Journal of Cancer* 104, no. 11 (May 24, 2011): 1797–1803.

344 A. Zucchetto et al., "Reproductive, Menstrual, and Other Hormone-Related Factors and Risk of Renal Cell Cancer," *International Journal of Cancer* 123, no. 9 (November 1, 2008): 2213–16.

345 K. Sachdeva et al., "Renal Cell Carcinoma."

346 J. Bacchetta et al., "Paraneoplastic Glomerular Diseases and Malignancies," *Critical Reviews in Oncology/Hematology* 70, no. 1 (April 2009): 39–58.

347 D. Gui et al., "Astragaloside IV Ameliorates Renal Injury in Streptozotocin-Induced Diabetic Rats through Inhibiting NF- ÐB-Mediated Inflammatory Genes Expression," *Cytokine* 61, no. 3 (March 2013): 970–77.

348 L. Liu et al., "[Astragalus Injection Ameliorates Cisplatin-Induced Nephrotoxicity in Mice]," *Zhongguo Zhong Yao Za Zhi* 35, no. 20 (October 2010): 2736–40.

349 B. H. Lau et al., "Chinese Medicinal Herbs Inhibit Growth of Murine Renal Cell Carcinoma," *Cancer Biotherapy* 9, no. 2 (Summer 1994): 153–61.

350 Ibid.

351 C. M. Gurrola-Díaz et al., "Inhibitory Mechanisms of Two Uncaria Tomentosa Extracts Affecting the Wnt-Signaling Pathway," *Phytomedicine* 18, no. 8–9 (June 15, 2011): 683–90.

352 J. Sonnenbichler et al., "Stimulatory Effects of Silibinin and Silicristin from the Milk Thistle Silybum Marianum on Kidney Cells," *Journal of Pharmacology and Experimental Therapeutics*, 290, no. 3 (September 1999): 1375–83.

353 H. R. Chang et al., "Silibinin Inhibits the Invasion and Migration of Renal Carcinoma 786-O Cells In Vitro, Inhibits the Growth of Xenografts In Vivo and Enhances Chemosensitivity to 5-Fluorouracil and Paclitaxel," *Molecular Carcinogenesis* 50, no. 10 (October 2011): 811–23.

354 R. A. Isbrucker and G. A. Burdock, "Risk and Safety Assessment on the Consumption of Licorice Root (Glycyrrhiza sp.), Its Extract and Powder as a Food Ingredient, with Emphasis on the Pharmacology and Toxicology of Glycyrrhizin," *Regulatory Toxicology and Pharmacology* 46, no. 3 (December 2006): 167–92.

355 S. Yamazaki et al., "Isoliquiritigenin Suppresses Pulmonary Metastasis of Mouse Renal Cell Carcinoma," *Cancer Letters* 183, no. 1 (September 8, 2002): 23–30.

356 W. Arjumand and S. Sultana, "Glycyrrhizic Acid: A Phytochemical with a Protective Role against Cisplatin-Induced Genotoxicity and Nephrotoxicity," *Life Sciences* 89, no. 13–14 (September 26, 2011): 422–29.

357 N. H. Jeong et al., "Preoperative Levels of Plasma Micronutrients Are Related to Endometrial Cancer Risk," *Acta Obstetrica Gynecologica Scandinavica* 88, no. 4 (2009): 434–39.

358 J. Yin, H. Xing, and J. Ye, "Efficacy of Berberine in Patients with Type 2 Diabetes Mellitus," *Metabolism* 57, no. 5 (May 2008): 712–17.

359 S. J. Lee et al., "Berberine Sensitizes TRAIL-Induced Apoptosis through

Proteasome-Mediated Downregulation of c-FLIP and Mcl-1 Proteins," *International Journal of Oncology* 38, no. 2 (February 2011): 485–92.

360   J. Li et al., "Isoangustone A Suppresses Mesangial Fibrosis and Inflammation in Human Renal Mesangial Cells," *Experimental Biology and Medicine* 236, no. 4 (April 1, 2011): 435–44.

361   N. Aksoy et al., "Protective and Therapeutic Effects of Licorice in Rats with Acute Tubular Necrosis," *Journal of Renal Nutrition* 22, no. 3 (May 2012): 336–43.

362   S. Sakr, A. El-Kenawy, and D. El-Sahra, "Metiram-Induced Nephrotoxicity in Albino Mice: Effect of Licorice Aqueous Extract," *Environmental Toxicology* 28, no. 7 (July 2013): 372–79.

363   H. K. Joh et al., "Predicted Plasma 25-Hydroxyvitamin D and Risk of Renal Cell Cancer," *Journal of the National Cancer Institute* 105, no. 10 (May 15, 2013): 726–32.

364   A. M. Mondul et al., "Vitamin D-Binding Protein, Circulating Vitamin D and Risk of Renal Cell Carcinoma," *International Journal of Cancer* 134, no. 11 (June 1, 2014): 2699–2706.

365   Garland et al., "Vitamin D Supplement Doses and Serum 25-Hydroxyvitamin D in the Range Associated with Cancer Prevention."

366   A. J. Monserrat et al., "Protective Effect of Coconut Oil on Renal Necrosis Occurring in Rats Fed a Methyl-Deficient Diet," *Renal Failure* 17, no. 5 (September 1995): 525–37.

367   J. J. Carrero and M. Cozzolino, "Nutritional Therapy, Phosphate Control and Renal Protection," *Nephron. Clinical Practice* 126, no. 1 (2014): 1–7.

368   Y. Shutto, "Inadequate Awareness among Chronic Kidney Disease Patients Regarding Food and Drinks Containing Artificially Added Phosphate," *PLoS One* 8, no. 11 (November 13, 2013): e78660.

369   S. Ash et al., "Nutrition Prescription to Achieve Positive Outcomes in Chronic Kidney Disease: A Systematic Review," *Nutrients* 6, no. 1 (January 22, 2014): 416–51.

370   T. Ishigami et al., "An Association between Serum Ð-Glutamyltransferase and Proteinuria in Drinkers and Non-Drinkers: A Japanese Nationwide Cross-Sectional Survey," *Clinical and Experimental Nephrology* 18, no. 6 (December 2014): 899–910.

371   C. Latchoumycandane, L. E. Nagy, and T. M. McIntyre, "Chronic Ethanol Ingestion Induces Oxidative Kidney Injury through Taurine-Inhibitable Inflammation," *Free Radical Biology and Medicine* 69 (April 2014): 403–16.

372   "Fight Kidney Disease with a Better Diet, Weight Loss and Smoking Cessation," *Harvard Health Letter* 38, no. 9 (July 2013): 8.

373   R. Bilton, "Averting Comfortable Lifestyle Crises," *Science Progress* 96, pt. 4 (2013): 319–68.

374   R. Matsuzawa et al., "Association of Habitual Physical Activity Measured by an Accelerometer with High-Density Lipoprotein Cholesterol Levels in Maintenance Hemodialysis Patients," *ScientificWorldJournal* 2013 (December 21, 2013): 780783.

375   K. Tsuruya et al., "Association of the Triglycerides to High-Density Lipoprotein Cholesterol Ratio with the Risk of Chronic Kidney Disease: Analysis in a Large Japanese Population," *Atherosclerosis* 233, no. 1 (March 2014): 260–67.

376   N. Mumoli and M. Cei, "Licorice-Induced Hypokalemia," *International Journal of Cardiology* 124, no. 3 (March 14, 2008): e42–44.

377   National Cancer Institute, "SEER Stat Fact Sheets: Thyroid Cancer," accessed August 2014, http://seer.cancer.gov/statfacts/html/thyro.html.

378   Ibid.

379   P. L. Horn-Ross et al., "Continued Rapid Increase in Thyroid Cancer Incidence in California: Trends by Patient, Tumor, and Neighborhood Characteristics," *Cancer Epidemiology, Biomarkers and Prevention* 23, no. 6 (June 2014): 1067–79.

380   L. Davies and H. G. Welch, "Thyroid Cancer Survival in the United States: Observational Data from 1973 to 2005," *Archives of Otolaryngology—Head and Neck Surgery* 136, no. 5 (May 2010): 440–44.

381   S. Sadetzki et al., "Risk of Thyroid Cancer after Childhood Exposure to Ionizing Radiation for Tinea Capitis," *Journal of Clinical Endocrinology and Metabolism* 91, no. 12 (December 2006): 4798–4804.

382   M. M. Gramatges et al., "Telomere Content and Risk of Second Malignant Neoplasm in Survivors of Childhood Cancer: A Report from the Childhood Cancer Survivor Study," *Clinical Cancer Research* 20, no. 4 (February 15, 2014): 904–11.

383   Y. M. Yang et al., "The Association between the C677T Polymorphism in MTHFR Gene and the Risk of Thyroid Cancer: A Meta-Analysis," *European Review for Medical and Pharmacological Sciences* 18, no. 15 (2014): 2097–2101.

384   A. C. Brehar et al., "Genetic and Epigenetic Alterations in Differentiated Thyroid Carcinoma," *Journal of Medicine and Life* 6, no. 4 (2013): 403–8.

385   M. Derwahl and D. Nicula, "Estrogen and Its Role in Thyroid Cancer," *Endocrine-Related Cancer* 21, no. 5 (October 2014): T273–83.

386   S. H. Kim et al., "Correlation between Obesity and Clinicopathological Factors in Patients with Papillary Thyroid Cancer," *Surgery Today*, July 25, 2014.

387   L. Xu et al., "Obesity and the Risk of Papillary Thyroid Cancer: A Pooled Analysis of Three Case-Control Studies," *Thyroid* 24, no. 6 (June 2014): 966–74.

388   Y. Yeo et al., "Diabetes Mellitus and Risk of Thyroid Cancer: A Meta-Analysis," *PLoS One* 9 no. 6 (June 13, 2014): e98135.

389   S. Dvorkin et al., "Differentiated Thyroid Cancer Is Associated with Less Aggressive Disease and Better Outcome in Patients with Coexisting Hashimotos Thyroiditis," *Journal of Clinical Endocrinology and Metabolism* 98, no. 6 (June 2013): 2409–14.

390   K. Hauser, "Low 25-Hydroxyvitamin D Levels in People with a Solid Tumor Cancer Diagnosis: The Tip of the Iceberg?" *Supportive Care in Cancer* 22, no. 7 (July 2014): 1931–39.

391   Garland et al., "Vitamin D Supplement Doses and Serum 25-Hydroxyvitamin D in the Range Associated with Cancer Prevention."

392   J. Jonklaas, M. Danielsen, and H. Wang, "A Pilot Study of Serum Selenium, Vitamin D, and Thyrotropin Concentrations in Patients with Thyroid Cancer," *Thyroid* 23, no. 9 (September 2013): 1079–86.

393   S. Rajoria et al., "Estrogen Induced Metastatic Modulators MMP-2 and MMP-9 Are Targets of 3,3'-Diindolylmethane in Thyroid Cancer," *PLoS One* 6, no. 1 (January 18, 2011): e15879.

394   S. Rajoria et al., "3,3'-Diindolylmethane Modulates Estrogen Metabolism in Patients with Thyroid Proliferative Disease: A Pilot Study," *Thyroid* 21, no. 3 (March 2011): 299–304.

395   K. Tadi et al., "3,3'-Diindolylmethane, A Cruciferous Vegetable Derived

Synthetic Anti-Proliferative Compound in Thyroid Disease," *Biochemical Biophysical Research Communications* 337, no. 3 (November 25, 2005): 1019–25.

396   F. De Amicis et al., "Epigallocatechin Gallate Inhibits Growth and Epithelial-to-Mesenchymal Transition in Human Thyroid Carcinoma Cell Lines," *Journal of Cellular Physiology* 228, no. 10 (October 2013): 2054–62.

397   G. Belcaro et al., "A Controlled Study of a Lecithinized Delivery System of Curcumin (Meriva®) to Alleviate the Adverse Effects of Cancer Treatment," *Phytotherapy Research* 28, no. 3 (March 2014): 444–50.

398   C. Y. Zhang et al., "Curcumin Inhibits Invasion and Metastasis in K1 Papillary Thyroid Cancer Cells," *Food Chemistry* 139, no. 1–4 (August 15, 2013): 1021–28.

399   C. Y. Zhang et al., "Curcumin Inhibits the Metastasis of K1 Papillary Thyroid Cancer Cells via Modulating E-Cadherin and Matrix Metalloproteinase-9 Expression," *Biotechnology Letters* 35, no. 7 (July 2013): 995–1000.

400   S. J. Oh et al., "Silibinin Inhibits TPA-Induced Cell Migration and MMP-9 Expression in Thyroid and Breast Cancer Cells," *Oncology Reports* 29, no. 4 (April 2013): 1343–48.

401   W. J. Mack et al., "Lifestyle and Other Risk Factors for Thyroid Cancer in Los Angeles County Females," *Annals of Epidemiology* 12, no. 6 (August 2002): 395–401.

402   P. K. Kandala and S. K. Srivastava, "Diindolylmethane Suppresses Ovarian Cancer Growth and Potentiates the Effect of Cisplatin in Tumor Mouse Model by Targeting Signal Transducer and Activator of Transcription 3 (STAT3)," *BMC Medicine* 10 (January 26, 2012): 9.

403   A. Ahmad et al., "3, 3'-Diindolylmethane Enhances the Effectiveness of Herceptin against HER-$_{2/N}$eu-Expressing Breast Cancer Cells."

CHAPTER 9

1   J. Tilan and J. Kitlinska, "Sympathetic Neurotransmitters and Tumor Angiogenesis—Link between Stress and Cancer Progression," *Journal of Oncology* 2010, article ID 539706, www.ncbi.nlm.nih.gov/pmc/articles/PMC2874925/.

2   O. Palesh et al., "Stress History and Breast Cancer Recurrence," *Journal of Psychosomatic Research* 63, no. 3 (September 2007): 233–39.

3   E. K. Sloan et al., "The Sympathetic Nervous System Induced a Metastatic Switch in Primary Breast Cancer," *Cancer Research* 70, no. 18 (September 15, 2010): 7042–52.

4   S. Ben-Eliyahu, "The Promotion of Tumor Metastasis by Surgery and Stress: Immunological Basis and Implications for Psychoneuroimmunology," *Brain, Behavior, and Immunity* 17, no. S1 (February 2003): S27–36.

CHAPTER 10

1   B. L. Andersen et al., "Psychological Intervention Improves Survival for Breast Cancer Patients: A Randomized Clinical Trial," *Cancer* 113, no. 12 (December 15, 2008): 3450–58.

2   Moshe Frenkel, "Integrative Oncology Exceptional Patients: Thoughts and Reflections," *Cancer Strategies Journal* 1 no. 2 (Spring 2013): 2–7.

RESOURCES

YOUR HEALTH SOLUTION

"Diet, appropriate supplementation, exercise, and stress management all powerfully affect the tumor micro-environment, and can have significant effects on clinical outcomes."

—DWIGHT MCKEE, MD

For additional expert resources and ongoing support
and to receive
YOUR PERSONAL HEALTH SOLUTION,
Visit us at YOURHEALTHSOLUTION.com

You can also follow us on:
Twitter.com/yourhealthsol
Facebook.com/YourHealthSolutionLLC
Pinterest.com/yhshealth
aftercancercare.com

Your Health Solution™

...Because YOU deserve to THRIVE

BIOS

GERALD M. LEMOLE, MD, is a pioneer in cardiology—he was a member of the surgical team that performed the first successful heart transplant in the United States; performed the first coronary bypass in the tristate area of Pennsylvania, New Jersey, and Delaware; and performed the first open heart operation in the state of Delaware. He was the medical director of Christiana Care's Preventive Medicine and Rehabilitation Institute and Center for Integrative Health from 2007 to 2010 and was previously the chief of cardiovascular surgery at the Medical Center of Delaware beginning in 1986. In 2006, Dr. Lemole was appointed the first W. L. Samuel Carpenter III Distinguished Chair of Cardiovascular Surgery, Christiana Care Health System. He is presently full professor of surgery at Temple University and Thomas Jefferson Medical College. Dr. Lemole has written over 150 articles, book chapters, and editorials for professional publications. He has also written several books on integrative medicine, including *Facing Facial Pain* and *The Healing Diet*.

PALLAV MEHTA, MD, is a medical oncologist/hematologist with expertise and interest in breast cancer and integrative oncology currently practicing in the Philadelphia area. He is currently an assistant professor of medicine at Cooper Medical School and the director of integrative oncology at the MD Anderson Cancer Center at Cooper. Previously, he served as the chief of the division of hematology and oncology and the medical director of the Charles A. and Betty Bott Cancer Center at Holy Redeemer Hospital. He is board certified in medical oncology, hematology, and integrative medicine. He has been the cancer liaison physician to the Commission on Cancer (COC) and authored several journal articles and clinical trials, in which he has served as a local principal investigator along with developing a broad integrative medicine initiative aimed at patients with cancer. He has been invited to speak nationally on the topic of exercise and cancer and serves as a consultant and speaker for several international oncology-related companies pertaining to breast cancer, genetics, and molecular profiling. He is a Castle Connolly "Top Doc" 2014 and resides in Philadelphia with his wife and three children.

DWIGHT MCKEE, MD, practiced complementary medicine with an emphasis in nutritional and body/mind medicine for 12 years prior to re-entering training in 1988 to complete a 3-year residency in internal medicine. This was followed by 3 years of subspecialty training in hematology and oncology and 2 years of immunology research at the Scripps Research Institute in La Jolla, California. He thus brings a comprehensive perspective to the practice of oncology and hematology and is at the forefront of the application of integrative medicine to the field of cancer care. Dr. McKee is board certified in medical oncology, hematology, nutrition, and integrative and holistic medicine. He serves as chairman of the scientific advisory board of the Mederi Foundation, which sponsors education and research in the application of botanical medicine to cancer therapy, and edited the *Cancer Strategies Journal* from 2012 to 2014. Dr. McKee is not currently involved in direct patient care but consults with other physicians in the design of treatment and research protocols. He also works as the scientific director of Lifeplus International, developing advanced nutraceutical formulations with an emphasis on support of the immune system, regulation of the cell cycle, and DNA protection.

INDEX

Underscored page references indicate boxed text.

C

Cabbage
  Rainbow Asian Slaw with Tangy
    Asian Dressing, 221
Cadmium, 129
Caffeine, 48
Calcium, 84
Calories, burned by
  aerobic *versus* anaerobic exercise, 85
  muscle and fat, 78, 89
CAM, 6, 40
Carcinoembryonic antigen (CEA), 114
Carcinogens, 93–95, 99–100. *See also*
    Toxins
Cardiac rehab, 30–34, 79
Cardiomyopathy, 69, 179
Cardiovascular exercise. *See* Exercise,
    cardiovascular
Carotenoids, 58
Carpets, 96
Carrots
  Carrot and Ginger Soup, 215
  Rainbow Asian Slaw with Tangy
    Asian Dressing, 221
  Salmon and Vegetable Curry, 228–29
  Salmon in Parchment, 231
Casein, 52
Catechins, 56. *See also* Green tea extract
Catheters, 84
Cat's claw, 166
CEA, 114
Celery, 59
  Blue Bell Inn Lentil Salad, 218
  Don't Worry Curry, 236
Cell phones, brain tumors and, 99
Chaga, 162
Checkpoint inhibitors, 40
Cheese, 52–53
Chemicals, carcinogenic. *See* Toxins
Chemo-brain, 69
Chemotherapy
  exercise precautions and, 83
  muscle atrophy with, 88
  supplements treating residuals, 69
Chickpeas
  Hector's Hummus, 240
Chile peppers, 60
  Cilantro-Walnut Pesto, 242
  Mariachi Guacamole, 239
  Snazzy Salsa, 238

Chili powder
  Grilled Shrimp with Salsa, 224
  The Very, Very Best Veggie Burgers,
    226
Chives
  Lemon Vinaigrette, 242
Chromosome, 37–38
Cilantro
  Fish Tajine, 234–35
  Moroccan Chicken Stew with
    Apricots and Plums, 232–33
  Salmon and Vegetable Curry,
    228–29
Cinnamon
  Sweet Zoe's Potatoes, 237
Classes, exercise, 91
Cleaning supplies, toxic, 96
Coconut oil
  benefits of, 52, 61
  Salmon and Vegetable Curry,
    228–29
Coconut water, 84
Coenzyme Q10, 69, 155–56
Coenzymes, 73
Colon (colorectal) cancer, 113–19
  basics, 113
  causes/contributing factors, 113–14
  diagnostic testing, 25, 114
  dietary action plan, 118–19
  endometrial cancer and, 142
  hereditary nonpolyposis colorectal
    cancer (HNPCC), 142
  increase with physical inactivity,
    81
  lifestyle interventions, 119
  mortality reduction with exercise,
    76–77, 82
  nutrient/drug interactions, 119
  staging, 114–16
  supplement program, 116–18
  0, 5, 10, 30, 150 rehab formula, 32
Colonoscopy, 114
Complementary and alternative
    medicine (CAM), 6, 40
Computed tomography (CT) scan
  lung cancer screening, 120
  procedure, 26
  radiation exposure, 24–25
Cooking, 45, 61
Coptis, 161
Cordyceps, 149

Stress management, 183–84, 188–92
    guided imagery, 191
    HeartMath, 190, 191
    individual preferences, 191–92
    meditation, 191
    progressive muscle relaxation, 189,
        191
    qigong, 190
    reiki, 190
    tai chi, 190
    yoga, 189–90
Stretching, 89–90
Sugar
    cancer risk link, 54
    immune system suppression by, 78
    refined sugars, 54–55
Sugar substitutes, 54
Sulfur, 58
Sunscreen, 97
Supplements, 65–69, 70–75
    absorption of micronutrients, 74
    career path for, 66–67
    decision to use, 66
    inflammation and, 69
    media editorials/bias, 70–73
    programs for specific cancers
        bladder cancer, 138–40
        breast cancer, 109–12
        colon (colorectal) cancer, 116–18
        endometrial cancer, 143–44
        leukemia, 148–50
        lung cancer, 125–27
        lymphoma, 154–56
        melanoma, 161–62
        prostate cancer, 132–34
        renal cancer, 166–67
        thyroid cancer, 173–75
    reasons for need, 65–66, 68
    research studies, 70–75
    treating chemotherapy residuals, 69
    types, 67–68
        herbs, 68
        micronutrients, 67–68
        phytonutrients, 68
Support system, 186–87, 193–98
    friends and family, 197
    high tech, 198
    pets, 198
    spiritual groups, 193–95
    support groups, 31, 195–96, 196

Surgery
    exercise after, 84
    immune suppression from, 181
Surveillance, 24, 28
Survivorship, increase in, 80
Sweet potatoes
    Fish Tajine, 234–35
    Sweet Zoe's Potatoes, 237
Swimming, 87–88
Sword of Damocles, 4, 14, 31

T

Tai chi, 90, 190
Takotsubo cardiomyopathy, 179
Tamoxifen, 76, 141–42
Tannins, 100
Taurine, 69
Taxol (paclitaxel), 83, 87
Telomere shortening, 169
Terrain, 6–8
Testosterone, prostate cancer and, 106
Tests. *See also specific cancers; specific tests*
    follow-up, 24–28
    radiation exposure, 24–25
    what to expect, 25–28
Thyme, 60
    Cream of Mushroom Soup, 216–17
    Jean Bean's Roma Pasta Sauce, 241
Thyroid cancer, 169–76
    basics, 169
    causes/contributing factors, 169–70
    diagnostic testing, 170–71
    dietary action plan, 175
    lifestyle interventions, 175–76
    nutrient/drug interactions, 176
    staging, 171–73
    supplement program, 173–75
Tissue polypeptide antigen (TPA), 114
TMAO, 63
Tocopherols, 111, 118, 126–27, 134, 138–39
Tomatoes
    Fish Tajine, 234–35
    Fresh Tomato Sauce, 240
    Jean Bean's Roma Pasta Sauce, 241
    Mariachi Guacamole, 239
    Portuguese Baked Wild Halibut
        with Rice, 227
    Snazzy Salsa, 238
    Zorba's Chopped Salad, 219